Mastering Rhinoplasty: A Comprehensive Atlas of Surgical Techniques with Integrated Video Clips

Rollin K. Daniel

Rollin K. Daniel

Mastering Rhinoplasty

A Comprehensive Atlas
of Surgical Techniques
with Integrated Video Clips

2nd Edition
With 259 Color Figures in 1408 Parts
and 146 Integrated Intraoperative DVD Clips

Jaye Schlesinger, Medical Illustrator
Chuck Cox, Videographer

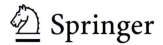 Springer

Rollin K. Daniel, MD
1441 Avocado Ave., Suite 308
Newport Beach, CA 92660, USA
rkdaniel@aol.com
and
Clinical Professor of Surgery
Department of Plastic Surgery
University of California, Irvine
Irvine, CA, USA

Medical Illustrator:
Jaye Schlesinger, MFA
School of Art and Design
University of Michigan
906 Miner St.
Ann Arbor, MI 48103, USA
jayes@umich.edu

Videographer:
Chuck Cox, WBV
SD Biomedical Communications
4127 Pallon Court
San Diego, CA, USA
chuckcoxepacbell.net

ISBN 978-3-642-01401-7   eISBN 978-3-642-01402-4

DOI 10.1007/978-3-642-01402-4

Springer Heidelberg Dordrecht London New York

Library of Congress Control Number: 2009931340

Cover design: eStudio Calamar, Figueres/Berlin

Printed on acid-free paper

Springer is part of Springer Science+Business Media (www.springer.com)

Dedication

To Beatrix Tirkanits, MD, FRCS (C)
Diplomat, American Board of Plastic Surgery
Both personal and professional partner whose sacrifice
and support made this book possible.

To Andrew Nicholas Daniel, PhD
Son, scholar and fellow adventurer.

Contents

Table of DVD Clips

Simplifying Rhinoplasty 1

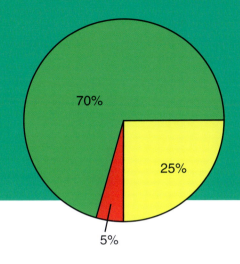

70%

25%

5%

Based on my 25-year experience of practicing, teaching, and writing about rhinoplasty surgery, I have come to the conclusion that we must simplify the rhinoplasty operation. For the average surgeon who performs less than 25 rhinoplasties a year, it makes no sense to try several new techniques each year and then discard them before attaining proficiency. Instead, one should master a fundamental rhinoplasty operation that can be adapted to a wide range of primary nasal deformities. Initially, the surgeon should operate within their comfort zone and gradually progress to more difficult cases. Over a period of 3–5 years, the operation's surgical cause and effect will become apparent. With this approach, the surgeon will attain proficiency and confidence in dealing with a variety of nasal deformities. Equally, an increasing number of happy patients will insure an expanding rhinoplasty practice.

Instead of writing an encyclopedic text of the various nasal procedures, this Atlas will emphasize a fundamental rhinoplasty operation and its application to a wide range of patients with various levels of difficulty progressing from minor (Level 1) to moderate (Level 2), to major (Level 3) deformities. The Atlas is divided into three sections. Chapters 1–7 provides the fundamentals of the rhinoplasty surgery, while Chapters 8 and 9 are an in-depth look at progressively more difficult primary rhinoplasties and Chapters 10–12 review the complex challenges of secondary and aesthetic reconstructive rhinoplasty. Since I believe strongly that rhinoplasty surgery should be learned in the operating room rather than in the library, the reader will find extensive DVD clips of surgical techniques throughout the book. These short 1–5 min DVD clips are referenced in the figures and provide a unique opportunity to see and experience how a specific technique is actually done. It is my hope that this text will represent a major advance in teaching a simplified approach to rhinoplasty surgery.

Introduction

A Foundation Rhinoplasty Operation

What would constitute the "P.E.R.F.E.C.T." rhinoplasty operation? I think the following attributes are important and perhaps acronymic.

Progressive. The surgeon should be able to use the operative technique for increasingly difficult cases by adding to the foundation operation (Fig. 1.1). Rather than learning an entirely new procedure, one merely adds additional steps as more demanding cases are encountered. For example, once the surgeon learns to master open tip suture techniques, then additional tip definition can be achieved with add-on Tip Refinement Grafts (TRG) of excised cartilage.

Expandable. Although one may begin with a certain patient population, it is inevitable that one will begin to see different types of patients who require modification of the basic technique. In Southern California, I saw a large number of Hispanic and Asian patients whose thicker skin and under-projecting tips forced me to expand my surgical repertoire. Rather than being a new operation, additions and modifications represent an expansion of the foundation operation.

Reproducible. Every surgeon wants to achieve reproducible results. The critical first step is to master a procedure in-depth and learn its surgical cause and effect. Many of the steps in this operation are consistently reproducible including radix grafts, tip sutures, and spreader grafts. The number of surprises and revisions can be quite low.

Functional. Form without function is not acceptable. I am convinced that 35% of patients requesting a cosmetic rhinoplasty have a significant *preexisting* anatomical nasal obstruction, which if not corrected will lead to postoperative nasal obstruction. Therefore, a clear understanding of septal, valvular, and turbinate function, as well as their surgical correction must be a critical component of a rhinoplasty operation.

Esthetic. The reality is that virtually all female patients want a more attractive nose, but one that looks natural. The younger the patient the greater the desire for a smaller cuter nose – nine times out of ten, they inherited their father's nasal features . In addition to being smaller, they often want a slightly curved bridge, a slightly rotated columellar, and a well-defined tip. This operation enables the surgeon to achieve these goals consistently.

Comfort Zone. Each surgeon has his/her own "rhinoplasty comfort zone." Following completion of their residency or fellowship, most surgeons have experience with one operative sequence. Initially, the surgeon should select those patients for whom they are confident that they can achieve a good result. The advantage of this operation is that the surgeon can progress to levels of greater difficulty from a solid foundation.

Tip Intentsive. One of the realities of cosmetic rhinoplasty surgery is that patients are convinced that "as the tip goes so goes the result." If the tip is not attractive, the patient will not be happy. Thus, tip surgery is emphasized heavily in this operation and through out the text.

The following operation is a relatively standard procedure that I use routinely, but with virtually unlimited variations. The operative sequence is individualized for each primary rhinoplasty with certain steps deleted or modified as indicated.

A Standard Operative Sequence

1) Essentials – 2.5× loupes, fiberoptic headlight, own instruments
2) Anesthesia – general with appropriate monitors
3) Local anesthesia injection followed by Prep – wait 10–15 min
4) Remove intranasal nasal pack and shave vibrissae
5) Open Approach using infracartilaginous and transcolumellar incisions
6) Elevation of skin envelope
7) Septal exposure via transfixion incision and extramucosal tunnels
8) Tip analysis and reassessment of operative plan
9) Creation of symmetrical alar rim strips
10) Incremental hump reduction – bone: rasp, cartilage: scissons
11) Caudal septum/ANS excision (optional)
12) Septal harvest/septoplasty
13) Osteotomies
14) Graft preparation
15) Spreader grafts (optional)
16) Columellar strut and suture
17) Tip sutures with optional add-on grafts of excised alar cartilage
18) Closure
19) Alar base modification (optional)
20) Alar rim grafts or Alar rim structure grafts (optional)
21) Doyle splints, external cast, and nasal anesthesia block

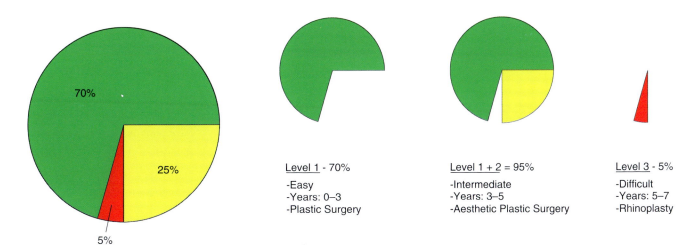

Fig. 1.1 Level of difficulty in primary rhinoplasty

Level of Difficulty: A Classification

Our assessment of how hard a rhinoplasty is involves integration of anatomy, aesthetics, patient's goals, and requisite operative techniques. Although each surgeon will have their own individual classification, I suggest dividing the range of primary rhinoplasties into three "levels of difficulty" based on the requested degree of change, requisite technical expertise, and complexity of the operative plan. I use a simple Levels 1–3 for classifying primary rhinoplasties – Level 1 (minor), Level 2 (moderate), and Level 3 (major).

Patient Request. The majority of Level 1 rhinoplasty patients have three basic complaints: the bump on profile, the wide dorsum, and the poorly defined tip. The challenge is to achieve an aesthetic result that the patient desires. The hallmark of a Level 2 case is that the complaints are similar to a Level 1 case, but the presenting deformity and requisite surgical maneuvers are more challenging. A boxy tip requiring alar rim support would be a Level 2 case. In contrast, Level 3 cases are truly "deformities" where the patient suffers from a significant loss of self-esteem. They are seeking to be "normal." Surgical correction requires an aggressive complex approach. Subtleties will not work.

Patient Deformity. Perhaps, the best method for assigning the level of difficulty to a specific nose is to use a classic "standard deviation" system based on deviation from normal. The simplest example is modification of the nasal base. Using a simple ruler or caliper, one measures intercanthal width, alar flare, and alar crease width. If the alar flare is within the intercanthal width, then no modification is usually necessary (Level 1). If the alar base is quite wide and exceeds the intercnathal width by 2 mm or more, then a combined nostril sill/alar base excision is necessary (Level 2). When one encounters extreme widths in ethnic noses or markedly retracted alars due to hypoplasia of the alar cartilages, then advanced techniques will be required (Level 3).

Surgical Techniques. After developing an individual set of "aesthetic" grading criteria for Level 1–3 cases based on presenting deformity, it can now be expanded by adding required operative techniques. A radix reduction is a magnitude harder than a radix augmentation. Ethnic noses are more challenging than the usual Caucasian nose. As regards the tip, an open structure tip graft signals a harder case than a tip suture. Yet, an open tip graft added to sutured domes is easier than one where the domes are excised to drop projection.

Operative Complexity. Each surgical technique included in the operative plan has both its range of results and risks. Therefore, one should keep the operative plan as simple as possible and do maneuvers only when necessary. Level 1 cases may not require grafts, while Level 3 always do. Lateral osteotomies may range from none for the narrow nose to as many as 8 for the wide nose. Thus, operative complexity is both how many maneuvers are required and how complex is the individual step.

Level 1: Form and Function

This patient has a typical Level 1 nasal deformity with the triad of a bump on profile, an unrefined tip, and a wide nose (Fig. 1.2). Many women will state that their nose is too masculine and request a more feminine one. All too often, it really is daddy's nose on the daughter. Cosmetic patients are most concerned about appearance and may be totally unaware of existing nasal obstruction. In this case, the patient stated that she had no functional impairment despite an obvious septal deviation and internal valve collapse due to the tension nose (see Fig. 2.22). The linkage between *form and function* is central to all of rhinoplasty surgery.

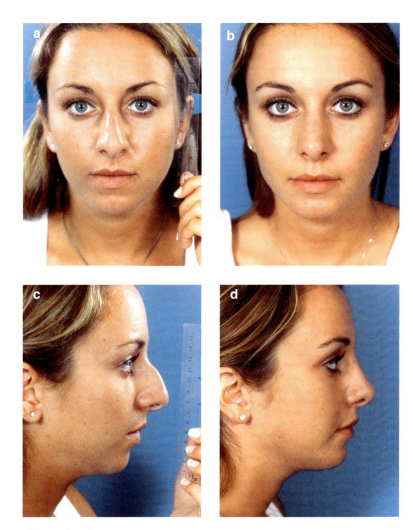

Fig. 1.2 (a–d)

Level 2:   Tip Challenges

The Level 2 patient has a *progressively* greater degree of complexity as compared to the Level 1 patient. As seen in the patient below (Fig. 1.3), any improvement in the tip must be achieved despite an unfavorable skin sleeve and weak alar cartilages. The critical step was a folded add-on tip graft of excised alar cartilage. In Level 2 cases, a wider array of techniques, both sutures and grafts, is required to achieve the desired tip. As regards the profile, one must often pursue a "balanced" approach – reducing prominences and building up deficiencies. As the surgeon expands their comfort zone, one will encounter patients with a thicker skin envelope, a wide nasal base, or dorsal deficiencies. All of a sudden, success or failure will depend on insertion of major tip grafts, alar base excisions, or diced cartilage grafts to the dorsum. Many surgeons will decide to limit their rhinoplasty practice at this level and do the 95% of patients who present with Level 1 and 2 deformities while referring the other 5% to a rhinoplasty specialist.

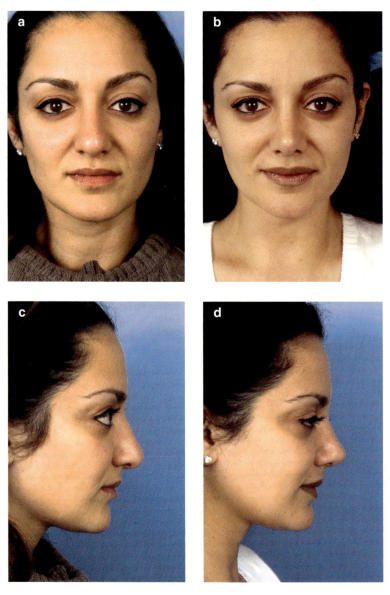

Fig. 1.3 (a–d)

Level 3:   Major Changes

Level 3 patients want a major change in their nose. These are not subtle finesse cases. The surgeon must achieve a significant change in the nose while giving it an attractive natural nonoperative look. As seen in Fig. 1.4, this 15-year-old girl desperately wanted to reduce the incessant teasing at school while her parents wanted to boost her self-confidence before she entered high school. The requisite surgical techniques are part of the basic rhinoplasty operation, but applied on an extreme scale. They included an 11 mm dorsal reduction, a 9 mm caudal septal shortening, and 7 asymmetric osteotomies. One must deal with the extremes of nasal anatomy and remodel the entire nose. Significant asymmetry intrinsic to the nose and within the face will limit the outcome. Often, techniques have to be executed in quantitative differences on the two sides to adjust for the asymmetry. Fortunately, these patients are often happy with a limited improvement.

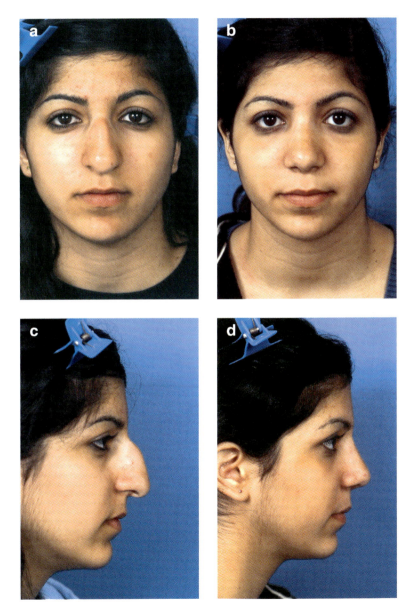

Fig. 1.4 (a–d)

Teaching Yourself Surgical Cause and Effect

No one is born a rhinoplasty surgeon. With one or two exceptions, no one finishes his/her residency or fellowship being very good at rhinoplasty surgery, myself included. However, most surgeons can become proficient at rhinoplasty surgery provided they are willing to take the time to teach themselves surgical cause and effect. Here are ten ways to improve your understanding of surgical cause and effect.

1) *Pre-op Photo Analysis.* With the advent of digital photography, there is no excuse not to have excellent *standardized* pre-op photographs in all views, static and smiling. It is important to develop a reproducible system with consistent lighting. Equally, large prints, scaled to life size, are easily available. Learning to do a sequential photographic analysis is the fastest way to train your eye to analyze clinical deformities. Go through the three-step progression of developing an operative plan – define the deformity, overlay the ideal aesthetics, and develop a realistic operative goal.

2) *Write Out the Op Plan.* Writing out a step-by-step operative plan, from anesthesia to dressing, and posting it in the operating room is the best way to simplify your surgery. As you write out each step you are forced to decide whether to do that step and more importantly how to do it. By asking and answering as many questions as possible preoperatively, one has a greater sense of clarity and certainty in the operating room.

3) *Nasal Aesthetics, Analysis, and Anatomy.* Nasal anatomy determines what is wrong with the nose and what must be modified surgically to achieve the aesthetic goals. One of the best examples is tip definition and its linkage to the domal notch and the domal creation suture. The open approach allows the surgeon to carefully study and record tip and dorsal anatomy in every case. If available, cadaver dissections provide an important learning opportunity, but nothing replaces assessing nasal anatomy in every case.

4) *Inrtaop Instruments and Photos.* It took me only one operation at the University with the residents to realize that you cannot do delicate surgery with bad instruments. Although a complete personalized set of rhinoplasty instruments is ideal, one should at least have their own set of cutting instruments (scissors, rasps, osteotomes) from the very beginning. It is extremely important to take a four-view set of the completed tip surgery before closing the skin. Then, review these photos at each post-op visit.

5) *Op Diagram and three Questions.* It is extremely important to keep a visual record of the final operation (see p.51). It is so important that I fill out the op diagram before I dictate the official op report. Although checking the boxes facilitates data retrieval, it is the numerous drawings that I add that are vitally important. At the bottom of the page, I record three questions to answer at the post-op visits. Typical questions are: Is tip definition sufficient? Should I have done a structure tip graft rather than add-on grafts? Does the patient need nostril splints?

6) *Frequent Post-op Visits and Photos.* The more frequently you see the patient post-op, the quicker you will learn surgical cause and effect. In my office, the patient's chart is opened to the op diagram and the intraop tip photos when I enter the exam room. I need to know what I did both diagrammatically and visually. At the end of the exam, I answer the three questions – sometimes suspicions are confirmed and other times I am pleasantly surprised, but I always learn something.

7) *Revisions.* Yes, you will have to revise your own cases, everybody does. You also have a choice – you can see it as a sign of failure or as a learning opportunity. Recently, I revised a nose to fix a small tip bossa. To my surprise, it was not a sharp domal cartilage point, but rather the cephalic end of an alar rim graft. From this experience, I learned to taper my ARG grafts even more, do not hesitate to shorten them, and check the soft tissue facet for any distortion. Learn from your revisions.

8) *Reading and Meetings.* Read everything you can about rhinoplasty surgery. Obviously, begin with the most pertinent recent articles and books. Do not hesitate to read the "classics." A familiarity with less popular techniques is valuable in secondary cases where recognition of a "Universal tip' or a "Goldman tip" allows one to reverse the primary procedure and reduce the number of grafts.

9) *Visit Other Surgeons or Find a Mentor.* Every year, I try to spend a few days in the O.R. observing a colleague. This experience is tremendously helpful as I learn lot of tricks and alternative ways of doing things as well as new operations – some I will do and some I won't. At the initial stages of one's practice, it would be ideal to find a mentor and some one close by that you could observe frequently and discuss your problems with. Experience is a dear teacher and takes time to acquire.

10) *Give a Presentation, Write a Paper.* Until one prepares a presentation, one may think that they know how to do a good rhinoplasty. All illusions are stripped away when the 1-year result photos are examined from all four views. Rather than accepting defeat, one should see where the mistakes are and keep working until you have enough good results to present. Writing a paper provides even greater understanding as one must clarify one's thoughts and put it within the context of prior work. I have always said that writing these books has made me a much better surgeon, but a poorer golfer.

The Most Important Step – Progress to the Next Level. With experience and a greater understanding of surgical cause and effect, one is ready to progress to the next level. The reality is that most surgeons will have inadvertently operated beyond their comfort zone, by underestimating the difficulty of a few cases. Also, the opportunity to do one's own revisions are part of the learning experience. Remember: it is hard work and a commitment to excellence that is critical in the evolution of a rhinoplasty surgeon.

Guiding Principles

As one enters practice and begins to learn rhinoplasty surgery in the real world, decisions have to be made and their consequences must be accepted. Hopefully, these principles will guide the younger surgeon through the challenges of learning rhinoplasty surgery.

- Rhinoplasty is the most difficult of all cosmetic operations for three reasons: (1) nasal anatomy is highly variable, (2) the procedure must correct form and function, and (3) the final result must meet the patient's expectations.
- Few surgeons do more than 25 rhinoplasties a year. Thus, one must maximize the learning experience of each case by careful documentation of the operative procedure and frequent follow-up visits – only you can teach yourself surgical cause and effect.
- Form without function is a disaster. Most postoperative nasal obstruction reflects a failure to diagnose and treat a preoperative subclinical condition. One must identify and correct preexisting anatomical deformities of the septum, nasal valves, and turbinates. There is no excuse for not doing a thorough preoperative internal exam and recording a specific operative plan.
- One must accept in advance that there is no magic operation that guarantees perfect results. Each surgical maneuver within an operation has its learning curve. Within an operative sequence, the individual maneuvers are additive, but their interactions and potential complications are geometric. Keep the operation simple – maximum gain, minimum risk. Expand what you know from your comfort zone. Do not incorporate every new fad.
- Early in your practice, select nice patients with obvious deformities that you can easily correct using surgical techniques that you know. With experience, begin to add new maneuvers and then take on cases of greater difficulty. Operate within your comfort zone early on.
- The preoperative course is finite, but the postoperative course is infinite, so pick your patients carefully. Postoperative problems are most often confirmations of intraop suspicions – if the tip did not look exactly right during the case, it rarely gets better later. Do not cut corners or you will go in circles. Once you operate on a patient, it is your result, regardless of how many previous operations were done or how noncompliant the patient. Select your patient's carefully.
- Once you have a complication or poor result, admit it directly to the patient and discuss how it can be improved. Do not pretend that it is not there or shame the patient into accepting a minimal improvement or make it financially impossible to correct the problem. Treat patients as family – at worst they will be disappointed, but not litigious.
- Understand your own limitations and progress through Level 1–3 primary cases before embarking on major secondaries. Secondary rhinoplasty is technically more demanding and requires greater surgical expertise that can only be gained through operative experience. In primary cases one often takes away the negatives to reveal the underlying attractive nose while in secondaries the surgeon must be capable of rebuilding a destroyed framework using numerous grafts.
- Rhinoplasty is the most rewarding of all cosmetic operations, both for the patient and the surgeon. Few operations can make as great a change in a young person's appearance or in their self-confidence. For the surgeon, rhinoplasty is the ultimate in artistic three-dimensional sculpturing. It is truly worth the patient's risk and the surgeon's commitment.

At this point in the text, the sophisticated reader will realize that this chapter is, in reality, the Preface to this book. It is my contention that very few surgeons ever read the Preface and therefore I have previewed within this chapter what is to come. Although reading this text in sequence is recommended, the reality is that most surgeons focus on that portion, which is most relevant to them at a particular moment. Thus, it is necessary to make each section complete in a stand-alone fashion, which leads to a certain repetition of important points throughout the text. I do think that is important for the reader to integrate the *DVD clips* into the learning experience. I consider the opportunity to actually be in the operating room and see how the technique are done to be of infinite value. Ideally, one should have their computer available with the appropriate DVD loaded – read the text, look at the drawings or intraop photographs, and then enter the OR to see how it is done in the real world. The overall experience should be as close to a Rhinoplasty Fellowship as possible. On another note, the number of cited references is low because this book was written from notes and diagrams made during and after surgery. Thus, it is one surgeon's approach to rhinoplasty and not an encyclopedic multivolume text on the entire subject. Once the text was completed, I did review the rhinoplasty literature and added a Reading List to each chapter. Certain references will be cited using the following format (Author, date). Once again, I have found that writing a book on rhinoplasty surgery has made me a much better surgeon and I can only hope that the same will be true for the reader.

How to Use This Book

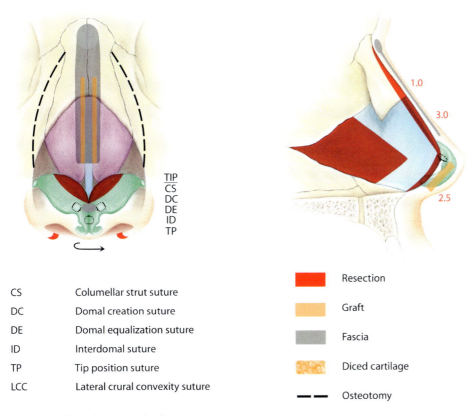

CS	Columellar strut suture
DC	Domal creation suture
DE	Domal equalization suture
ID	Interdomal suture
TP	Tip position suture
LCC	Lateral crural convexity suture

Resection

Graft

Fascia

Diced cartilage

Osteotomy

Fig. 1.5 Codex of case study diagram

A Basic Rhinoplasty Operation 2

*W*hy is rhinoplasty so difficult? The answer is the wide variation in the patient's nasal anatomy and aesthetic desires. For the surgeon, the challenge is mastering the endless number of operative techniques available. Thus, the question becomes can one devise a basic rhinoplasty operation? A former resident who was 3 years into private practice made the following request: "Can you give me a basic rhinoplasty operation with which I can get good results and have few revisions?" My answer was quick and blunt – "It is impossible because both the anatomy and the requisite techniques are too varied." Despite my negativity, the desire to develop a basic rhinoplasty operation has continued to intrigue me. Gradually, the fundamentals of a standard rhinoplasty operation began to crystallize. The following operation is intended for the average well-trained plastic surgeon. It can be expanded to fit a large range of nasal deformities. However, it requires that the surgeon accepts two principles. First, the surgeon must begin by doing only those cases which fit within their surgical comfort zone. Second, the surgeon must implement a progressive approach for learning rhinoplasty surgery. One begins with easier Level 1 cases and then advances to the more challenging Level 2 deformities before ultimately taking on the most difficult Level 3 problems. Distribution wise, perhaps 70% of the primary cases are Level 1, 25% are Level 2, and only 5% are Level 3. A fundamental operation will be presented in a step-by-step fashion in this chapter and its progressive adaptations for the three levels of deformities will be detailed in the rest of the text. It is important to select only those steps that are appropriate for a specific case.

Remember the 95% rule – 95% of rhinoplasty articles and lectures deal with the most esoteric 5% of noses, yet 95% of surgeons do not want to do the most difficult 5% of noses. This basic rhinoplasty operation is designed to allow the surgeon to do surgery for 95% of primary patients seen by a surgeon in the private practice of aesthetic surgery.

Consultation During the initial consultation, I ask myself two critical questions about the patient. First, will a rhinoplasty make a significant improvement in this patient's nose? Second, do I want this person in my practice? If the answer is no to either question then I do not do their surgery. Rhinoplasty is not a frivolous operation; the procedure must be considered carefully by both the patient and the surgeon. The patient's goals should be to get a realistic assessment of the surgical risk to reward ratio and evaluate whether they feel comfortable with you being their surgeon. Unfortunately, surgeons too often concentrate on the technical challenge and the economic benefit of doing every nose, yet the risks of selecting the wrong patient is very real for the surgeon ranging from frustration to misery to physical abuse.

Nasal Deformity. In primary cases, patients are usually very accurate in defining what is wrong with their nose, but often very nonspecific about what they want. The easiest patients are those requesting elimination of obvious deformities (bump on profile, round tip), while the most difficult are those who are unable to say exactly what they desire or those who demand a specific "look." Essentially, one must get patients to commit to what they want. For this reason, I have the patient tell me what three things should be improved in the order of importance. Next, I examine the nose in detail and make my list of what must be done to make the nose attractive and to achieve balance with the face. Perhaps 90% of all the primary consultations have a correctable nasal deformity on evaluation. The other 10% are attractive females with minimal deformities, males seeking "model" refinements, and patients wanting a "major change" when only a limited improvement is realistic.

Patient Factors. It is important to assess the patient's motivation. Open-ended questions should be asked as they will often reveal the patient's motivation. "What do you not like about your nose?" "Why do you want surgery at this time?" "What effect will a rhinoplasty have on your life?" It is extremely important to "hear" what the patient is saying psychologically rather than merely listening to the words. Which patients do I reject for primary rhinoplasty? These would include the overly narcissistic male, the perfectionistic female who will never be satisfied, and the unhappy patient who thinks that the operation will change his or her life. Once you choose to operate, you must provide the care and concern that the patient requires, not the amount that is reasonable. I have learned the hard way that "the pre-op course is finite, but the post-op course is infinite."

Analysis. Given the choice, would most surgeons rather be a master technician with golden hands or a strategic tactician with a critical aesthetic eye? In rhinoplasty as in chess, it is the thought process before the manipulation of the pieces that is critical. If one fails to recognize that the radix is low, then the dorsum will be lowered excessively resulting in a nose job appearance. In contrast, the simple addition of a fascia graft to the radix allows a more limited dorsal reduction producing a more natural, elegant, unoperated look. The difference is not surgical skill, but rather the design of the operative plan based on preoperative analysis.

Prior to my evaluation, I hand the patient a mirror and ask them to show me what bothers them the most, preferably in the order of importance. I write these down on the operative planning sheet and they become the cornerstone of the operative plan assuming they are correctable. After a thorough internal and external exam, I do a top-down region exam.

Radix and Dorsum. The radix is analyzed on lateral view for both the radix area (from glabella to lateral canthus level) and nasion (the deepest point in the nasofrontal angle). The critical decision is whether the radix needs to be maintained, augmented, or reduced. Fortunately, no modification is necessary in most cases (82%). Next, the dorsum is evaluated for height and width, while the bony base is assessed for width. The key determinant of dorsal height is the nasofascial angle, which is measured from nasion to tip. The desired profile line is slightly curved for females, straight for males. On anterior view, the width of the parallel "dorsal lines" is roughly the same as the philtral columns or tip-defining points, 6–8 mm for females, 8–10 mm for males. The maximum base bony width of the nose is marked as the "X-point" and should be less than the eyes' intercanthal width.

Tip. Tip analysis is complex and will be discussed in great depth in Chapters 4 and 8. The following is a basic overview. The "lobule" is the entire area overlying the alar cartilages, whereas the "intrinsic tip" incorporates just the area between the tip-defining points transversely and between the columella breakpoint and supratip point vertically. I focus on these characteristics: (1) the intrinsic factors of volume, definition, and width; (2) the extrinsic/intrinsic factors of rotation and projection; and (3) the overall factors of tip shape and skin envelope. I assign a "value" to each: ideal, minor, moderate, or major deformity in both a positive and negative direction. Then, I make a critical decision: is the tip inherently attractive or do I need to change it. As will be discussed extensively in the chapters on tip surgery, I feel that most surgeons should learn an open tip suture technique which can be expanded to fit a wide range of tip deformities. At the consultation, I draw the anticipated tip surgery procedure including the various sutures and any tip refinement grafts (TRG).

Base. The base of the nose consists of alar bases, nostrils, and columella. Numerous factors must be assessed including caudal septum, anterior nasal spine, and maxilla. The most common decision is whether to reduce alar base width or nostril size. In general, the alar bases should be narrower than the intercanthal width and the nostril sills should not be excessively visible on anterior view. I have evolved a simplified approach of three procedures – nostril sill excision, alar wedge excision, or combined to deal with these problems. Although conservative in the amount of excision, one should not limit their application. Preexisting nostril asymmetry should be pointed out to the patient preoperatively as only a slight improvement is realistic.

Operative Planning

Formulation of an operative plan involves selecting specific surgical techniques which are combined to produce the optimal *individualized* operative sequence for the specific patient (Fig. 2.1). The first step is to define the patient's goals and the surgeon should write out the proposed operative sequence following a thorough internal and external exam (Op Plan #1). Nasal photographs are taken and individual views are printed to allow detailed planning using classic landmarks and angles defining actual, ideal, and realistic goals (Op Plan #2). When the patient returns for the pre-op visit, the nose is examined from the surgeon's perspective with the questions being: What do I not like about the nose (the negatives)? What are the aesthetic possibilities for this nose (the upside goal)? What will the patient's tissue and my experience allow me to achieve (the reality check)? (Op Plan #3) Then I review the photographs of the desired noses that the patient has brought. At the end of the pre-op visit, the final operative plan has evolved (Op Plan #4). A step-by-step operative plan is written out and it will be posted in the operating room with the photographic analysis of the patient. During the actual operation, changes may occur on a "sliding scale" but rarely is a step dropped. The final operation is recorded both by a check box table database plus drawings and dictated (Final Operation). The data table with drawings is checked at each post-op visit with emphasis on surgical cause and effect.

Operative Sequence

The advantage of a standard operation is that the operative sequence is largely predetermined (Table 2.1). I favor a dorsum to tip sequence. I first establish the ideal profile line and then fit the tip to it. I do the dorsal reduction prior to the septal surgery as it minimizes disjunction of the critical septal strut. Alar base modifications are done after all incisions are closed and alar rim grafts (ARG) follow any alar base modification. Initially, the surgeon should write out an operative sequence for each patient prior to surgery and then post it in the operating room below the patient's photographs.

Markings

On the day of surgery with the patient sitting up, I mark the following: ideal dorsal profile line, x-point, lateral osteotomies, ideal tip point, transcolumellar incision, and any alar base incisions.

PRINCIPLES

- One must correct the deformities that bother the patient or they will not be happy.
- The more detail the pre-op planning is, the smoother the operation.
- The simpler the operative plan is, the smaller the risk. Always design an operative plan with maximum gain and minimum risk.
- Write out your operative sequence step by step and put it up in the operating room – know what you are going to do.

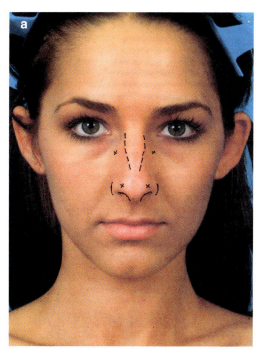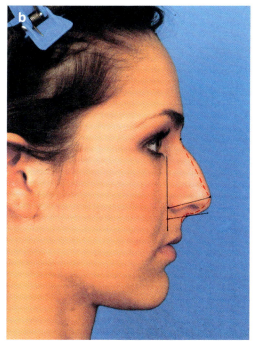

Fig. 2.1 (**a**) Patient analysis (**b**) Operative planing

Table 2.1 Operative sequence of a basic rhinoplasty operation

1. Essentials – 2.5x loupes, fiberoptic headlight, own instruments

2. Anesthesia – General with appropriate monitors

3. Local injection followed by preparation – wait 10–15 min

4. Remove intranasal nasal pack and shave vibrissae

5. Open approach using infralobular and transcolumellar incisions

6. Elevation of skin envelope

7. Septal exposure via transfixion incision and extramucosal tunnels

8. Reassess operative plan based on alar and septal anatomy

9. Creation of symmetrical alar rim strips

10. Incremental hump reduction – rasp:bone, scissors:cartilage

11. Caudal septum/ANS excision (Optional)

12. Septal harvest/septoplasty

13. Osteotomies

14. Graft preparation

15. Spreader grafts (Optional)

16. Columellar strut and suture

17. Tip sutures with optional add-on grafts (excised alar cartilage)

18. Closure

19. Alar base modification (optional)

20. Alar rim grafts (ARS) (optional)

21. Doyle splints, external cast, and nasal block

The basic operation is a relatively standard sequence that I use routinely, but with virtually unlimited variations. The operative sequence is individualized for each primary rhinoplasty with certain steps deleted as indicated. Although every step of the basic rhinoplasty operation does not need to be done in each patient, I am convinced each step will be needed in your first 25 rhinoplasties.

Anesthesia

I do the vast majority of my rhinoplasties under general anesthesia because this is what the patient and I prefer. Certain precautions have improved the safety record of general anesthesia: (1) a Raye tube is used and the tube is marked with tape at the lip line, (2) alarm sensors can determine any disconnection of the tube within 5 seconds, and (3) oxygen and carbon dioxide monitors are routinely used. Additional precautions include ointment in the eyes to prevent corneal abrasion and a throat pack of wet 2 in. gauze to prevent ingestion of blood. In nonallergic patients, 1 g of Ancef is given intravenously during the operation.

Once intubation is complete, the external and internal areas of the nose are thoroughly scrubbed with Betadine paint by the surgeon. Then, the local anesthesia with its vasoconstrictive agent (1% xylocaine with epinephrine 1:100,000) is injected (Fig. 2.2). The injections are done in two components: a picture frame block to reduce the regional blood supply and then the specific areas of surgery. This method also produces an effective sensory block. Specifically, the five areas for injection consist of (1) tip and columella, (2) lateral wall, (3) dorsum/extramucosal tunnels, (4) incision lines, and (5) septum if appropriate. First, the needle is inserted from the vestibule toward the infraorbital foramen with injection occurring on withdrawal. Three sites are injected: infraorbital foramen (infraorbital vessels), lateral nasofacial groove (lateral facial vessels), and alar base (angular vessels). The columella base is injected extending outward below the nostril sills (columellar vessels). The needle is then inserted along the top of the septum in the area of the extra mucosal tunnels (anterior ethmoidal vessels). On withdrawal, the needle passes along the dorsum to facilitate future dissection and terminates in the radix area on either side (infratrochlear vessels). Next, the access incisions are injected with minute amounts of local anesthesia. The septum is blocked from posterior to anterior. For an open approach, I inject the lobular skin envelope over the alar cartilages from the tip extending laterally and down the columella. The nasal vibrissae are most easily trimmed with a scissors. The internal nose is packed with 18 in. strips of 0.5 in. gauze wetted with 4 cc of one of the three solutions: 4% cocaine, 1% xylocaine with epinephrine 1:100,000, or Afrin. I prefer 4% cocaine, but any of the three is effective.

PRINCIPLES

- Use general anesthesia with appropriate monitors and a throat pack.
- Do a thorough intranasal prep with Betadine prior to injection.
- Do a five-area injection of local anesthesia based on the vascular anatomy.
- With an open approach, do not hesitate to hydrodissect the entire lobule (1.5–2 cc). It will disappear quickly.
- Pack the nose with 0.5 in. gauze soaked in a topical vasoconstrictive agent.
- Once injected, wait 15 min. Do the definitive prep and drape.

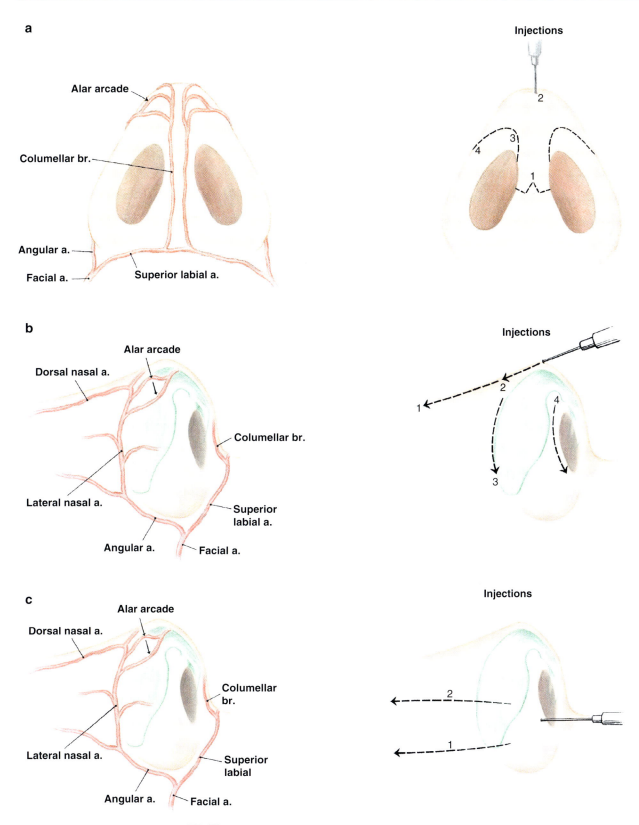

Fig. 2.2 (**a-c**) Local anesthesia

Open Approach   Immediately prior to the incisions, I redraw the transcolumellar incision and reinject the columellar with local anesthesia. Over the years, I have tried virtually all the standard columellar incisions, but I still prefer Goodman's original inverted-V with wings. A small 3 mm equilateral inverted-V is drawn whose apex is at the narrowest point of the columellar (Fig. 2.3a–d). The transverse wings are drawn across and behind the columellar pillars. The standard infracartilaginous incision consists of three parts: lateral crura, dome, and columella. It must be emphasized that this incision *follows the caudal border of the lateral crura* and not the nostril rim. Using a 10 mm double hook, the surgeon retracts the alar rim and then provides counterpressure with the ring finger. The #15 blade is then placed at the dome and the lateral cut is done following the caudal border of the lateral crura. Then the double hook is readjusted and counterpressure is placed on the dome allowing the incision to be carefully "scratched" high in the vestibule from the dome down onto the columellar to the level of the transcolumellar incision. Holding the columella with the nondominant hand, a #11 blade is used to make the inverted-V incision and then a #15 blade is used to make the transverse wings being careful to "scratch" through the skin overlying the cartilage.

Columella-to-Tip Exposure. With the incisions completed, a "columella to tip" dissection technique is used with three-point traction (Fig. 2.3e, f). The assistant retracts the alar rim upward with a small double hook while retracting the dome downward with a single double hook. The surgeon then elevates the columellar skin with a small double hook and dissects upward using the angled converse scissors. It is often necessary to switch back and forth between the two sides, and to use extreme caution as one approaches the domes. The skin envelope is retracted upward with a Ragnell retractor and the area overlying the septal angle is entered to expose the glistening cartilaginous vault. Hemostasis is done as required.

Bidirectional Exposure. Although the "columella to tip" exposure method is the classic one, the "bidirectional" exposure technique is easy to learn and extremely useful in scarred secondary tips (Fig. 2.3g, h). Essentially, one makes the standard infracartilaginous incision and then dissects over the lateral crura using blunt tip tenotomy scissors. Then the scissor tips are turned perpendicular and spread to allow rapid avascular dissection which is continued toward the domes. The soft tissue is elevated from the transcolumellar incision upward. The bidirectional exposure allows the dome to be preserved.

PRINCIPLES

- The location of the transcolumellar incision is more important than its shape. It's apex is at the narrowest point of the columellar.
- The infracartilaginous incision follows the caudal border of the alar cartilage – a true nostril rim incision can be a disaster.
- Do not hesitate to inject 1–2.0 cc of local anesthesia into the tip lobule – it facilitates dissection and will dissipate quickly.

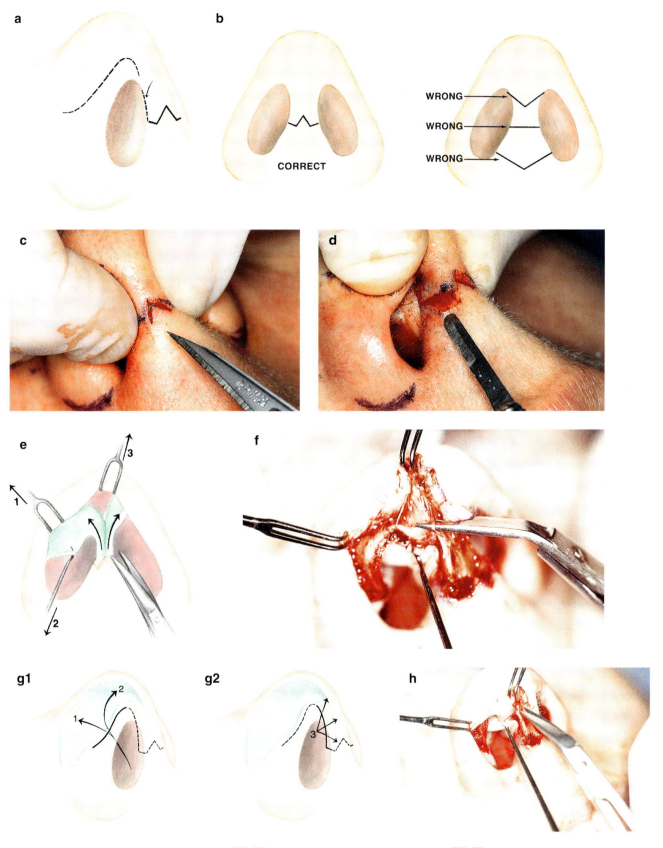

Fig. 2.3 (**a–d**) Open approach: incisions **DVD** (**e**, **f**) columellar to tip exposure **DVD** (**g**, **h**) bidirectional exposure **DVD**

Tip Analysis and Symmetrical Rim Strips

Tip Analysis. With exposure completed, it is important to take a "surgical time out" and review the operative plan based on the newly revealed nasal anatomy, especially the alar cartilages (Fig. 2.5a–c). One should reconcile the planned tip surgery with the actual crural configuration, especially the domes and lateral crura. Sometimes, one will encounter unexpected anatomical variations including marked domal asymmetry (solution: a concealer graft of excised alar cartilage) or significant concavity of the lateral crura (solution: a lateral crural fold rather than excision). Also, the tip cartilages may be flimsy (preserve more than 6 mm) or thicker (more sutures may be required). Also, one should reassess the dorsum and caudal septum/anterior nasal spine (ANS). At this point, the surgeon should have an idea as to the degree of septal deviation and the amount of cartilage available for harvest.

Symmetrical Rim Strips. Attention is then directed toward resection of the cephalic portion of the alar cartilages. A portion of the cephalic lateral crura is excised in virtually all cases to reduce the volume of the nasal tip and to increase the malleability of the cartilage for shaping with sutures (Fig. 2.5d–f). In addition, the excision causes significant changes in the convexity of the lateral crura. The line of incision is marked on the alar cartilage using a caliper and marking pen. A 6 mm strip of cephalic lateral crura is left as this width facilitates insertion of sutures and retains sufficient support for the rim while minimizing any alar retraction. However, three points are important in drawing the incision line: (1) the initial 6 mm width is drawn at the widest point of the lateral crura, (2) medially, the line is tapered to preserve the natural width of the domal notch, and (3) laterally, the line follows the caudal border of the lateral crura preserving a 6 mm width. Once the line is drawn, the underlying mucosal surface of the alar cartilage is injected with local anesthesia to facilitate dissection. The cartilage is then held with forceps and a #15 blade is used in incise the lateral crura along the marked line. The actual excision of the cartilage is usually done from the domal notch area laterally. The excision follows the scroll junction with the upper lateral cartilages cephalically. Every effort is made to remove the cartilage intact as it is often used for add-on grafts.

One of the advantages of doing the excision at this point in the operative sequence is that it improves visualization of dorsal reduction. One can easily elevate the mucosa over the septal angle by dissecting upward from the exposed caudal septum thus having a bidirectional exposure. Then, the Cottle elevator is inserted longitudinally beneath the dorsum making sure that the extramucosal tunnels are adequate.

PRINCIPLES

- Volume reduction of the tip is achieved by excising the lateral crura.
- Excising the lateral crura creates symmetrical rim strips which will be sutured.
- Keep a 6 mm wide rim strip for support and suturing.
- It is rarely necessary to narrow the domal notch area.
- Follow the caudal border of the lateral crura, tapering your excision at either end.

a   Tip Diamond

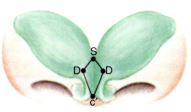

Projection
Rotation

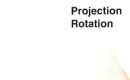

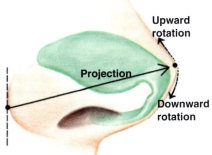

Upward
rotation

Projection

Downward
rotation

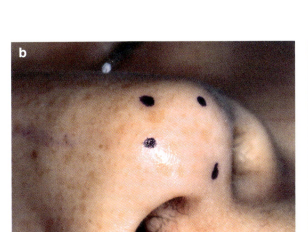

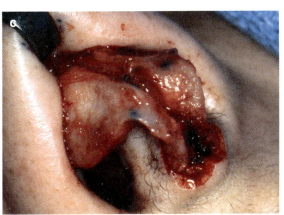

Fig. 2.5 (a–c) Tip analysis **DVD**

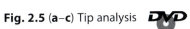

d

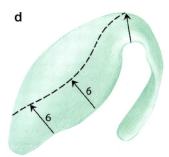

6

6

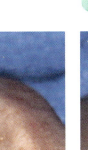

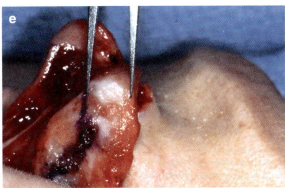

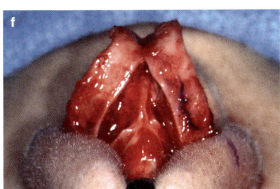

Fig. 2.5 (d–f) Symmetrical rim strips **DVD**

Dorsal Modification

Preoperatively, decisions must be made as to dorsal height (reduction, augmentation, or preservation), width (narrower, wider, or asymmetric correction) and length (shorter or longer).

Incremental Dorsal Reduction. The most common selection is dorsal reduction which is done incrementally using rasps for the bony hump and scissors for the cartilaginous hump (Figs. 2.6 and 2.7). The bone is done first using puller rasps to reduce the midline and then each nasal bone individually on an angle. Once the bony dorsum matches the ideal profile line drawn on the skin preoperatively, then the cartilaginous hump is reduced. I prefer the "split hump technique" in which the cartilaginous hump is separated into three parts (septum and two upper lateral cartilages). Straight blunt tip-serrated scissors are inserted vertically into the extramucosal tunnels. Then the cartilage is cut perpendicular to the septum thus splitting the hump. The dorsal septum is reduced incrementally with the scissors. The skin is redraped and the dorsal line checked by pulling the nasal skin laterally. Any additional lowering of the septum is done in minuscule amounts with a broken off #11 blade. Next, the upper lateral cartilages are excised conservatively. One must be cautious in this excision as the simple act of retracting the skin upward can cause the upper laterals to appear higher than they really are. In general, upper lateral excision is 33–50% of the dorsal cartilage reduction (3 mm of septum, 1–1.5 mm of upper lateral). Also, the goal is different for the two excisions – excision of the dorsal septum *reduces profile height* while excision of the upper laterals *narrows dorsal width*. At this point in the operation, it is extremely important to check the cartilaginous dorsum near the anterior septal angle. Any remaining prominence is easily removed with scissors. Finally, the dorsal line is carefully checked and micro adjustments if any are made.

Why do I prefer bony vault reduction before the cartilaginous vault and why not an osteotome? In most hump reductions, the bony vault is quite thin (<1 mm) and rasping reveals the underlying cartilaginous hump that extends 8–10 mm cephalically beneath the bone. Thus, rasping is effective and conservative while an osteotome has little margin of error and a very real risk of too much excision. Removing the bone first reveals the true dimensions of the necessary cartilaginous hump removal.

PRINCIPLES

- Ninety-five percent of patients want a smaller nose which implies dorsal reduction.
- Incremental reduction using a rasp for the bony hump and scissors for a split cartilage hump excision is the most controllable and conservative method.
- Upper lateral excision (dorsal width reduction) is usually 33–50% of the dorsal septal excision (dorsal height reduction).

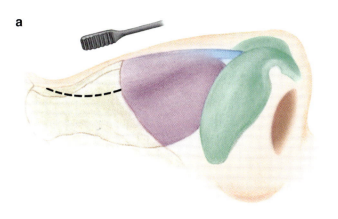
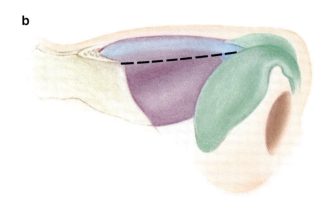

Fig. 2.6 (**a**, **b**) Bony reduction **DVD**

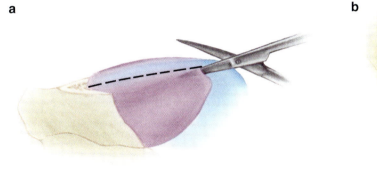
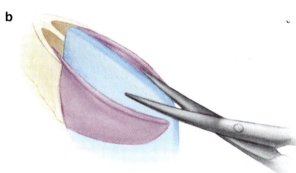

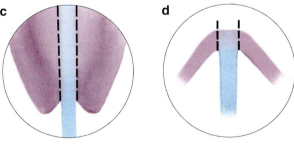
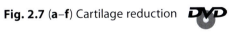
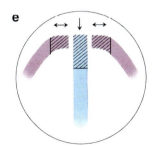
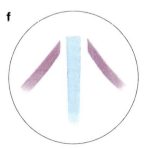

Fig. 2.7 (**a**–**f**) Cartilage reduction **DVD**

Caudal Septum and Anterior Nasal Spine

Resection. Modification of this area should be done conservatively. Preoperative assessment, both visual and palpable, in repose and on smiling is essential. Although the region can be approached through a "tip split" of the alar cartilages, greater control and flexibility is possible through the transfixion incision. Three changes are considered: (1) rotating the tip by resecting the upper half, (2) shortening the nose by resecting the lower half, and (3) altering the columellar labial segment by contouring or resecting the anterior nasal spine (Fig. 2.8). Minor changes usually consist of cartilage only resections (2–3 mm) cephalically angled for rotation or alternatively a full-length parallel resection for shortening which maintains the double break. Moderate changes tend to be slightly wider (3–5 mm), but rarely include the overlying mucosa bilaterally. For maximum change, resections can be wider and may include a portion of the mucosa. In the vast majority of the cases, one should avoid excising the membranous septum. The anterior nasal spine can be either reduced (excising its prominence while maintaining its contour) or resected to deliberately change the contour of the columella labial segment.

Grafting. Augmenting the columellar base is usually done in the form of a columellar strut to push down the columella inclination or small "plumping" grafts placed beneath the columella labial segment. Only in severe secondary cases or certain ethnic groups would diced cartilage grafts be placed in a subperiosteal transverse position across the pyriform aperture.

Caudal Septal Relocation. Correction of the deviated caudal septum is most easily achieved by relocation (Fig. 2.9). The caudal septum is freed from its bony/fibrous attachments, brought to the midline, and then sutured to the ANS. This method works extremely well if one respects three factors: (1) the caudal septum must be completely released and totally mobile, (2) fixation to the ANS must be rigid, and (3) the structural integrity of the caudal septum must not be compromised by incisions or excisions. The cartilaginous caudal septum is freed from ANS and a hole is drilled through the ANS. A 4–0 polydioxanone suture (PDS) is placed through the ANS from the nondeviated side, then through the septum, and looped on itself. The knot is then tied on the nondeviated side of the ANS. When completed, the caudal septum is rigidly fixed on the nondeviated side of the ANS midline.

PRINCIPLES

- Conservative excision of the caudal septum allows tip rotation and shortening of a long nose with a dependent tip.
- Avoid excision of the membranous septum as it often leads to disastrous upward rotation and shortening.
- Relocation of the deviated caudal septum is often necessary for both functional and aesthetic reasons.
- Caudal septal relocation is easily mastered. One should not do incisions of the caudal septum as it will weaken it.

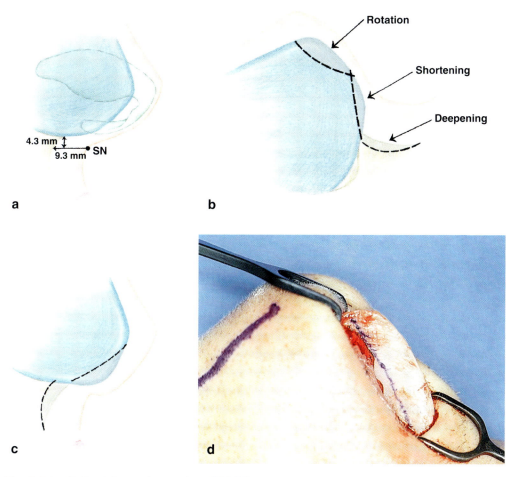

Fig. 2.8 (a–d) Caudal septal resection

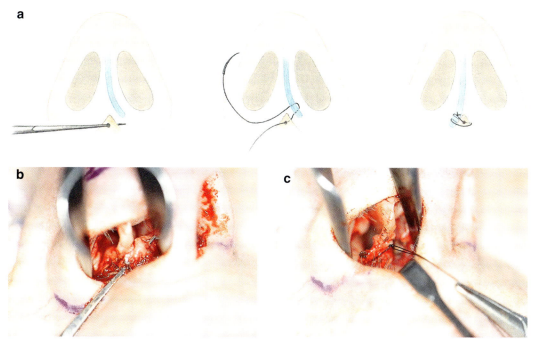

Fig. 2.9 (a–c) Caudal septal relocation

Septal Harvest and Septoplasty

Once the desired nasal profile is established, septal correction and harvesting can be done safely without compromising septal support or risking a septal disruption. In a septal harvest procedure, one tends to take as much cartilage as required while maintaining the essential 10 mm L-shape strut (Fig. 2.10). Common variations include: (1) the lower half of cartilage for a columella strut and/or spreader grafts, (2) the available quadrilateral cartilage for multiple grafts, and (3) extensive cartilage and bone en bloc especially in Asian rhinoplasty. In all practical aspects, a septal harvest is the equivalent of a septoplasty of the septal body.

Definitive Septal Exposure. At this point in the operation, it is often wise to inspect the internal nose and reinject the septum with local anesthesia for hydrodissection. Elevation of the septal mucosal lining is usually quite easy as one has a *bidirectional approach* – top down from the dorsal resection and straight back from the transfixion incision. The dissection planes are already defined from creation of the extra mucosal tunnels. The mucosa is elevated from caudal to cephalic over the upper portion of the cartilage using the round sharp end of a Cottle elevator. Then, a vertical sweep is done back over the perpendicular plate of ethmoid and downward onto the vomer. The inferior mucosa is elevated from the posterior vomer forward which allows easier separation of the fused perichondrial/periosteal fibers. In significant deviations, it is always best to start on the easier concave side and get a feel for the tissues before doing the more challenging convex side.

Septal Harvest. Once satisfied with the exposure, the quadrilateral cartilage can be harvested which simultaneously corrects any septal body deviation. With the mucosa reflected laterally, cuts are made parallel to the dorsal and caudal portions of the desired L-shape strut. The caudal cut is extended down to the cartilaginous vomerine junction while paralleling the caudal septal border, thus preserving a 10 mm strut. The dorsal cut is easily completed under direct vision from the dorsal approach while preserving a 10 mm strut. Then the septal body is dissected out of the vomerine groove as far back as possible using the round sharp end of the Cottle elevator. One separates the cartilage from the bone vertically along the cartilage's junction with perpendicular plate of ethmoid. The "extension" of the cartilaginous septum is usually removed with the body of the septum. I do not use a septal mucosal suture to approximate the mucosal space, but rather rely on sutured Doyle splints to compress the dead space. Note: it is rarely necessary to excise large osseocartilaginous portions of the septum which increases the risk of septal collapse.

PRINCIPLES

- A 10 mm L-shaped septal strut is always maintained.
- A septal harvest implies excision of quadrilateral cartilage (no bone) and is also an effective septoplasty for body deviations.
- One must be able to do a caudal septal relocation.

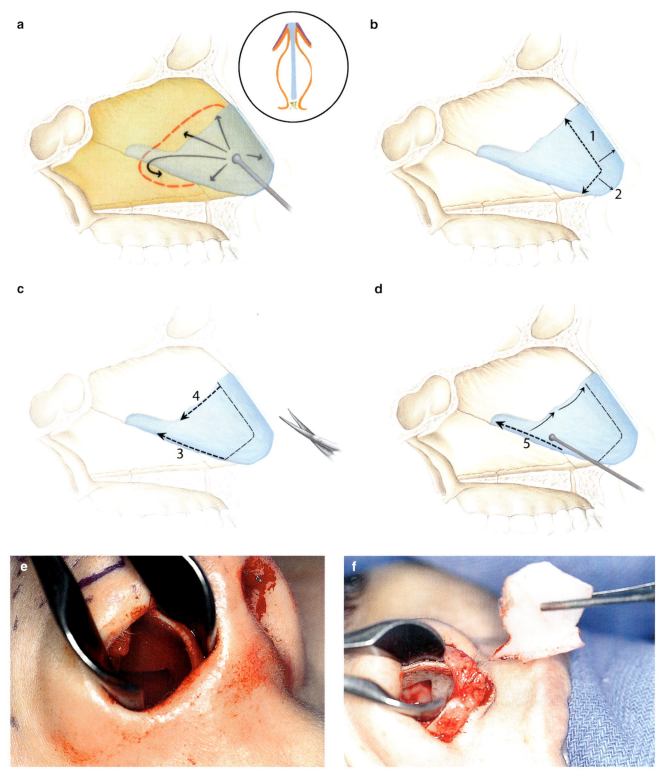

Fig. 2.10 (**a**–**d**) Septal harvest, (**e**) transfixion approach, (**f**) dorsal approach

Osteotomies

Types of Osteotomies. The purpose of lateral osteotomies is to narrow the base bony width (x-x) of the nose as measured at its widest point; not merely to close the open dorsal roof. The two most common methods are the low-to-high and low-to-low osteotomies which differ in their direction, degree of bony fracture, and movement. The *low-to-high osteotomy* begins at the pyriform aperture on the nasal process of maxilla and passes tangentially across it to the nasal bone suture line at the level of the medial canthus (Fig. 2.11a, b). Next, digital pressure on the lateral wall results in a greenstick fracture of the transverse portion and a gentle tilt of the lateral nasal wall. In contrast, the *low-to-low osteotomy* is done in two steps (Fig. 2.11c, d). First, a transverse osteotomy is done with a 2 mm osteotome placed through a small vertical stab incision just above the medial canthus. The osteotome is gently tapped to insure a complete vertical osteotomy in the lateral nasal wall. Second, a low-to-low lateral osteotomy is done using a straight osteotome. It begins at the pyriform aperture on the nasal process of the maxilla and passes straight up the lateral wall to end at the level of the medial canthus. Digital pressure produces complete mobilization of the lateral wall and definite narrowing of the nose. The primary difference is that a low-to-high osteotomy preserves bony contact at the transverse greenstick fracture which limits movement. In contrast, the low-to-low osteotomy incorporates a complete osteotomy transversely allowing total movement of lateral nasal wall.

Osteotomy Techniques. The type of osteotomy selected is determined by the base bony width of the nose (X-point), which should be narrower than the inter-eye distance. The osteotomy site is reinjected with 0.5 cc of local anesthesia, both subcutaneously and submucosally. A small speculum is inserted vertically in the nostril and straddles the pyriform aperture. A transverse cut is made in the mucosa using a cautery. The osteotome is inserted with the guard outward to facilitate palpation. The surgeon holds the *curved* osteotome in the dominant hand and palpates the guard with the other hand. The lateral osteotomy continues to the level of the medial canthus or the base of the previous transverse osteotomy. For a low-to-high osteotomy, the osteotome is withdrawn and digital pressure is used to create a transverse greenstick fracture which produces the desired tilt. For a low-to-low osteotomy, the *straight* osteotome is rotated 90° with the blade pushing against the maxilla which forces the lateral nasal wall inward.

PRINCIPLES

- Determine the indication for osteotomies on anterior view: base bony width is the key.
- Determine the method of osteotomy by the amount of movement required: tilt (low-to-high) or complete lateral wall narrowing (low-to-low).
- Although I prefer a continuous internal osteotomy, other surgeons prefer a percutaneous method – use whichever method you are comfortable with.

Table 2.2 Open tip suture technique

Step	Surgical technique	Effect	Frequency
Step #1	Symmetrical rim strips	Decrease volume	99%
	Cephalic lateral crura excision	More suturable	Leave 6 mm
Step #2	Columellar strut with strut suture	Increases projection	99%
		Prevents drooping	
Step #3	Domal creation suture R & L	Increases definition	95%
Step #4	Interdomal suture	Decreases tip width	90%
		Creates tip diamond	
Step #5	Domal equalization suture	Increase symmetry	75%
Step #6	Lateral crural convexity suture	Decreases convexity	20%
		of lateral crura	
Step #7	Tip position suture	Increase projection	75%
		Increase rotation	
Step #8	Add-on grafts	Increases definition	40%
		Increase projections	
Step #9	Alar rim grafts	Supports alar rims	10–15%

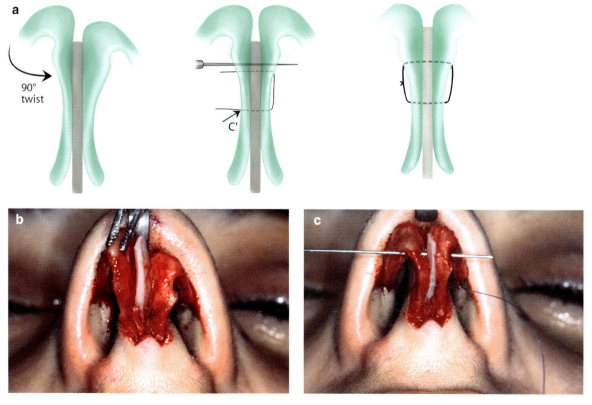

Fig. 2.13 (a–c) Columellar strut and suture

2) Domal Creation Suture

The domal creation suture produces tip definition by creating the ideal domal anatomy, even from flat or concave cartilages. Essentially, one inserts a horizontal mattress suture across the domal segment at the domal notch and cinches it down to create a convex domal segment next to a concave lateral crura (Fig. 2.14). This anatomical configuration produces the most attractive tip once the skin is redraped.

Although conceptually simple, the surgeon must become facile with this suture. The domal notch is determined and gently squeezed with an Adson-Brown forceps to determine the desired amount of convexity. The new dome defining point is marked.

Then a horizontal mattress suture is placed from medial to lateral with the knot tied medially. The tension is gradually tightened until the desired domal convexity is achieved. Although one focuses on the domal convexity, the reality is a gradually increasing domal convexity next to a gradually increasing lateral crura concavity. The following five suture errors are to be avoided: (1) too tight can result in a sharp point under thin skin, (2) too loose fails to achieve the desired definition, (3) too medial a placement snubs off the tip, (4) too lateral a placement makes the infralobule lengthy, and (5) do not try to modify the entire lateral crura, just the area comprising the dome. Unlike incision and excision techniques, which weaken the rim strip and often lead to bossa, the domal suture is initially reversible and can be replaced several times depending upon the rigidity of the cartilage. In contrast to tip grafts with their disadvantages, tip sutures achieve definition without visibility, cartilage atrophy, or thinning of the skin.

3) Interdomal Suture

The interdomal suture controls tip width both at the domes and in the infralobule. It is a simple vertical suture that begins on one crura adjacent to the domal creation suture, exits above the crural suture, then enters the opposite crura at the same level, and exits adjacent to the domal creation suture (Fig. 2.15). The knot is gradually tightened until the ideal width is achieved. The simplicity of inserting this stitch is due to its place in the tip suturing sequence. Since the columellar strut suture and domal creation sutures are already in place, the location of the interdomal suture is virtually predetermined. The suture enters just below the domal creation knot on the left and exits just above the sutured middle crura. Then the suture enters the right crura directly across on the middle crura and exits just below the domal creation knot. The only decisions are how far back from the caudal border to insert the suture and how tight to tie the knot. In general, the suture is placed 2–3 mm back from the caudal border of the crura. If placed too close to the caudal edge then excessive narrowing of the columellar occurs. The suture is gradually tightened to reduce the interdomal width not to create a single pointy tip. Remember the "tip diamond" concept. Also, the columellar flares at its base, narrows at its mid point, and gradually widens in the infralobule.

4) Tip Position Suture

The tip position suture achieves both tip rotation and increases projection which in turn creates the *supratip break* that most patients desire. It is a simple transverse suture between the infralobular mucosa and the anterior dorsal septum (Fig. 2.16a–c). As the knot is tightened the tip rotates upward and projects above the dorsal line creating a supratip set off. Early on, one should do a single throw, redrape the skin, and assess its effect – be careful, over rotation is a disaster.

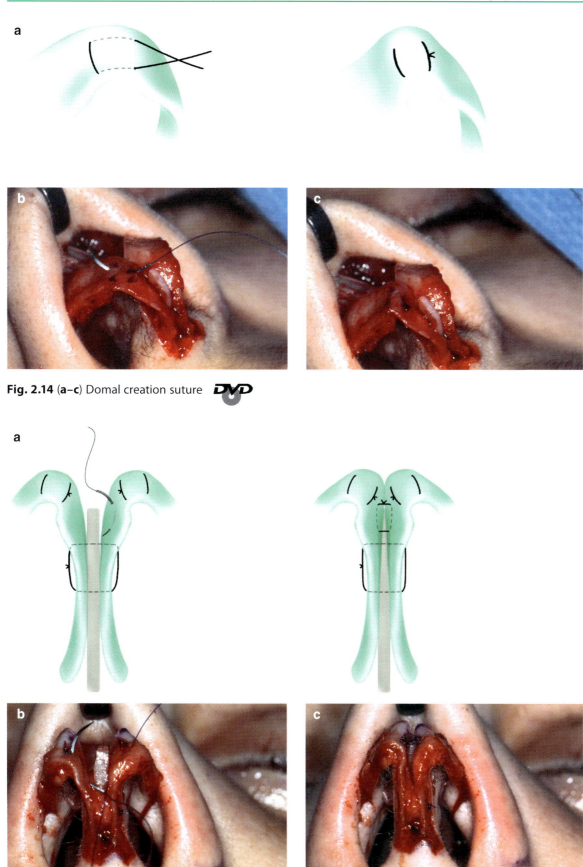

Fig. 2.14 (**a–c**) Domal creation suture

Fig. 2.15 (**a–c**) Interdomal suture

The tip position suture is inserted as follows. A 4–0 PDS suture on an FS2 needle is used. The surgeon stands at the top of the table. The suture is transverse beginning with a pass through the mucosa of the infralobule with optional inclusion of the columellar strut. The next pass is through the dorsal septum about 3–4 mm back from the anterior septal angle usually avoiding the spreader grafts. In general, I will do a single throw, redrape the skin, and asses the changes before adding additional ties. It is never tied rigidly tight, but rather serves as a loop bringing the tip above the anterior septal angle. The goal is to rotate the tip slightly while giving additional support to the tip which in turn creates the desired super tip break. I find this method of suturing more effective and with less risk of columellar distortion than Gruber's columellar-septal suture. Equally, I am not a fan of the tongue-in-groove technique where the alar cartilages are rotated on either side of the caudal septum and then fixed with sutures. The problem with the latter suture is that fine-graded adjustments in rotation and projection cannot be made once the alars are sutured to the septum. In contrast, the tip position suture is inserted after the ideal tip is created and the tension can be tightened incrementally.

5) Add-On Tip Refinement Grafts

Once suturing is completed, small tip grafts can be added to provide additional refinement (Daniel, 2002, 2009). Ideally, these grafts are made from excised alar cartilage and can be placed in different locations and combinations (Fig. 2.16d–f). Initially, I used these grafts as "concealer" grafts to hide tip asymmetry or bifidity under thin skin. However, their application has been expanded to include greater infralobular curvature (infralobule position) and tip definition (transdomal position). They are truly "added on" to the final sutured tip to enhance tip refinement with minimal risk. Whenever possible, excised alar cartilage is used as it is quite pliable, easily shaped, and can be layered. These grafts have minimal risk of showing through the skin in contrast to rigid grafts of septal or conchal cartilage. The two most common locations are transdomal (Peck-type graft) and infralobular (Sheen-type graft). The *transdomal onlay* graft is placed over the domes to increase tip definition or used as a double layer to slightly increase tip projection. The grafts are sutured to the underlying alar cartilages at the graft's four corners. The *infralobular* graft is cut in a tapered Sheen "shield" style and sutured to the alar cartilages at the domal notch and midcolumellar points. Prior to suturing, the top of the graft can be raised to the edge of the cartilage or slightly above to either increase projection or accentuate caudal tip position. If the top edge is raised more than 1 mm above the cartilage then a "cap" graft must be placed behind it to provide ridge support. These grafts can be either a transdomal or a vertical wedge depending upon where tip refinement is desired. Inherently, these grafts are also concealing any asymmetries. If the grafts are too visible, the first choice is to remove them. If the grafts are absolutely essential as in an asymmetric tip with thin skin, then one can consider adding a fascia graft to provide thicker soft tissue coverage.

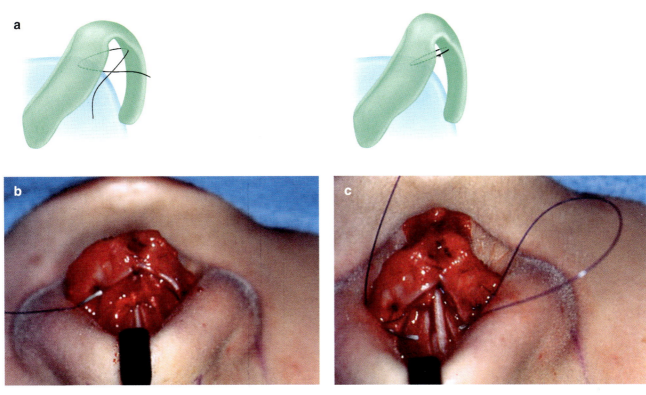

Fig. 2.16 (**a–c**) Tip position suture DVD

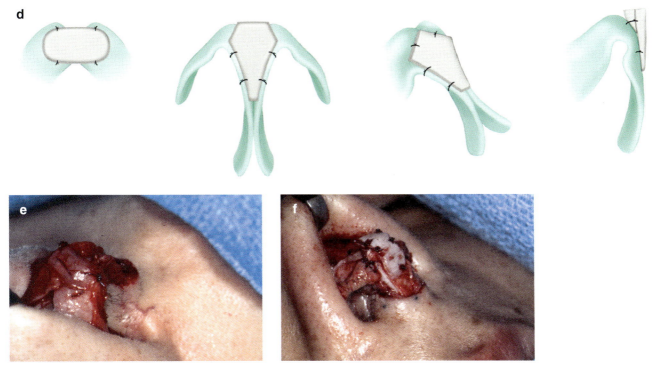

Fig. 2.16 (**d–f**) Add-on tip refinement grafts DVD

Alar Base Modification

Alar base modification should be carefully planned preoperatively, and executed very conservatively; aggressive excisions can be disastrous and virtually irreparable. The decision as to the type and amount of the excision is based upon nostril shape and sill width. The critical factor is the relationship between alar flare and alar width as regards intercanthal width. Alar width (AC-AC) is measured at the alar crease, whereas alar flare (AL-AL) is measured at the widest point of the alar, usually 3–4 mm above the crease. These two distances as well as the intercanthal width (EN-EN) are easily measured with a sliding caliper directly on the patient. The critical decision is whether alar width (AL-AL) is greater than intercanthal width (EN-EN) preoperatively or will become greater as dorsal support and tip projection are reduced intraoperatively. There are basically three surgical techniques: (1) a simple nostril sill excision to reduce nostril show, (2) an alar wedge excision to reduce nostril flare, and (3) a combined sill/wedge excision with components that can reduce flare as well as alar width.

Nostril Sill Excision. For nostril sill excisions, a 2.5–3.5 mm wide inverted trapezoid is drawn (Fig. 2.17a, b). The sides are vertical and then triangular with equal extension into the vestibule and onto the skin surface. After injection with local anesthesia, the wedge is excised. The sill/vestibule component is closed with a horizontal mattress suture of 4–0 plain catgut which everts the edges and prevents a depressed scar. The skin is closed with 6–0 nylon.

Alar Wedge Excision. For alar wedge excisions, it is important that the line of incision be placed in the alar crease; too high produces a visible scar. The line of excision is drawn using a caliper (2.5–4 mm average) with quantitative variance on the two sides to accommodate asymmetries (Fig. 2.17c, d). The base is injected with local anesthesia; a fresh #15 blade is used. With the area stabilized on a skin hook, a V-wedge excision is made without penetrating the underlying vestibular skin. Following hemostasis, the edges are closed with 6–0 nylon and the knots placed on the more dependent side.

Combined Sill/Wedge Excision. In more severe cases, a combined excision of nostril sill and alar wedge is necessary (Fig. 2.17e, f). These are complex advanced excisions which are most common in ethnic rhinoplasty cases and will be discussed later.

PRINCIPLES

- Alar base modification must be done precisely and conservatively.
- One should master isolated alar wedge and nostril sill excisions before doing combined excisions.
- Alar rim grafts are often necessary as alar base excisions accentuates alar rim notching.

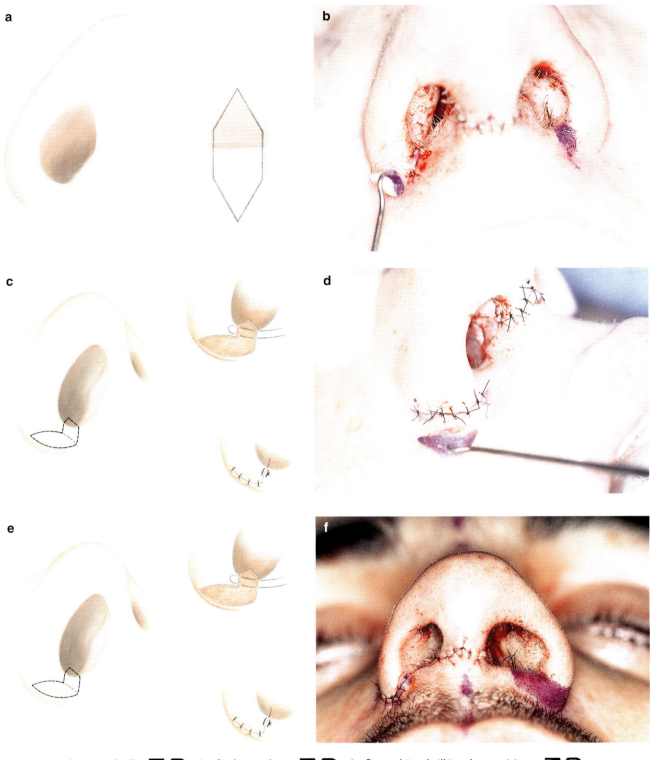

Fig. 2.17 (**a**, **b**) Nostril sill 🔵DVD (**c**, **d**) alar wedge 🔵DVD (**e**, **f**) combined sill/wedge excision 🔵DVD

Closure, Cast, and Post-op Management

All incisions are sutured. I begin with the transcolumellar incision: first, the midline suture at the apex of the V for alignment; second, the lateral corner sutures to insure redraping of the skin; and third, the columellar pillar sutures. Additional interrupted sutures of 6–0 nylon are added as indicated. Then the infracartilaginous incisions are closed with two sutures of 5–0 plain catgut. Rather than lining up predetermined dots, I favor two angulated sutures from lateral to dome. However, one must avoid notching the alar rim by suturing the mobile alar rim to a retracted alar cartilage. This problem can be treated by insertion of an alar rim graft. The transfixion incision is closed with 2–3 sutures of 4–0 plain catgut.

The classic nasal packing is not used It is not necessary, and patients hate it. If septal or turbinate work was done, then Doyle splints lubricated with polysporin ointment are inserted into the nasal airways (Fig. 2.18a, b). The splints are sutured together to compress the mucosal leaflets with a single horizontal mattress suture of 4–0 nylon which is always tied on the left side. These splints minimize the risk of a septal hematoma and prevent synechiae formation. The tubes are left on the Doyle splints when major septal straightening has been done and removed in other cases to facilitate breathing. The nose is then taped with 0.5 in. wide Steri-strips which compress the skin envelope, reduce edema, and model the tip (Fig. 2.18c). The tapes are applied in the following sequence: (1) three slightly overlapping transverse tapes on the bridge from radix to supratip, (2) two longitudinal tapes placed along the edges of the bridge of the nose and then pinched together to both narrow the tip and support it, and (3) another transverse tape to compress the supratip skin. A small piece of Telfa gauze (4 × 1 cm) is placed along the dorsum which will facilitate subsequent removal of the nasal splint. The plastic polymer splint is placed in boiling water to become flexible, molded over the bony portion of the nose, and then instantly "set" by pouring ice water over it.

The surgeon immediately dictates the operative report and fills out the operative flow sheet and diagrams. The smoothness of the postoperative course is directly proportional to the amount of time spent at the preoperative visit explaining to the patient what to expect. The post-op medications are confirmed (Vicodin for pain, cephalosporin antibiotic for 5 days). The patient is reminded to clean all suture lines free of crusts – two to three times a day with hydrogen peroxide and apply polysporin ointment. At 6 days, the dressings are removed in the following sequence: (1) the external cast is rocked side to side and comes off easily because of the Telfa sheet on the dorsum, (2) Steri-strips, (3) internal splints after cutting the suture on the left side, and (4) columellar and alar sutures,

PRINCIPLES

- The ease of the postoperative course is directly related to the thoroughness of the pre-op visit.
- Eversion of the nostril sill closure is critical, thus the horizontal mattress of 4–0 plain that everts the edges.
- After the cast is removed, the nose is taped using same taping method as intraop. The patient tapes at night for 3 weeks.

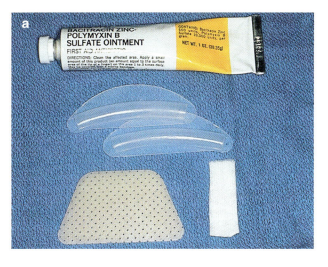

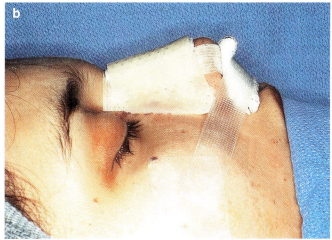

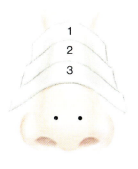

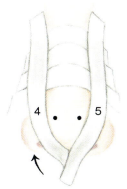

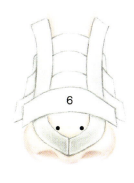

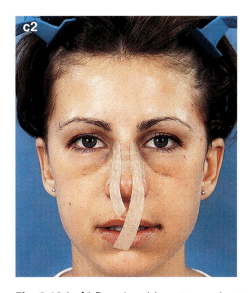

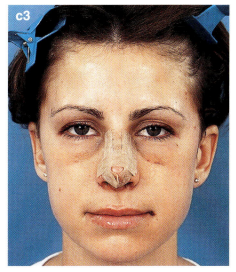

Fig. 2.18 (**a**, **b**) Dressing, (**c**) postoperative taping

The Basic Rhinoplasty Operation: A 95% Solution

This fundamental rhinoplasty operation allows surgeons to achieve very good results with an excellent margin of error. It is assumed that the surgeon has basic rhinoplasty skills acquired during their residency training. Building from their own foundation, one should assimilate the various parts of this standard operation. The surgeon does not need to use every step in every nasal surgery. However, one can be sure that every step might be required in the actual case one is doing that day. One cannot avoid correcting the anatomical causes of nasal obstruction that preexist in 35% of the cosmetic cases. As the surgeon gains experience, the operation can be expanded to an ever widening variety of cases and specific techniques added. A good example is incorporation of add-on grafts to get greater tip definition in thick skin patients and the use of alar rim grafts to minimize alar retraction. Some surgeons will question various aspects of this basic operation and I will attempt to address their concerns.

Q. Originally, you thought that a basic rhinoplasty operation was impossible because of the diversity of patients and operative techniques. What is different now?

A. I have concluded that a surgeon who does less than 35 rhinoplasties a year should learn one expandable operation well, select cases that are within their comfort zone, and commit to learning surgical cause and effect by keeping meticulous records of each procedure. Over a 3-year period, the surgeon can then expand their comfort zone and case profile from Level 1 to Level 2 which will cover 95% of the primary patients seen in a normal practice.

Q. Why the open approach in all cases?

A. A rhinoplasty is much easier to do open than closed. The variety of available tip procedures is much greater and 95% of the major secondary cases are done open. Therefore, it makes sense to master the open approach. If one is comfortable with the endonasal approach and wants to use it in some cases with limited tip deformities, that approach is certainly appropriate. However, for those with the usual limited residency experience, it makes sense to concentrate on one approach and that is the expandable open approach.

Q. Are you suggesting a septal harvest on all patients?

A. Yes, I am doing a septal harvest in most cases to obtain graft material. It is important to realize that a rhinoplasty is really an "*aesthetic septorhinoplasty*" and one must deal with all the functional aspects of a cosmetic case. I am convinced that 35% of the pure cosmetic rhinoplasty patients have a fixed anatomical nasal obstruction that will cause postoperative obstruction unless it is fixed during the operation. Thus, a septal harvest is also a septoplasty of the septal body that will improve nasal function in many cases. If one is going to do rhinoplasty surgery, one must become comfortable with all aspects of septal surgery including caudal septal relocation.

Q. How often do you do spreader grafts?

A. The percentage is around 75% with half for function and half for aesthetics. The larger the reduction is, the more frequent the use of spreader grafts to avoid an inverted-V deformity. Certainly, any reduction over 2 mm converts the Y-shape dorsum at the rhinion into an I-shape central septum with potential collapse of the upper lateral cartilages and blockage of the internal valve. Fully, half of my spreader grafts are made asymmetric in width to correct preoperative asymmetries. I have never regretted inserting spreader grafts, but I have regretted not doing them. It is my opinion that "spreader flaps" can be used for minimal problems, but are not a full-service solution.

Q. Why the columellar strut?

A. The columellar strut is almost magical in its beneficial effects on the tip. The columellar strut and its suture serve three purposes: tip stability, tip projection, and columellar shape. The strut fosters verticality and projection of the tip while eliminating plunging of the tip on smiling. Suturing the alars to the strut creates a unified tip complex and improves symmetry. It is this tip that can be positioned with the tip position suture to create a supratip set off. Equally important, the strut provides a rigid intrinsic shape for the columellar thus reducing the influence of a deviated caudal septum.

Q. How flexible is the tip suture operation?

A. The tip suture technique that I advocate is essentially a "sew until its perfect" procedure. One normally sets the foundation of the tip with the strut (strut suture), then creates tip definition (domal creation suture), narrows tip width (interdomal suture), reduces asymmetry (domal equalization suture), and then achieves the desired supratip break as well as projection and rotation (tip position suture). One stops when the tip looks great with the skin closed. Only those steps are done which the anatomy mandates. For example, one may not need a domal creation suture on both sides, or the symmetry is excellent and a domal equalization suture is not done. There are no special sutures or instruments required. All of this is done with off the shelf sutures of 5–0 and 4–0 PDS.

Q. Why should I follow the Level approach and learn the basic operation?

A. If you have just entered practice, both your clinical experience and surgical skill set are finite, while the variety of noses is infinite. If every good result brings you three referrals and every bad result loses you nine, why start with the hardest cases? Obviously, one of the goals of this text is to teach you to recognize the various levels of difficulty and help you select appropriate patients. Surgically, most residents finish their training having done less than 20 cosmetic rhinoplasties with minimal follow-up. Their understanding of surgical cause and effect is marginal at best. For the first few years in practice, one should concentrate on learning a single expandable operation. Meticulous records must be kept as they allow the surgeon to evaluate their results at each postoperative visit. Although every step of the basic operation does not need to be done in every patient, I am convinced that each step will be needed in your first 25 rhinoplasties. Thus, it makes sense to learn the basic operation as a collection of surgical techniques which the surgeon selects from to design the optimal operative plan for the individual patient.

Decision Making Level 1: Planning a Rhinoplasty

Step #1: The Consultation. A rhinoplasty will be successful only if it achieves what the patient wants. Therefore, you must have the patient point in the mirror at what three things bother him or her the most. Write them down on the operative planning sheet. Most women want a smaller more feminine nose with a lower profile, narrower width, and a more refined tip. Next, it is your turn to examine the nose externally and internally. Decide what the negatives are and what can be achieved realistically given the patients anatomy. Sketch out a proposed operative plan – how much reduction, what type of osteotomies, tip surgery, any base modification, and functional factors. Assess the level of difficulty and whether this case fits within your comfort zone. After talking with the patient, determine whether you want this patient in your practice. Standard nasal photos of the patient are taken assuming you both wish to proceed. The patient is asked to bring photos of noses they like to the next appointment. As shown in the DVD of Fig. 6.2, the importance of the intranasal exam cannot be over emphasized.

Step #2: The Pre-op Visit. Early in one's practice you should do a photo analysis on all patients as it trains you to "see" the deformity and the solution. The critical sequence is to define the deformity, to superimpose the ideal, and then determine what is surgically feasible. When the patient returns, examine the nose again without looking at your notes – you want to see what is wrong with the nose and visualize what a rhinoplasty can achieve. Then open your notes, give the patient a mirror and ask her to tell you what bothers her the most in the order of importance. Check her requests against your operative plan. Then look at the pictures of the noses that the patient likes. Then review the operative plan and make any necessary changes. Write out a step-by-step individualized operative plan.

Step #3: The Operation. The advantage of spending the time to write out a detail step-by-step operative plan is that the vast majority of operations go according to plan. You can concentrate on surgical execution and efficiency rather than surgical decision making. Yes, slight changes may be necessary based on actual anatomy (add-on graft, alar rim graft, etc.), but you are not staring at the nose wondering what to do next. It is wise to take a four-view set of photos of the exposed finished tip before closing. At the end of the operation, a detailed op diagram is made which records every step and any questions you might have as to surgical cause and effect (Fig. 2.20).

Step #4: Postoperative Follow-Up. The patient is seen a week later and the cast removed. The chart is opened to the op diagram page which allows you to assess surgical cause and effect. With the patient holding a mirror, the patient is taught how to tape their nose for compression. They are urged to wear the tapes for another 2–3 days and then tape at night for 3 weeks. They are given a set of their preoperative photographs. Return visits are scheduled at 1, 3, and 6 weeks with additional visits at 4 and 12 months.

A Basic Rhinoplasty Operation: Operative Sequence

  1) Essentials – 2.5x loupes, fiberoptic headlight, own instruments.

  2) General anesthesia with appropriate monitors.

  3) Local anesthesia injection, then preparation – wait for 10–15 min.

  4) Remove intranasal nasal pack and shave vibrissae.

  5) Open approach using infralobular and transcolumellar incisions.

  6) Elevation of skin envelope.

  7) Septal exposure via transfixion incision and extramucosal tunnels.

  8) Reassess operative plan based on alar and septal anatomy.

  9) Creation of symmetrical alar rim strips.

10) Incremental hump reduction – rasp:bony, scissors:cartilage.

11) Caudal septum/ANS excision.

12) Septal harvest/septoplasty.

13) Osteotomies.

14) Graft preparation.

15) Spreader grafts.

16) Columellar strut and suture.

17) Tip sutures.

18) Closure.

19) Alar base modification.

20) Alar rim support grafts (ARS).

21) Doyle splints and external cast and nasal block.

Note: all steps are considered, but only those steps indicated are actually used.

What Are the Most Common Variations?

1) Cartilaginous dorsal *reduction* is achieved primarily by excising the isolated dorsal septum, while *dorsal narrowing* is achieved by excision of upper lateral cartilage. The ratio is often 3:1 with minimal ULC resection.

2) The caudal septum is altered in less than 50% of the cases and the ANS in less than 5%.

3) The majority of septal problems in cosmetic cases are deviations of the septal body or caudal septum. A septal harvest often corrects the former while a relocation fixes the caudal septum.

4) Osteotomies are not done in 10% of the cases as the bony vault is quite narrow preoperatively and one does not want to reduce the nasal airway.

5) Spreader grafts are not done in 25% of the cases because the dorsum was reduced less than 2 mm. The majority of paired grafts are asymmetric and 50% are inserted for aesthetic reasons.

6) Tip sutures are sufficient in 75% of the patients with 20% having add-on grafts of excised alar cartilage. A true tip graft of septal cartilage is used in less than 5% of Caucasian patients, but 95% of Asian patients.

7) Initially, alar base modification should be something that the patient requests (smaller nostrils) rather than something that the surgeon suggests. Conservatism is essential.

8) Alar rim grafts may be necessary to minimize alar rim weakness. They are easily placed in subcutaneous pockets that parallel the alar rim.

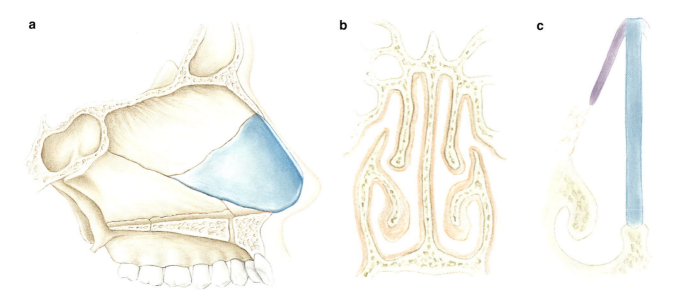

Fig. 2.19 (a–c)

Table 2.3 Photographic analysis

Anterior	Lateral	$N\text{-}T_i = 0.67 \times MFH$ $AC\text{-}T_i = 0.67 \times N\text{-}T_i$ $C\text{-}N_i = 0.28 \times N\text{-}T_i$		$N\text{-}T_i =$ $AC\text{-}T_i=$ $C\text{-}N_i=$	
EN-EN =	C-N =				
X-X =	AC-T =		Actual	Ideal	Change
AL-AL =	N-C' =	N			
AC-AC =	N-SN =	T			
IDD =	N-FA =	SN			
MFH =	TA =	NFA			
LFH =	CIA =	TA			
SME =	CLA =	CIA			
		C-N			
		N-T			
		AC-T			

Septorhinoplasty - Operative Procedure

Rollin K. Daniel, MD

LAST NAME   CASE NUMBER   DATE

INCISIONS AND APPROACH

Incisions: ☐ INTER ☐ INTRA ☐ INFRA ☐ Trans-columellar

☐ Transfixion-Unilateral ☐ Transfixion-Bilateral ☐ Killian

Approach: ☐ Closed ☐ Open ☐ Closed/Open

☐ Retrograde ☐ Trans-cartilagenous ☐ Delivery

NASAL TIP   ☐ UNTOUCHED

Cephalic Resection: ☐ Retrograde ☐ Trans-cartilage ☐ Delivery ☐ Open

Delivery: ☐ Cephalic resection ☐ Incisions ☐ Lateral seg. excision ☐ Domal excision

Sutures: ☐ Intradomal ☐ Transdomal ☐ Creation

☐ Other:

Tip Graft: ☐ Peck ☐ Juri ☐ Other:

Sheen Graft: ☐ Type I - crushed ☐ Type II - bruised ☐ Type III - solid ☐ Type IV - backstop

Open Structure: ☐ Suture ☐ Graft ☐ Domal excision ☐ Other:

Comment:

DORSUM   ☐ UNTOUCHED

Dorsum: ☐ Untouched ☐ Lowered ☐ Augmented ☐ Smoothed

☐ Other:

Radix: ☐ Reduction - rasp ☐ Reduction - osteotome ☐ Augmented - single graft ☐ Augmented - mutliple graft

☐ Other:

Bone: ☐ Rasp ☐ Osteotome ☐ Other:

Cartilage: ☐ Lowered ☐ Augmented ☐ Shortened ☐ Spreader

☐ Other:

OSTEOTOMIES   ☐ UNTOUCHED

		Right	Left
LATERAL	None		
	Low-high		
	Low-low		
	Double level		
TRANSVERSE	None		
	Digital		
	Osteotome		
MEDIAL	None		
	Medial		
	Medial Oblique		
CONTINUOUS			
MOVEMENT	Greenstick		
	Complete		

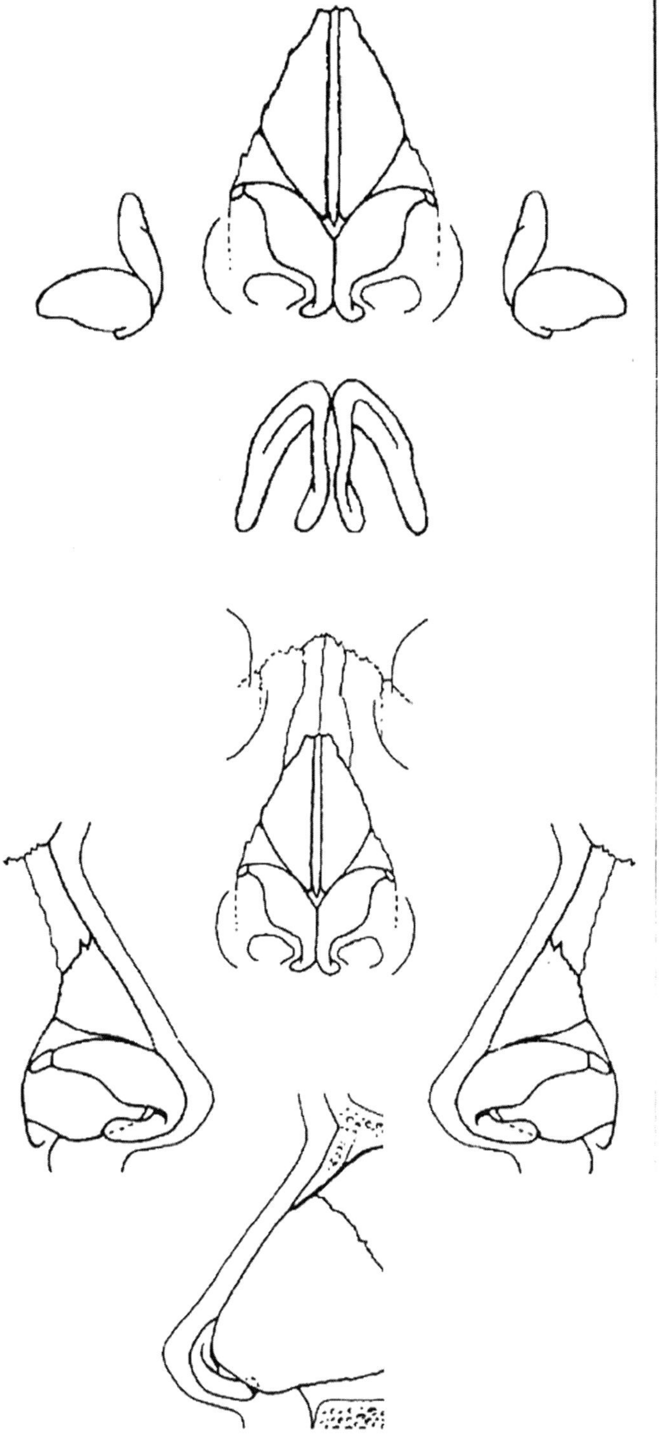

© Copyright 1992, Rollin K. Daniel, MD and Ronald G. Zelt, MD.

Fig. 2.20

Case Study: Aesthetic Septorhinoplasty (Level 1)

Analysis. A 16-year-old girl presented for a rhinoplasty (Fig. 2.21). She stated that she did not like her profile and that her breathing was normal. The external exam revealed a deviation of the caudal septum to the left. On profile and oblique view, she had a "tension nose" and a high potential for an inverted-V deformity. On internal exam, the septum totally blocked the right airway while the caudal deflection blocked the left external valve. Aesthetically, this is an easy case to obtain an excellent result. An incremental dorsal reduction (2 mm bone, 4 mm cartilage) and 4 mm of caudal septal resection was done. In addition, a chin implant gave better balance to the face. Yet the case illustrates the necessity of being able to correct septal deviations and doing spreader grafts for functional and aesthetic purposes. Thus, both techniques are part of the basic rhinoplasty operation.

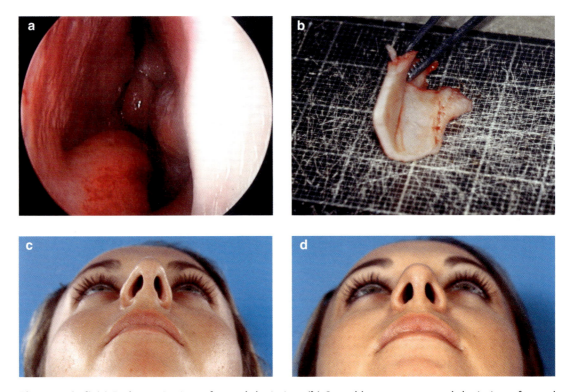

Fig. 2.21 (a-l) (**a**) Endoscopic view of septal deviation, (**b**) Septal harvest corrected deviation of septal body, (**c,d**) caudal septal relocation

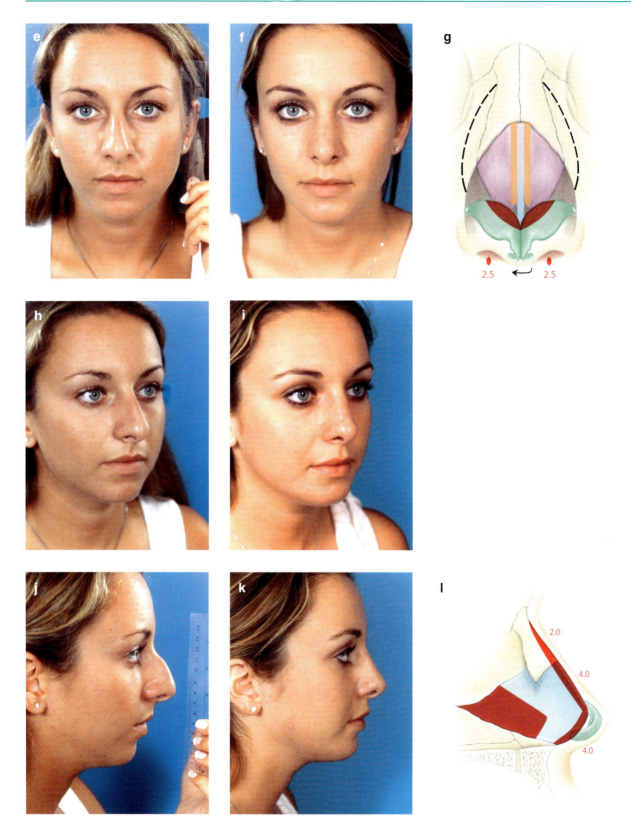

Fig. 2.21 (continued)

Decision Making Level 2: The Harder Nose

Each surgeon must develop their own criteria for assigning a degree of difficulty to each nose, from Level 1–3. Perhaps, the best method is to use a classic "standard deviation" system based on deviation from normal (Fig. 2.22). Each of the six tip criteria can be analyzed as well as skin thickness. After assessing the tip, a degree of difficulty is assigned for the dorsum, base, and septum. Added to the mix are patient factors and history of trauma or nasal obstruction. Here are a few of my own criteria and concerns.

Patient Factors. Is this patient psychologically a candidate for surgery and would a rhinoplasty make a real difference in their appearance? How would this patient cope with a complication? What is my margin of error? How close can I come to achieving what the patient wants? Am I comfortable with this patient and the operative plan?

Surgical Factors.

1. **Tip.** In most Level 2 cases, the challenge is bringing the tip back into the normal range without having to fundamentally change its shape. An example is the difference between a broad tip (Level 2) which requires aggressive suturing and perhaps add-on grafts versus an over projecting ball tip (Level 3) which may require alar transposition plus lateral crura strut grafts.
2. **Dorsum.** Level 2 cases often differ from Level 1 cases quantitatively – the amount of reduction and its cephalic extent are often greater. Spreader grafts are now a necessity. Any radix graft will be fascia and occasionally have diced cartilage beneath it. All full-length augmentations or major radix reductions are Level 3.
3. **Base.** Assigning a level for the base is most easily determined from the surgical plan. For example: Level 1 (nostril sill or alar wedge), Level 2 (combined nostril sill/alar wedge with alar rim graft), or Level 3 (major combined excisions in the ethnic nose). In Level 2 cases, one must be comfortable with all types of base excision and the standard alar rim grafts (ARG, ARS).
4. **Septum.** The more difficult septums are those with severe deviations due to developmental or traumatic etiologies. Correction may require dorsal splinting and division which can be challenging. Once comfortable with restoring dorsal stability and replacing the caudal septum, one can do a total septoplasty – a very frightening maneuver when done for the first time. Severe posttraumatic and secondary septums are considered Level 3 as there is no certainty as to how complex the surgery will become including possible rib grafts.

PRINCIPLES

- The simpler the operative plan is, the greater the chance of success.
- Transition from Level 1 to Level 2 cases by picking cases where only one or two areas of the nose are harder – not all aspects.
- Make sure the nose looks significantly better at the end of the operation – continue until it is as good as you can do.
- Never hesitate to take out sutures or grafts that are not perfect.

Tip width (Level 1–3)

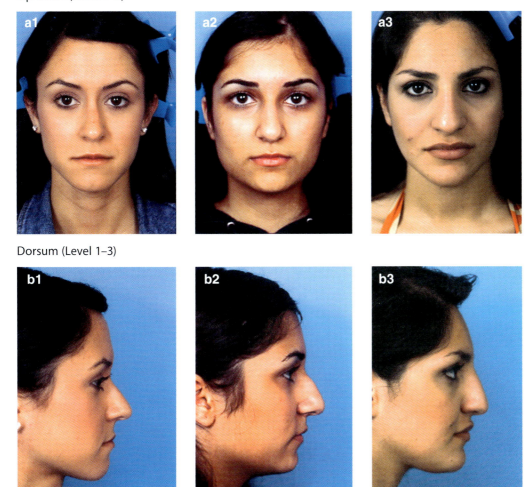

Dorsum (Level 1–3)

Nasal base (Level 1–3)

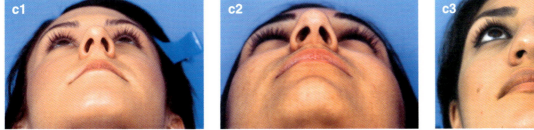

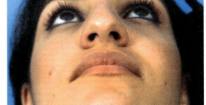

Septum (Level 2+)

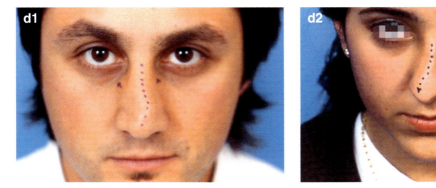

Fig. 2.22 (a–d) (Level 1–3) cases

Case Study: The Plunging Tip (Level 2)

A 17-year-old Hispanic girl complained of her profile view and that the nose plunged when she smiled (Fig. 2.23). On lateral view, the dorsum was normal height while the radix was low. On anterior view, the dorsum was wide both dorsally and laterally. A "balanced approach" was used with radix augmentation and tip support. The caudal septum was shortened 6 mm which eliminated downward pull on the tip when smiling. The ability to rotate the tip upward was achieved with the columellar strut and a dorsal positioning suture. Narrowing of the dorsal and lateral width without lowering the dorsum was achieved using parallel dorsal and lateral osteotomies. At 4 years post-op, the patient has done well.

Operative Technique Highlights

1) Exposure of the nose – no dorsal reduction
2) Caudal septal resection of 6 mm and septal harvest
3) Paramedain and low-to-low osteotomies
4) Crural strut and tip sutures: CS×2, DC, ID, DE, C-S
5) Radix graft of diced cartilage in fascia (0.5 cc)
6) Nostril sill excisions 2.5 mm
7) Small chin implant

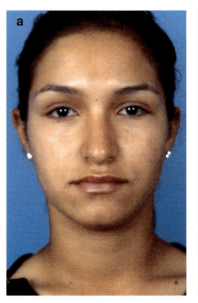
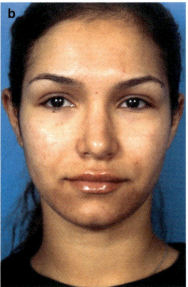
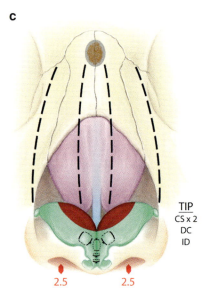

Fig. 2.23 (a-j)

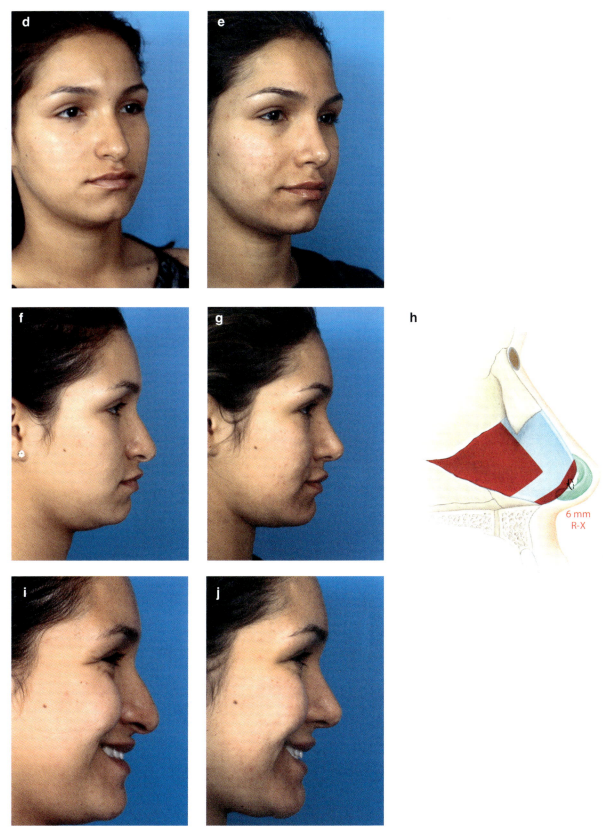

Fig. 2.23 (continued)

Decision Making Level 3: The Difficult Nose

Level of Difficulty. Put simply, a Level 3 nose is one whose anatomical deformity limits the achievement of an excellent result. Often, the skin will be too thick, the alars too asymmetric, or the entire nose is unattractive. Early in my practice, I could always recognize these cases because I did not sleep well the night before surgery. The result was that I spent hours in the operating room sweating the details and then months in the exam room listening to the patients complain. A smarter surgeon would have recognized them at consultation and passed on doing them until their surgical skill set had expanded. What should you do?

First, you have to develop your own individual set of "*aesthetic*" criteria for grading Level 1–3 cases based on the presenting deformity. You must reconcile both the patient's deformity and requests with your surgical ability to achieve the patient's goal. In the first few years of practice, there is nothing wrong with a "one third distribution" for each level of difficulty. Second, as you gain experience and progress from Level 1 to Level 2 cases you can shrink the percentage of cases assigned to Level 3. Third, experience will give you the judgment and confidence to do more difficult cases.

Expansion of Operative Techniques. Level 3 cases demand both *excellence* of the fundamental steps in a rhinoplasty operation and *expansion* of the skill set. For example, virtually all types of grafts may be required from columellar struts to tip grafts to alar grafts. A radix reduction is a magnitude harder than a radix augmentation. A combined nostril sill/alar base resection is a grade more difficult than an alar base resection. Ethnic noses are more challenging than the usual Caucasian nose. As regards the tip, an open structure tip graft signals a harder case than a suture tip. Yet, an open tip graft added to sutured domes is easier than one where the domes are excised to drop projection. One may encounter severe alar malposition under thin skin which requires alar transposition and coverage with a fascial blanket graft.

Transitioning from Level 2 to Level 3. For most surgeons, the transition from Level 2 to 3 cases will be gradual and sometimes unplanned. For example, when dealing with a combined large nose and tip, it becomes necessary to reduce both. The dorsum is reduced first in increments and suddenly the tip looks relatively enormous. The planned open tip suture procedure will not reduce the tip. Rather, domal excision and tip grafting becomes obligatory. Yes, it would have been ideal to have decided on this op plan first, but the unexpected happens. Obviously, preoperative planning is better and identification of a subset of patients that require more sophisticated techniques is the goal. In my own practice, the transition from Level 2 to 3 was possible by operating on easier Asian and Type II Hispanic noses. Preoperatively, one knows that the skin envelope will be thick, the need for structure great, dorsal augmentation frequent, and alar base reduction demanding. These cases require sophistication and are probably Level 2.5 which makes them ideal for transitioning to Level 3 (Fig. 2.24).

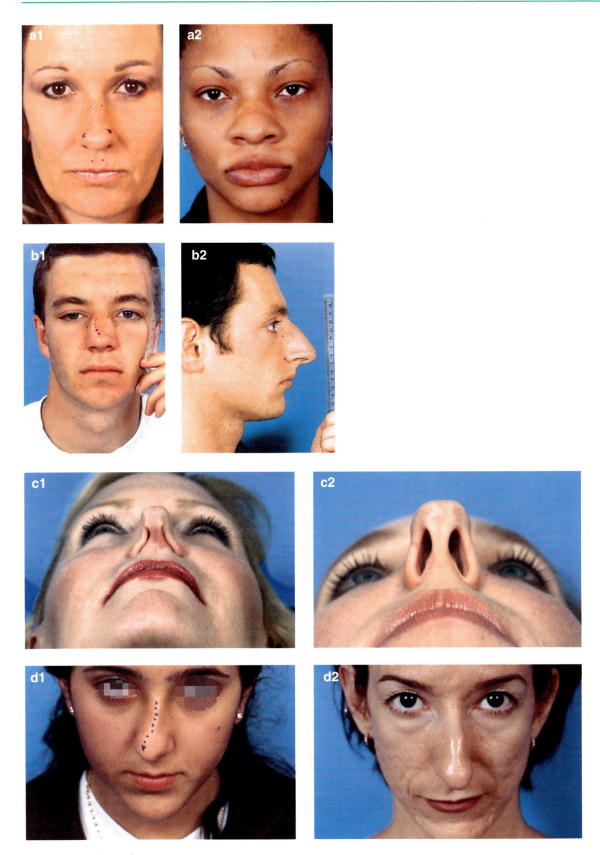

Fig. 2.24 (a–d) Level 3 cases

Case Study: The Ball Tip (Level 3)

A 44-year-old woman wanted a rhinoplasty because she hated her large round tip (Fig. 2.25). The size of the tip was compounded by the juxtaposition of a narrow dorsum. There was no alar malposition. She had a deep alar cartilage – A1 junction compressing the vestibular valve that collapsed on deep inspiration. After extensive discussion, she made it clear that she wanted a "smaller model's tip."

There was nothing simple about this nose from either an aesthetic or a functional perspective. One had to excise the strong ball-shaped alar cartilages in the presence of vestibular and nostril valve collapse. Six functional steps were done to provide structure: (1) a columellar strut, (2) lateral crural strut grafts, (3) the septoplasty aspect of the septal harvest, (4) major spreader grafts, (5) out fracture of the turbinates, and (6) the decision not to do lateral osteotomies. By comparison, direct excision of a domal segment and coverage with a tip graft of excised cartilage was straightforward.

Operative Technique

1) Exposure disclosed round alar cartilages 14 mm in width.
2) Incremental dorsal reduction (bone 1 mm, cartilage 4 mm).
3) Septal and fascial harvest.
4) No osteotomies.
5) Bilateral spreader grafts.
6) Create 6 mm rim strips.
7) Insertion of crural strut. Excision 5 mm domal segment.
8) Repair of domal excision. Coverage with an alar concealer graft.
9) Excision of alar – A1 junction. Insertion of lateral crural strut grafts Type I.

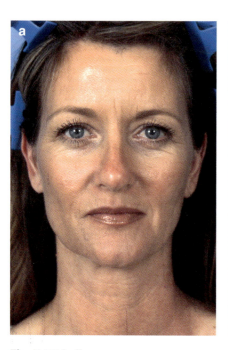
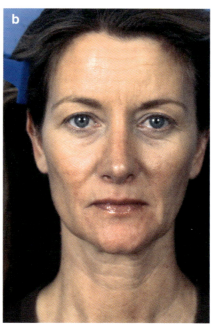
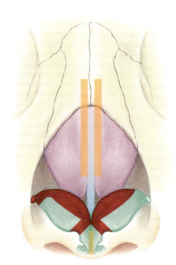

Fig. 2.25 (a-j)

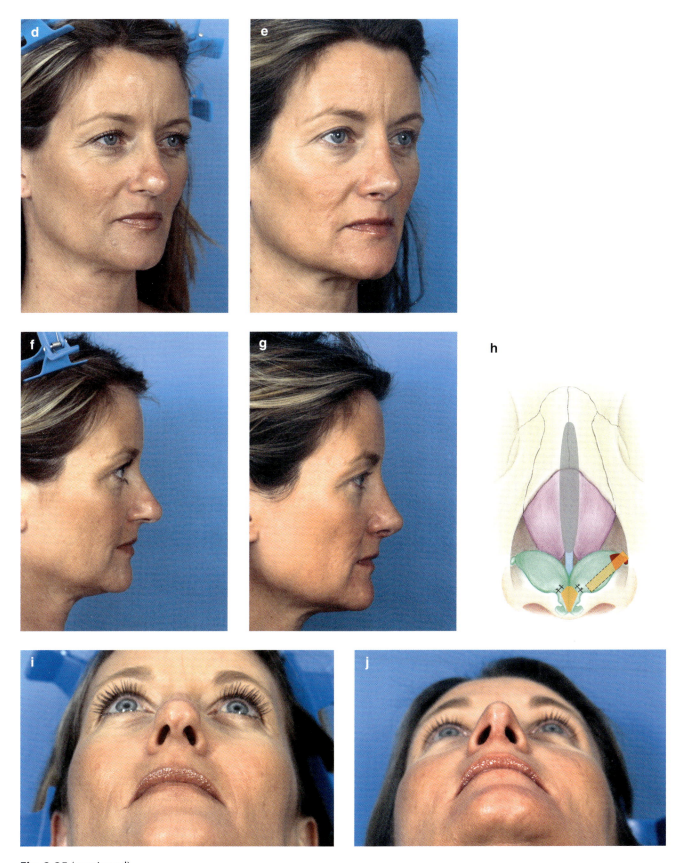

Fig. 2.25 (continued)

Postoperative Management

The smoothness of the postoperative course is directly proportional to the thoroughness of the preoperative preparation. Another copy of the "10 Most Frequently Asked Post-Op Questions" is given to the patient's caregiver. The patient is instructed to begin pain medication and oral antibiotics (Ciprof 500 mg BID for 5 days). Head elevation and ice compresses over the eyes for 36 h are recommended. The drip pad is changed as necessary. Meticulous cleaning of all suture lines two to three times a day with hydrogen peroxide and coverage with antibiotic ointment is stressed. The patient is seen 1 week later. On the morning that the cast is to be removed, the patient is instructed to take a shower and get the cast and nose wet. They are also told to take a pain pill 30 min before coming to the office. The sequence of removing the dressing is as follows: (1) the acrylic cast is lifted off by gentle rocking (the Telfa dorsal strip allows it to come off without pulling the skin), (2) the Steri-strips are removed, (3) the intranasal splints are extracted after the suture is cut on the left side, (4) all external sutures are removed, and (5) the nose is gently cleansed with hydrogen peroxide. The patient is allowed to see the nose with a mirror; especially the profile view with the preoperative lateral photograph held beside the head for comparison. Then the patient is taught how to tape and also given a step-by-step "taping diagram" plus a roll of tape. The technique is as follows: (1) four 2 cm pieces, one 4 cm piece, and one 6 cm piece of 0.5 in. flesh-colored paper tape are cut, (2) three short pieces are slightly overlapped on the dorsum, (3) the medium and long piece are placed longitudinally along the edge of the dorsum, (4) the distal ends are pinched together to narrow the tip and the longer piece rotated to the opposite side, and (5) the final short piece is placed transversely to set off the tip. The patient is encouraged to tape the nose at night for 3 weeks to reduce swelling. In patients with thick skin, taping may be done for 4–6 weeks. If the nostrils have been narrowed extensively or I am concerned about their shape then "nostril splints" are inserted prior to the taping. Patients will use the nostril splints at night, unilateral or bilateral, for 1–3 weeks. When turbinates and complex septal surgery are done, the patient is encouraged to irrigate the nose with a generic salt water spray. The patient is seen 2 weeks later and then at regular intervals: 3, 6, and 12 months and then annually, thereafter. The usual concerns include bruising, swelling, breathing, smiling, numbness, and initial appearance.

Ecchymosis and Edema

Bruising and swelling are a normal occurrence following a rhinoplasty. Since the patient must be off aspirin for 2 weeks prior to surgery, bruising rarely persists for more than 1 week. Some patients do have a residual bruising in the malar area that can be covered up with makeup and an unfortunate few do get scleral hemorrhage that may persist for 3–6 weeks. Very rarely, a patient of Mediterranean descent will get dark circles beneath their eyes which require a course of 4% solaquin forte. Patients are told preoperatively to expect swelling and that it will regress in two stages. Stage I is a generalized swelling that reduces uniformly over the first 2–3 weeks. Stage II is a more gradual period of scar remodelling that follows a constant pattern: bony dorsum 3 months, cartilaginous dorsum 6 months, supratip area 9 months, and tip 12 months. I emphasize to the patient that they loose one third of their tip swelling by 2 months, the next third between 3 and 9 months, and the final third between 9 and 12 months.

Breathing

Most patients breathe well, especially after removal of the intranasal splints. They are warned that the splints have been compressing the mucosa and that a rebound swelling may occur for a week or so. They are encouraged to use a nasal spray to replace normal nasal secretions and mechanical cleansing, both of which are often reduced temporarily following surgery. During the winter, a humidifier and coating the vestibule/caudal septum with vaseline is often encouraged to counteract the drying of forced air heating.

Initial Appearance

Before the cast is removed, the patient is reminded of the preoperative admonitions: (1) the nose will be swollen, (2) the nose will look swollen on front view, but the lines of the nose will be visible on profile view, and (3) the tip may appear a bit turned up at first. The patient is reassured that their nose will look better the minute the cast is removed than it did preoperatively and that it will gradually get better and better. Also, they are told that the nose will swell on recumbency and not to be surprised if the nose swells more on one side than the other depending on which side they sleep on. Night time taping is encouraged.

Smiling

When extensive septal work is done including relocation of the caudal septum, it is not uncommon for the patient to complain of a weak smile and limited exposure of their upper teeth. Release of the depressor septi nasalis is the cause and complete return usually occurs by 4–6 weeks. It is best to warn the patient of this potential occurrence preoperatively.

Numbness

Many patients complain that their nose is numb postoperatively. Its occurrence is due to the severance of the continuation of the anterior ethmoidal nerves. Although most surgeons consider it a minor problem and one that always resolves within 6 months, my experience has been different. It is my impression that the return is often much longer (12–18 months) and often partial rather than complete. Again, a prepared patient will more easily accept some reduction in sensation.

Reading List Aiach O. Atlas of Rhinoplasty (2nd ed). St. Louis: Quality Medical Publishing, 1996

Daniel RK. Rhinoplasty: Creating an aesthetic tip. Plast Reconstr Surg 80: 775, 1987

Daniel RK. (ed) Aesthetic Plastic Surgery: Rhinoplasty. Boston: Little, Brown, 1993

Daniel RK. Open tip suture techniques. Part I: Primary rhinoplasty. Part II: Secondary rhinoplasty. Plast Reconstr Surg 103: 1491, 1999

Daniel RK. Rhinoplasty: Nostril/tip disproportion. Plast Reconstr Surg 107: 1454, 2001

Daniel RK. Rhinoplasty: An Atlas of Surgical Techniques. Berlin: Springer-Verlag, 2002

Daniel RK. Rhinoplasty: Septal saddle nose deformity and composite reconstruction. Plast Reconstr Surg 119: 1029, 2007

Daniel RK, Calvert JC. Diced cartilage in rhinoplasty surgery. PlastRreconstr Surg 113: 2156, 2004. Follow-up in: Daniel RK. Diced cartilage grafts in rhinoplasty surgery: Current techniques and applications. Plast Reconstr Surg 122: 1883, 2008

Daniel RK. Tip refinement grafts: the designer tip. Aesth Surg J 29: 528, 2009

Goodman WS. External approach to rhinoplasty. Can J Otolaryngol 2: 207 (Entire Issue devoted to Open Rhinoplasty) 1973

Gorney M. Patient selection in rhinoplasty: Practical guidelines. In: Daniel RK (ed) Aesthetic Plastic Surgery: Rhinoplasty. Boston: Little, Brown, 1993

Gruber RP, Nahai F, Bogdan MA, et al Changing the convexity and concavity of nasal cartilages and cartilage grafts with horizontal mattress sutures. Part I. Experimental results. Plast Reconstr Surg 115:589, 2005. Part II Clinical Results. Plast Reconstr Surg 115: 595, 2005

Gruber R, Chang TN, Kahn D, et al Broad nasal bone reduction: an algorithm for osteotomies. Plast Reconstr Surg 119:1044, 2007

Gubisch W. Twenty-five years experience with extracorporeal septoplasty. Facial Plast Surg 22: 230, 2006 (Note: entire journal issue is devoted to septal surgery)

Gunter JP. Secondary rhinoplasty: The open approach. In: Daniel RK (ed) Aesthetics Plastic Surgery: Rhinoplasty. Boston: Little, Brown, 1993

Gunter JP, Rohrich RJ, and Friedman RM. Classification and correction of alar-columellar discrepancies in rhinoplasty. Plast Reconstr Surg 97: 643, 1996

Gunter JP, Rohrich RJ, and Adams WP. (eds) Dallas Rhinoplasty: Nasal Surgery by the Masters. QMP,757, 2007

Guyuron B. Dynamic interplays during rhinoplasty. Clin Plast Surg 23: 223, 1996. (Entire Issue)

Guyuron B. Precision rhinoplasty. Part I: The role of life-size photographs and soft-tissue cephalometric analysis. Plast Reconstr Surg 81: 489, 1988

Johnson CM Jr. and Toriumi DM. Open Structure Rhinoplasty. Philadelphia: Saunders, 1990. Additional information in Johnson CM, Wyatt CT. A Case Approach to Open Structure Rhinoplasty. 2nd ed. New York: Elsevier, 2006

Meyer R Secondary Rhinoplasty. Berlin: Springer, 2002

Sheen JH. Rhinoplasty: Personal evolution and milestones. Plast Reconstr Surg 105: 1820, 2000

Sheen JH, and Sheen AP. Aesthetic Rhinoplasty (2nd ed.) St. Louis: Mosby, 1987

Tardy ME. Rhinoplasty: The Art and the Science. Philadelphia: Saunders, 1997

Tebbetts JB. Rethinking the logic and techniques of primary tip rhinoplasty. Clin Plast Surg 23: 245, 1996. (Entire Issue)

Toriumi DM and Johnson CM. Open structure rhinoplasty: Featured technical points and long-term follow-up. Facial Plast Clin 1: 1, 1993. (Entire Issue)

Toriumi, DM. New concepts in nasal tip contouring. Arch Facial Plast Surg 8: 156, 2006

Thomas JR. The relationship of lateral osteotomies in rhinoplasty to the lacrimal drainage system. Otolaryngology 94: 362, 1986

Radix and Dorsum 3

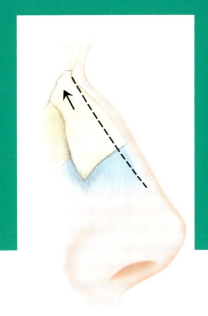

The radix and dorsum are fused anatomically, aesthetically, and surgically. For the vast majority of patients, their three main complaints in order of importance are the "bump" on profile, the lack of tip definition, and the wide nose. Thus, two of three complaints are located in the radix and dorsum. Anatomically and embryologically, the bony vault and the cartilaginous vault are a single entity – the osseocartilaginous vault (hereinafter the dorsum). The key to designing the optimal surgical solution is the nasofacial angle (NFA), which most surgeons consider to be the most important aesthetic angle in the entire face. The setting of the ideal nasion point determines the nasofacial angle and also whether the radix area needs to be augmented or reduced. Equally, the line connecting the nasion to the tip reveals the need for dorsal modification. This linkage is expressed in the "balanced approach" to the dorsum. For example, a radix augmentation decreases the amount of dorsal reduction required thereby preserving a more natural profile. Osteotomies to narrow the bony vault are neither an automatic maneuver nor a single technique. The cartilage vault requires equal emphasis with spreader grafts done to preserve function and to improve aesthetics. Failure to stabilize the midvault can lead to a visible inverted-V deformity with internal valve collapse. The importance of understanding the dorsum and selecting the optimal operation is obvious in examining a large number of secondary rhinoplasty patients where the sign of a "nose job" is now dorsal deformities rather than tip problems.

Introduction

Overview   Approximately 90% of my Caucasian rhinoplasty patients want a smaller natural nose which leads to dorsal reduction. The actual amount of dorsal reduction can be limited if one uses a "balanced approach." The combination of a radix graft and greater tip projection minimizes the amount of dorsal height reduction. The surgeon does not reduce the dorsum to fit the tip, but rather seeks the ideal dorsum and then fits the tip to the dorsum.

Level 1

Radix. In reviewing 100 primary rhinoplasties, I modified the radix as follows: (1) nothing to the radix (80%), (2) augment it with fascia (12%) (3) augment it with fascia plus diced cartilage (4%), and (4) reduce it (4%) (Fig. 3.1). Early on, one should be able to do a basic fascia graft to the radix – do not use solid cartilage grafts as they always show.

Dorsum. I feel strongly that an incremental dorsal reduction using rasps and straight scissors is the most controlled, flexible, and safest method of dorsal reduction (Fig. 3.2). In addition, one must perfect a method of doing lateral osteotomies. I prefer the endonasal approach as it allows me to do both low-to-high and low-to-low osteotomies. Spreader grafts are done for both aesthetic and functional reasons. There is no way to avoid learning and doing spreader grafts.

Level 2

Radix. As the radix deficiency increases in depth and/or extends caudally into the dorsum, it becomes necessary to add diced cartilage below the fascia graft. For significant defects, diced cartilage is placed on the bone and covered with a fascial graft (DC+F). As the defect extends onto the bony vault, a true diced cartilage in fascia graft is used (DC−F) for these half-length dorsal defects. When the radix is full due to soft tissue, excision of muscle tissue can reduce the radix.

Dorsum. Management of the asymmetrical, deviated dorsum mandates modifications in the spreader graft design and the selection of osteotomies. When confronted with the wide dorsum, medial oblique or even paramedian osteotomies may be necessary. Changes in lateral wall convexity may require double-level osteotomies.

Level 3

Radix. Bony reduction of the radix is never easy and is less effective than one would want. Minor to moderate reductions imply either soft tissue excision or extension of the hump reduction cephalically. In contrast, major reductions require a total excision of the bony radix as a separate entity using a double-guarded osteotome or burr.

Dorsum. Due to the advances in diced cartilage in fascia (DC−F), augmentation of the dorsum can be done successfully and with few problems. Previously, solid dorsal grafts of septum or layered conchal grafts were always disappointing due to either visibility or displacement. As the number of ethnic rhinoplasties has increased, the use of DC−F grafts has provided a wonderful solution to the challenge of dorsal augmentation.

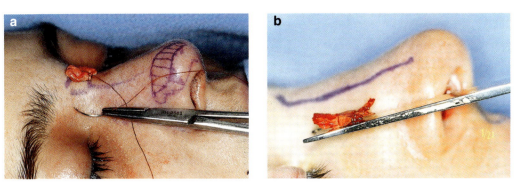

Fig. 3.1 Radix, (**a**) augmentation, (**b**) reduction

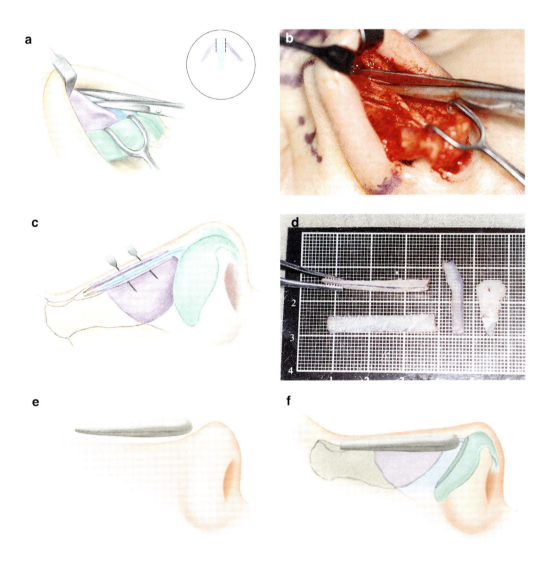

Fig. 3.2 Dorsum, (**a, b**) incremental reduction, (**c, d**) spreader grafts, (**e, f**) dorsal augmentation

Anatomy   **Radix.** The soft tissue of the radix area is often heavy and consists of thicker skin, subcutaneous fat, and muscle (7.2 mm in adults, range 3.5–9.5 mm). In contrast, the skin of many adolescent patients is a tight yoke which reveals any underlying cartilage graft. The bone in the radix area is a fused solid triangle of multiple bones which can be reduced only with difficulty (Fig. 3.3c). The bone has the contour of the nasofrontal angle within it. Preoperatively, it is important to differentiate by palpation whether radix fullness is due to soft tissue or bone.

Dorsum. The anatomy of the osseocartilaginous vault reflects its embryology. The laying down of the nasal bones over the cartilaginous vault is reflected in their broad overlap, which measures 11 mm in the midline and 4 mm laterally (Fig. 3.3a, b). Thus, the bony and cartilaginous vaults are not simply joined at a seam, but rather have an overlapped integration. The importance of this overlap is evident in reduction rhinoplasty – the hump is far more cartilaginous than bony. Technically, the implication is that rasping the bony hump first brings the larger underlying cartilaginous hump into relief and avoids overresection of the bony dorsum. In childhood, nasal height is mainly due to the nasal bones. During puberty, the nose undergoes radical changes due to the foreword thrust of the maxilla and the absorption/deposition along the nasal profile line. Thus, lateral osteotomies are done within, or pass across, the frontal process of the maxilla in order to narrow the base bony width.

Perhaps, the greatest anatomical misunderstanding in the entire nose concerns the *cartilaginous vault* – it is a single anatomical entity, not a septum with two juxtaposed upper lateral cartilages. Reduction of the cartilaginous dorsum destroys the normal architecture permanently and creates a tripartite entity, which can be visible as an inverted-V deformity. Spreader grafts are an attempt to recreate normal nasal anatomy. Another important point is the change in the shape of the *cartilaginous dorsum* as it progresses from a broad "T" shape beneath the bony dorsum, to a "Y" shape at the midvault (Fig. 3.3d), and to a narrower "I" near the septal angle (Fig. 3.3e).

The overlying soft tissue envelope varies dramatically from its thickest portion in the radix area, to its thinnest at the rhinion, and to its most unpredictable in the supratip area (Fig. 3.4). The rhinion is the thinnest because there is minimal subcutaneous fat, and the transverse nasalis muscle fibers have given way to an aponeurosis. The supratip area is often filled with subcutaneous fat which masks the downward descent of the cartilaginous dorsum. These soft tissue layers constitute a Superficial Muscular Aponeurotic System (SMAS). Surgically, the most avascular and the least traumatic plane of dissection is supraperichondrally in the subaponeurotic space. As one elevates the soft tissue envelope, one should see the shining white cartilage underneath.

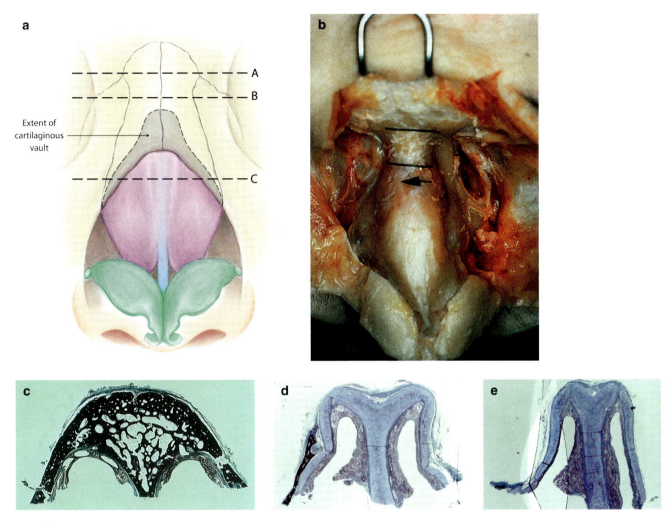

Fig. 3.3 (a–e) Osseocartilaginous vault

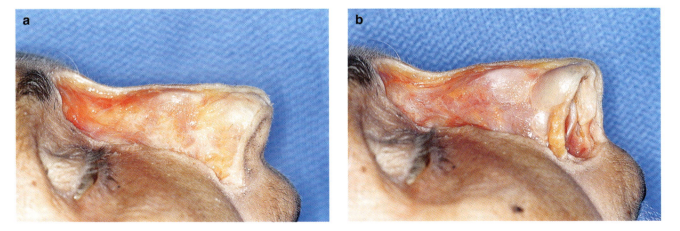

Fig. 3.4 (a, b) Soft tissue coverage

Aesthetics

Radix. Nasion (N) refers to a specific point – the deepest point of the nasofrontal angle. The ideal *nasion level* or vertical position is set between lash and crease line of the upper eyelid (Fig. 3.5). The *nasion height* or projection can be measured from the vertical tangent to the cornea or glabella. These two factors determine the nasion *location*, which in turn sets the critical starting point of the nose with regard to the nasofacial angle and the nasal length. Thus, setting the nasion is often the first step in planning a rhinoplasty.

Dorsum. On anterior view, one assesses the dorsal lines, base bony width, and lateral wall inclinations (Fig. 3.6). The parallel dorsal lines begin at the supraorbital ridge, narrow at the radix, and continue down to the tip defining points. The ideal width of the dorsal lines often corresponds to the width of the tip defining points and philtral columns. A general rule of thumb is 6–8 mm for females and 8–10 mm for males. A visual break in the continuity of the dorsal lines creates the inverted-V deformity that one can see following a rhinoplasty. The base bony width (X-point on either side, X-X for total width) is the widest point of the nose at the level of the maxilla. It is easily measured with a caliper. One compares base bony width (X-X) to the intercanthal width (EN-EN) to determine the need for, and the type of, lateral osteotomies. If the bones are wider than the intercanthal width, then I usually perform transverse and low-to-low osteotomies to achieve complete movement. Otherwise a simple low-to-high osteotomy is done plus a gentle greenstick fracture. The inclination of the bony vault is checked and only rarely is excessive bowing or verticalization noted. However, asymmetries are seen in over 25% of the primary cases, and these differences are always pointed out to the patient preoperatively.

On lateral analysis, the key determinant is the nasofacial angle. In classical art, a nasofacial angle of approximately 34° for females and 36° for males is the accepted standard. The nasofacial angle (NFA) is measured from a vertical through the ideal nasion (Ni) and a line dawn from the nasion to the ideal tip (Ti). If a hump is present, the line is drawn through it. The final aesthetic line is often concave for females and straight for males. Patients with too great an angle complain that their noses stick out too far and those with a low angle do not like their flat noses. One must be careful in using this angle rigidly for operative planning. In certain cases, the nasion/radix may be wrong and perhaps even noncorrectable which in turn will limit the angle's value. Second, there is a relatively ideal dorsal height which is independent of the angles. A classic example is the patient with a low radix and underprojecting tip whose intervening dorsum appears quite prominent. The balanced approach is to graft both the radix and the tip with minimal reduction of the dorsum. The importance of maintaining a high natural dorsum is seen in recent changes in operative technique away from "make the dorsum fit the tip" to "make the tip fit the ideal dorsum."

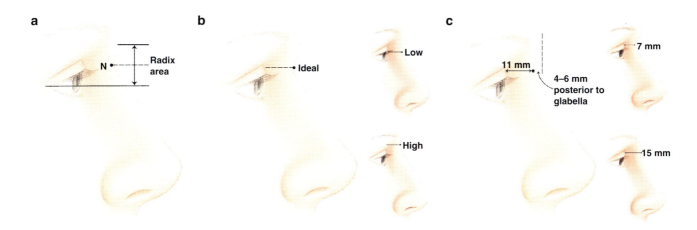

Fig. 3.5 (a–c) Radix aesthetics

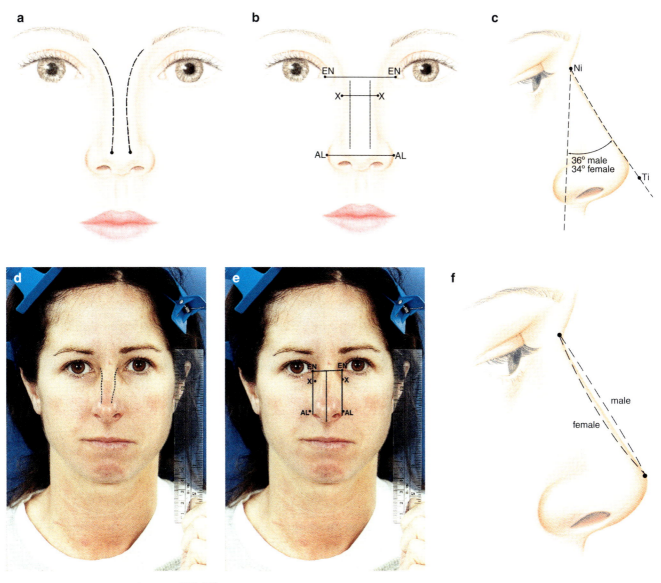

Fig. 3.6 (a–f) Dorsal aesthetics

Radix Reduction

The author has developed a new approach to radix reduction by dividing the radix components into soft tissue and bone based on preoperative palpation. It is important to assign a relative importance to each component in selecting the best operative technique (Fig. 3.10).

Soft Tissue Reduction. Preoperatively, one must assess both the soft tissue fullness that blunts the nasofrontal angle and the width of the medial orbital lines that continue into the dorsal lines. In younger patients, one can excise the soft tissue fullness using the following technique: (1) elevate the skin over the radix and glabellar region, (2) then dissect upward on top of the dorsal bones, (3) excise the intervening soft tissue, and (4) place a drain and compressive dressing (Fig. 3.11). In older patients, one may need to do a concurrent endoscopic central forehead lift.

Bony Reduction. The first step is to visually separate radix from dorsum using a transverse line through the lateral canthus. Then the ideal nasion is determined and the nasofacial angle set, which reveals the new dorsal line. Since both areas are usually excessive, dorsal reduction is necessary and it is done first. Contrary to the classic en bloc osteotome excision which often resulted in dorsal destruction, a two-step technique is preferred (Fig. 3.12). First, the dorsum is lowered using rasps for the bony vault and a scissor for the cartilage vault. Once satisfied with the dorsal line, the radix area is undermined extensively using a Joseph elevator. Complete freeing of the soft tissue facilitates subsequent removal of the bone. Then a 12 mm wide, sharp, double-guarded osteotome is inserted until it catches on the dorsal/radix junction, which often marks the upper limit of effective rasping. The handle of the guard is rotated upward 45–60° depending on the amount of bone to be excised. With multiple strikes, the osteotome is engaged and the bony radix becomes palpable on top of the osteotome. The amount of bone being removed may seem frighteningly large. The osteotome is driven upward to the glabella where a distinct change in sound occurs as the guards strike the skull. Then the osteotome is rotated upward and twisted, which disarticulates the bone from the nasofrontal suture line. If the bone cannot be dislodged, then a 2 mm osteotome is inserted beneath the medial eyebrow and "walked across" the nasofrontal suture line going down to the guarded osteotome, which has been left in place. In major cases involving both the radix and dorsum, it is necessary to use either spreader grafts or a full-length dorsal graft to fill the dorsal void. Following a radix reduction, bleeding is significant and I routinely drain the nose with a 7 Fr suction drain. A curved trochar is inserted from the nose and made to exit in the hairline. The drain is removed after 3 days.

PRINCIPLES

- The radix area is made of solid bone and its reduction requires significant removal – often 10–12 mm long, 4–8 mm thick.
- Never try to do an en bloc dorsum/radix reduction as you will remove too much dorsum and too little radix.

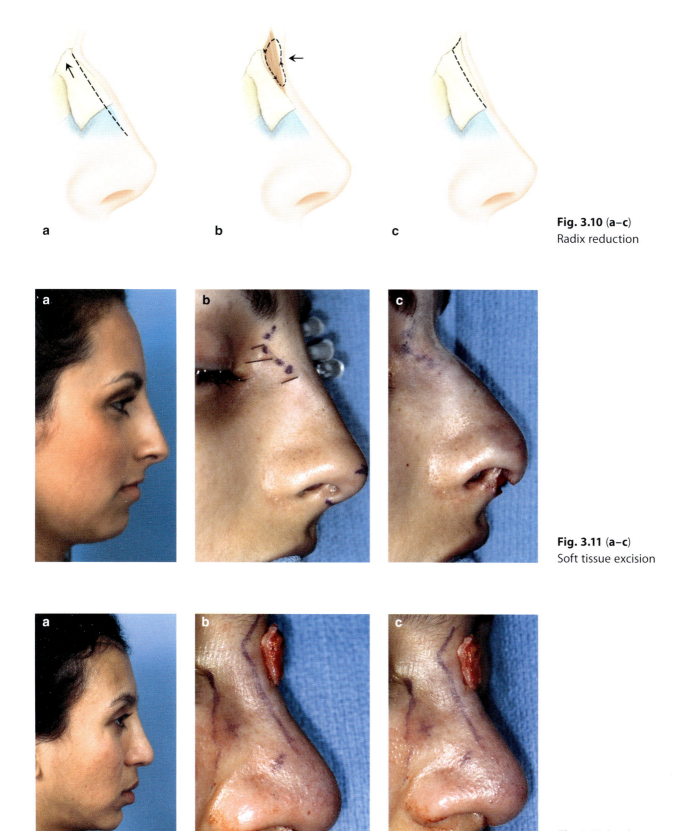

Fig. 3.10 (a–c)
Radix reduction

Fig. 3.11 (a–c)
Soft tissue excision

Fig. 3.12 (a–c)
Bony excision

Dorsal Reduction

The first step in operative planning is to decide whether the dorsum should be reduced, augmented, balanced, or maintained. Excluding ethnic patients, primary rhinoplasties are reduced (89%), modified (7%), or augmented as part of a balanced approach (4%). Although numerous instruments and sequences are possible for dorsal reduction, I have found graded incremental bony rasping followed by a split-hump cartilaginous excision using scissors to be the most effective method with the least risk. The incremental approach allows one to fine tune the dorsal reduction at least three times: during the initial resection, then the graded adjustment, and finally following the osteotomies.

Bony Vault Reduction. The soft tissue envelope is elevated in two stages. First, scissor dissection is done in close contact with the cartilage over the cartilaginous vault. Second, a Joseph elevator is used in the subperiosteal plane over the bony vault. In most cases, *extramucosal tunnels* are then made to avoid transecting the underlying mucosa when the cartilaginous hump is excised. A sharp puller rasp is used first in the midline and then progressively on either side (Fig. 3.13). As the rasping continues, two changes occur – the cartilaginous hump becomes more obvious, and one needs to rasp each nasal bone separately and on an angle. The rasping continues until one is satisfied with the height of the bony dorsum as it relates to the nasion, i.e., the upper half of the ideal dorsal line has been achieved. Then the cartilaginous dorsum is lowered.

Cartilaginous Vault Reduction. Two methods are available for reducing the cartilaginous vault: a split-hump technique using scissors or a transverse en bloc reduction using a broken-off #11 blade (Fig. 3.14). The classical vertical split-hump reduction involves making paraseptal vertical cuts with straight scissors on either side of the septum following the creation of extramucosal tunnels. The scissor blades vertically straddle the cartilaginous vault. The cut produces a narrow septum with two upper lateral cartilages often with curved dorsal edges. Then, the scissors are turned transversely and each of the three components of the cartilaginous vault is lowered incrementally. Excision of the dorsal septum *lowers* dorsal height, while excision of the upper lateral *narrows* dorsal width. In absolute terms of height reduction, excision of the upper laterals is much more conservative than the dorsal septal resection. One must be aware that upward traction on the soft tissue envelope tends to raise the upper lateral cartilages artificially high. Once the osteotomies are completed, additional rasping of the bony vault and minimal excision of both septum and upper lateral cartilages may be necessary. The one method which I do not recommend for routine use is en bloc hump removal using an osteotome because of the risk of overresecting the bony vault and underresecting the cartilaginous vault.

PRINCIPLES

- *Exposure* consists of two steps – soft tissue elevation above and extramucosal tunnels below.
- A cartilaginous hump reduction of more than 1 mm requires extramucosal tunnels while one greater than 3 mm requires spreader grafts.
- A rasp is much easier to control than an osteotome.
- Excision of cartilaginous septum reduces *height*, and excision of upper laterals reduces *width*.

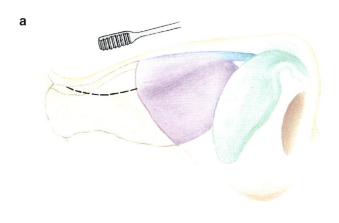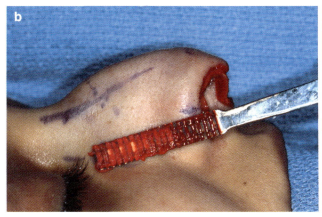

Fig. 3.13 (a, b) Bony reduction: rasp

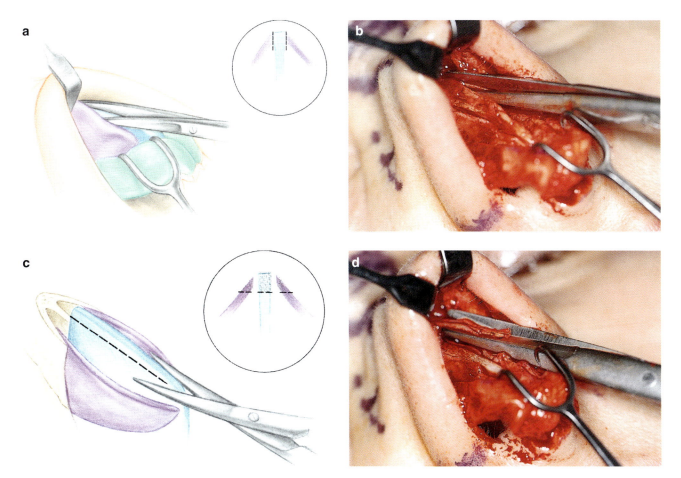

Fig. 3.14 (a–d) Cartilage reduction: split hump

Osteotomies

With few exceptions, the type of osteotomies can be decided upon preoperatively and executed without change intraoperatively. For years, lateral osteotomies were classified according to their location or level rather than their purpose. The critical factor is how much movement of the lateral nasal wall is required to narrow the base bony width. If a great deal of movement is necessary, then one needs complete osteotomies with bony separation. In contrast, if one only needs a more limited narrowing, then a greenstick fracture along the transverse component is sufficient. Second, the lateral osteotomy should go beneath the widest point of the base bony width (X-point). With these parameters, 95% of my osteotomies can be divided into two types: (1) a low-to-high osteotomy followed by a digital compression to produce a transverse greenstick fracture (limited movement), and (2) a transverse osteotomy followed by a low-to-low osteotomy which results in a continuous osteotomy (complete movement). I perform the lateral osteotomies intranasally because I have found the intraoral approach to be too low and inflexible, while the percutaneous method results in too many segmental bony bridges and mucosal perforations. There are no medial osteotomies nor "outfractures." Eliminating medial osteotomies has reduced dramatically bony irregularities and major bleeds. The classical outfracture leads to excessive mobility and verticalization of the nasal bones, and thus has been eliminated.

Low-to-High Osteotomy. I inject the area with local anesthesia immediately prior to the osteotomies. I do *not* create a subperiosteal tunnel as it damages blood vessels and increases bruising. The pyriform aperture is straddled with a small speculum and a transverse mucosal cut is made. When doing a low-to-high osteotomy, I use a slightly curved osteotome and place it low on the pyriform aperture (Fig. 3.15a, b). Then, with the assistant tapping at a sequenced pace, the osteotome is driven from low on the pyriform aperture across the frontal process of the maxilla to end high at the nasal bone suture line at the level of the medial canthus. There is no need to drive the osteotome up to the skull base. Then, I use my thumb to make a transverse fracture across the thin nasal bone extending from the lateral osteotomy into the open roof. The lateral nasal wall does two things: it hinges along the transverse greenstick fracture while moving medially, and it tilts with the dorsal portion closing the open roof.

Low-to Low Osteotomy. When greater movement is required, I do a two-part combined osteotomy: first a transverse percutaneous osteotomy followed by a low-to-low osteotomy (Fig. 3.15c, d). A vertical stab incision is made just above the medial canthus with a #15 blade and then a 2 mm osteotome is used to completely fracture the lateral wall transversely from just above the medial canthus upward. Next, the low-to-low lateral osteotomy is done using a straight osteotome. Essentially, the osteotome is driven along the base of the frontal process of maxilla, not across it in an ascending fashion as with the low-to-high osteotomy. Once the level of the preceding transverse osteotomy is reached, the osteotome is rotated medially forcing the lateral wall medially and achieving maximum movement. The reason for the transverse osteotomy is to insure that the thick frontal process of maxilla breaks at the desired level and separates to allow complete movement.

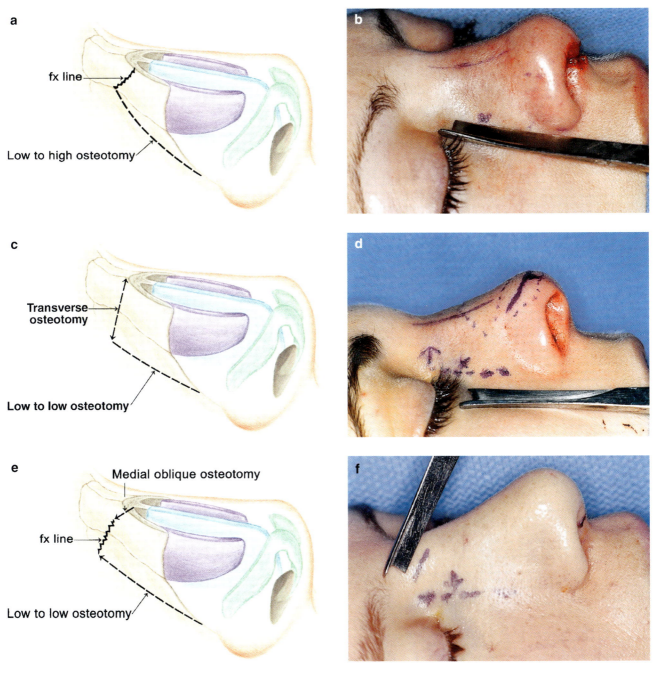

Fig. 3.15 (**a–f**) Osteotomy, (**a, b**) Low-to-high osteotomy **DVD** (**c, d**) low-to-low osteotomy **DVD** (**e, f**) medial oblique osteotomy

Specialized Osteotomies

On occasion, other osteotomies will be required including the medial oblique, the double-level, the paramedian, and the microosteotomy. The *medial oblique osteotomy* is designed to narrow the broad bony dorsum and is coupled with a low-to-low lateral osteotomy (Fig. 3.15e, f). A curved osteotome is placed at the cephalic end of the open roof and driven downward toward the medial canthus. The *double-level osteotomy* consists of an osteotomy along the inferior border of the nasal bone parallel to, and combined with, a low-to-low osteotomy (Fig. 3.15g–i). The goal is to reduce the convexity of the lateral wall. The higher osteotomy must be done first. The *paramedian osteotomy* is used in the broad nose when one does not wish to change dorsal height. These are essentially straight osteotomies made 3–5 mm parallel to the dorsal midline. *Microosteotomies* are done with the 2 mm osteotome and are used to correct asymmetries or irregularities intrinsic to the bones.

Spreader Grafts

Spreader grafts are used to treat or prevent internal valve collapse in primary cases (Fig 3–15j–l). Currently, I am using spreader grafts in the majority of my primary cases with equal emphasis on function and aesthetics. I have found spreader grafts to be extraordinarily valuable for maintaining the width of the cartilaginous vault and also reducing asymmetries. Technical considerations are as follows: (1) the grafts are 15–20 mm long, 3 mm high, and the width is determined by aesthetic requirements, (2) extramucosal tunnels are made beginning near the junction of the upper lateral cartilage with the septum and extending beneath the bony vault, (3) the tapered end of the spreader grafts is inserted into the pocket and then the grafts are held in place with two percutaneous #25 needles, and (4) two horizontal sutures of 4–0 polydioxanone suture (PDS) are used to fix the grafts in place. The cephalic portion rests beneath the intact bony vault or within a defined submucosal tunnel, which avoids postoperative displacement and visibility. In general, I prefer to suture upper lateral cartilages, spreader grafts, and septum (five layers). A three-layer suture is required high in the bony vault. Failure to suture the grafts in place can result in subsequent extrusion at the time of dressing application.

PRINCIPLES

- Tailor the osteotomies to fit the bony vault deformity. No osteotomies are done in 7% of the primary cases.
- Movement and stability of the lateral walls are critical factors in the decision process.
- There is no need for medial osteotomies nor dramatic outfractures.
- Consider spreader grafts as an integral part of a rhinoplasty for both functional and aesthetic reasons. They prevent internal valve collapse and the inverted-V deformity.

g

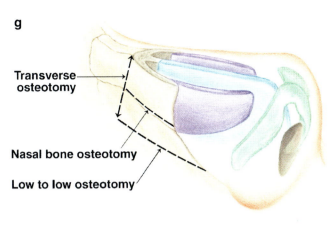

Transverse osteotomy

Nasal bone osteotomy

Low to low osteotomy

h

i

Fig. 3.15 (**g–i**) Double-level osteotomy note narrowing of bony walls

j

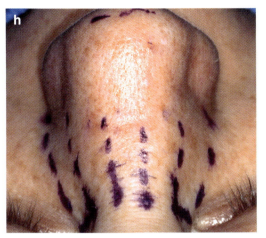
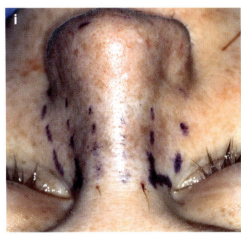

k

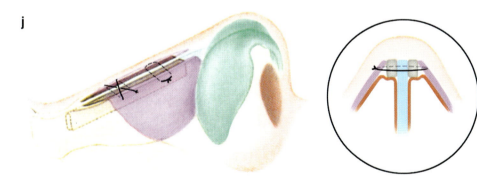
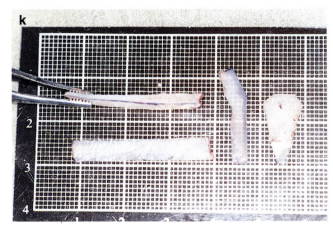

l

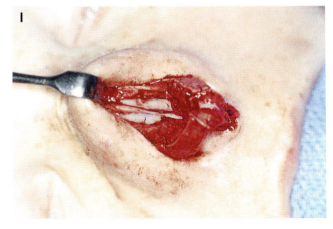

Fig. 3.15 (**j–l**) Spreader grafts

Dorsal Modification

Approximately, 5–7% of the primary noses do not require reduction. Modification of asymmetry and width are the primary issues.

Narrow Asymmetric Dorsum. The narrow asymmetric dorsum must be carefully analyzed as problems can occur in any of the following three areas: (1) the dorsal or lateral wall component of each vault, (2) the septum, and (3) adjacent lateral crura (Fig. 3.16). The operative sequence is as follows: (1) dorsal modification, (2) septal straightening, (3) osteotomies, (4) asymmetric and occasionally unilateral spreader grafts, (5) anatomical onlay grafts over the upper lateral cartilages, and (6) tip modification. The critical step is to achieve as straight a septum as possible and harvest cartilage for grafts. In most minor cases, asymmetric spreader grafts of differing widths will achieve improved symmetry in the dorsal lines. For moderate cases, one often has to add an anatomically designed lateral wall graft which replicates the upper lateral cartilage and is sutured onto the hypoplastic cartilage. The difficulty with these grafts is excessive thickness and visibility. For major deformities, one often has to do asymmetric and sophisticated osteotomies to achieve more symmetrical lateral walls. The goal is to meet in the middle of the discrepancy as it is impossible surgically to make one side match its unoperated counterpart.

Wide Dorsum. A wide dorsum is corrected in most rhinoplasties by reducing the wide hump and infracturing the lateral nasal walls. For minor width excesses, I achieve narrowing with hump reduction plus transverse and low-to-low osteotomies. For moderate width problems, I do the hump reduction and then a medial oblique osteotomy coming from the open roof and angling out about 45° followed by a low-to-low lateral osteotomy. The reason for the medial oblique osteotomy is that it insures that narrowing will occur at the dorsum. For major width deformities and especially those with a normal dorsal height, I have devised the following procedure (Figs. 3.17 and 3.18): (1) the dorsum is exposed through an open approach and extramucosal tunnels are made, (2) the midline is marked, (3) the ideal dorsal width is marked on the osseocartilaginous vault (5–8 mm), (4) paramedian cuts are made along the cartilaginous vault up to the keystone area, (5) these cuts are extended through the bone as paramedian osteotomies using a straight guarded osteotome, (6) lateral osteotomies are done usually consisting of transverse and low-to-low osteotomies, (7) after the infractures, excessive height of the upper lateral cartilages is excised (often 3–6 mm), and (8) the upper lateral cartilages are sutured adjacent to, or underneath, the T-shaped septum.

PRINCIPLES

- The asymmetric dorsum requires asymmetric spreader grafts.
- The asymmetric nose usually has a deviated septum.
- The wide nose with *normal dorsal height* can be easily narrowed with multiple osteotomies, including the paramedian.

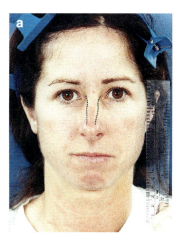
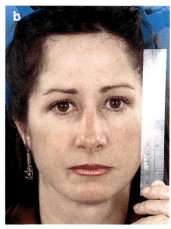
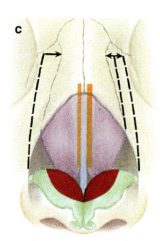

Fig. 3.16 (**a–c**) Narrow asymmetric nose

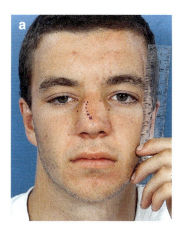
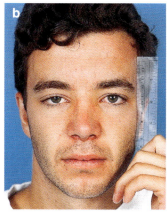
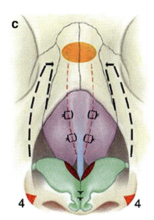

Fig. 3.17 (**a–c**) Wide dorsum

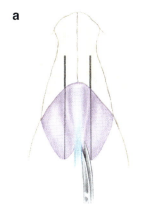
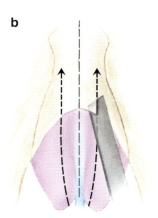
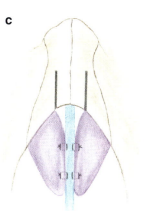

Fig. 3.18 (**a–c**) Narrowing wide dorsum

Dorsal Augmentation

I use only autogenous tissue for dorsal augmentation, and am adamantly opposed to alloplastic grafts, especially in secondary cases. Any alloplastic material or cadaver cartilage put over the nasal dorsum is essentially subdermal and prone to visibility, extrusion, infection, or absorption. It is in the patient's best interest to use autogenous tissues. In primary cases, most dorsal grafts are done for aesthetic reasons, whereas in secondaries they are used for aesthetic, functional, and structural reasons.

Fascia Grafts. When one wants to insure a smooth dorsum or create a more natural curvature under thin skin, then I will often insert deep temporal fascia as a single sheet or folded for double thickness (Fig. 3.19). The graft is guided into the pocket up to the radix with percutaneous sutures and then sutured caudally in the supratip area to the cartilaginous vault. The dorsal skin is then taped down with external Steri strips.

DC–F Grafts. Traditionally, a straight piece of septal cartilage measuring 35 mm in length and 5–6 mm in width was the gold standard of dorsal grafts. These grafts can be difficult to obtain in secondary cases and prone to visible edges. Due to the ease of diced cartilage grafts, I have not used a septal dorsal graft for the last 7 years and they are no longer a part of my surgical armamentarium. Instead, I employ diced cartilage in fascia grafts which are extremely variable in shape and efficient in donor material (Fig. 3.20). The cartilage is diced to 0.5 mm cubes and then placed in fascia which is sutured with 4–0 plain catgut. The *construct* is "made to measure" on the back table and guided into the dorsal pocket using percutaneous sutures. Any excess cartilage is milked out at the caudal end and then the graft is closed and sutured to the cartilaginous dorsum.

Structural Osseocartilaginous Rib Grafts. Although cranial bone enjoyed a decade's preference for nasal augmentation, I quickly found its disadvantages very real (complex harvest, only bony tissue, and limited patient acceptance). When major structural support is essential, I find the osseocartilaginous rib graft to be extremely flexible for the nasal dorsum and the cartilaginous rib tip is used for the columella (Fig. 3.21). A straight osseocartilaginous segment of the ninth rib is harvested and then shaped circumferentially using a power burr. Most of the grafts are 40–45 mm in length, 5–8 mm in width, and a tapered thickness of 4 mm at the nasion to 7–10 mm in the supratip area. The graft is fixed cephalically with percutaneous K-wires which are removed at 10 days post-op. These grafts provide excellent structural support with little risk of warping.

PRINCIPLES

- Dorsal grafts are infinitely easier than a decade ago.
- Fascia is the ideal camouflage material under thin skin.
- DC-F grafts allow variations in length and height to fill any dorsal defect using all types of cartilage pieces.

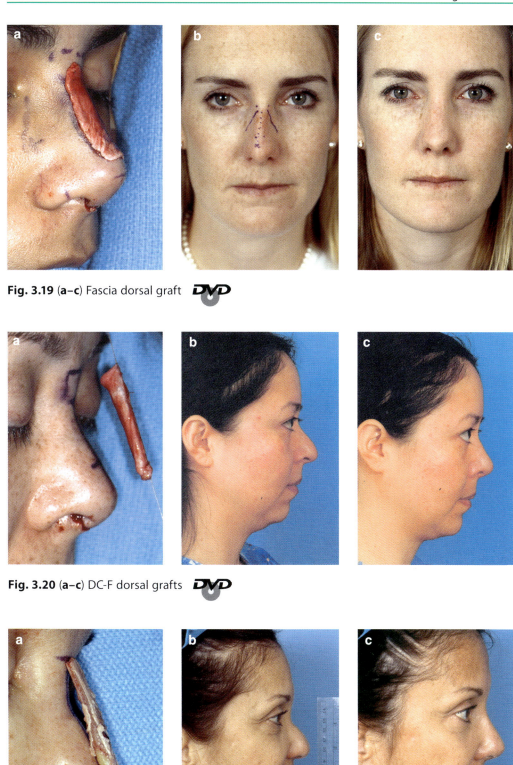

Fig. 3.19 (**a–c**) Fascia dorsal graft **DVD**

Fig. 3.20 (**a–c**) DC-F dorsal grafts **DVD**

Fig. 3.21 (**a–c**) Structural osseocartilaginous rib grafts **DVD**

**Decision Making
Level 1**

Operative Planning. As always, operative planning begins with "what does the patient want and what will her tissues allow me to achieve?" Next comes a relatively simple photo analysis. On lateral view, the nasion, as well as its level and height, usually at the eyelash level is marked (Fig. 3.22). When in doubt, do not attempt major radix changes. Any change greater than 4 mm is unrealistic in either direction. Next the ideal profile line is drawn through any preexisting dorsal hump. One must decide whether the dorsum should be reduced, augmented, balanced, or maintained. On anterior view, the dorsal lines are drawn and the X-X distance measured. One should decide on the aesthetic indications for spreader grafts and type of osteotomies.

Technique

Step #1. Radix changes are done out of necessity with reduction rarely performed (<5%). Radix augmentation (15%) is frequently done as part of a balanced approach. The dorsum is reduced first and then fascia is placed in the radix area (Fig. 3.23).

Step #2. Excluding ethnic noses, dorsal reduction is done in almost 90% of the cases as most female patients want a smaller cuter nose. An incremental approach to dorsal reduction is the safest and easiest approach. Sequentially, the bony dorsum is reduced first with rasps and the cartilaginous dorsum is then reduced using a "split hump" technique with scissors. Note: the septal harvest is always done after the dorsal reduction, but before the osteotomies.

Step #3. Osteotomies are employed to narrow the base bony width and close the open roof, although spreader grafts can also achieve the latter. The options for osteotomies are as follows: (1) none (7%), (2) low-to-high (45%), (3) low-to-low plus transverse (45%), and (4) double level (3%).

Step #4. Spreader grafts are always considered as their functional and aesthetic benefits far exceed any technical demands (Fig. 3.24). Avoidance of internal valve collapse and inverted-V deformity justifies any tediousness of inserting spreader grafts.

Lessons Learned

1) Think "balance" rhinoplasty and especially a balanced reduction.
2) The ideal nasion is at the lash line ±2 mm.
3) When in doubt, do not change the radix.
4) Print out two lateral photos. Have the patient draw their desired profile change and compare it to your analysis when planning a major profile change.
5) Incremental dorsal reduction with rasps and scissors is the safest and easiest technique to master.
6) Begin with bony vault reduction as it exposes the true cartilaginous hump deformity.
7) A "split hump" reduction of the cartilaginous vault is very precise.
8) Reduction of the septal component decreases dorsal *height*. Upper lateral excision decreases *width*. Septal excision is often 3 × upper lateral cartilage (ULC) excision.
9) Osteotomies narrow base bony width (X-X width on anterior view).
10) Spreader grafts are a functional and aesthetic necessity.

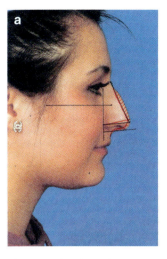
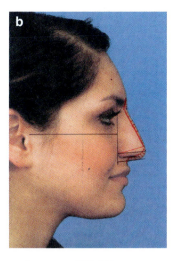
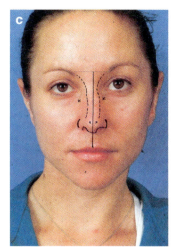

Fig. 3.22 (**a–c**) Analysis/operative planning   **DVD**

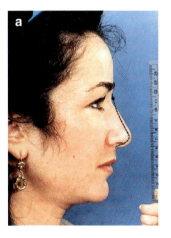
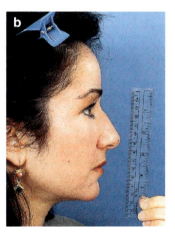
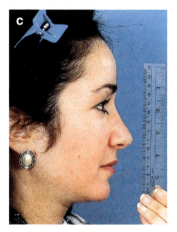

Fig. 3.23 (**a–c**) "Balanced" reduction with radix augmentation

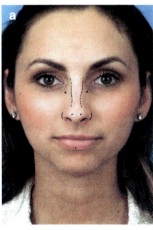
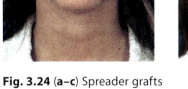
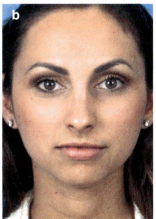
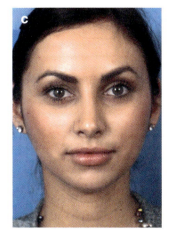

Fig. 3.24 (**a–c**) Spreader grafts

Case Study: Profile Correction

Analysis

A 19-year-old 5' 3" girl wanted a smaller, cuter nose (Fig. 3.25). She felt that her profile was too much of a beak, especially when she smiled. Incremental dorsal reduction and shortening of the caudal septum resulted in a smaller cuter nose. Supporting the tip on a columellar strut prevents it from plunging when she smiles. Different types of lateral osteotomies reduced the preexisting asymmetry of the bony vault. Functionally, the patient breathed fine, but the caudal septum was deviated. Surgically, the goal was to achieve a "functional reduction" – make the nose significantly smaller without compromising the airway.

Operative Technique Highlights

1) Open exposure of nose and septum including extramucosal tunnels
2) Incremental dorsal reduction: bony (1.5 mm), cartilage (4 mm)
3) Caudal septum shortening (4 mm) and contouring of anterior nasal spine (ANS)
4) Major septoplasty/septal harvest including 7 mm bony spur
5) Caudal septum relocation, R to L
6) Asymmetric osteotomies: R (low-tolow), L (low-to-high)
7) Columellar strut plus tip sutures: CS, DC, ID, DE, and TP

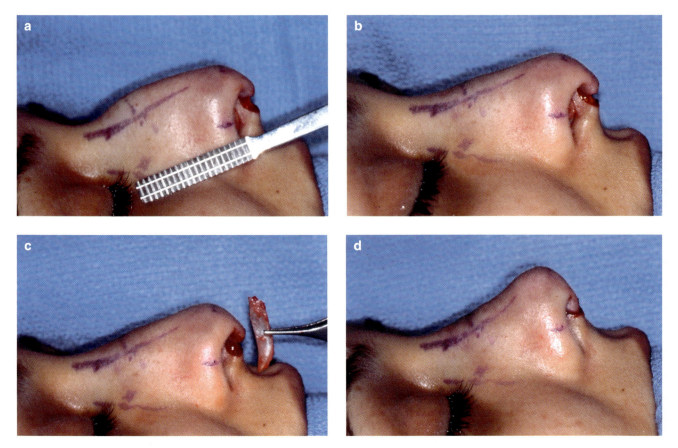

Fig. 3.25 (**a,b**) Incremental dorsal reduction, (**c**) caudal septul shortening, (**d**) tip projection and position

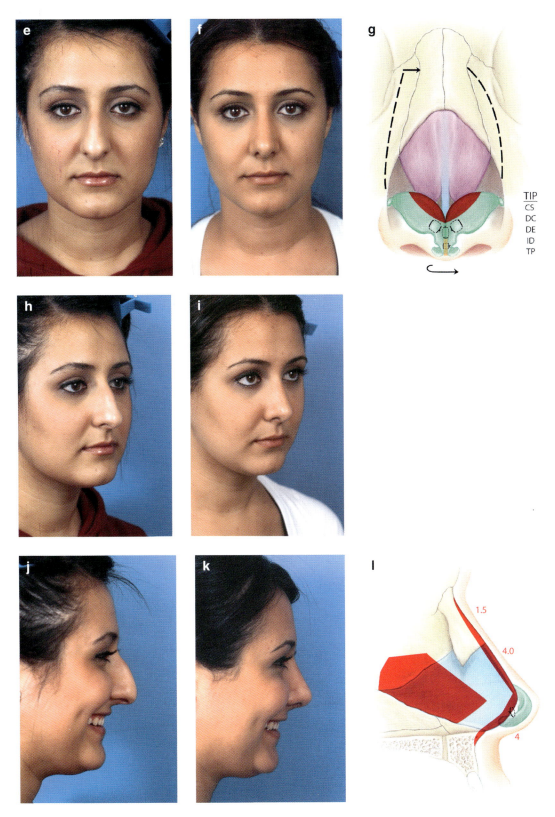

Fig. 3.25 (e–l)

Decision Making Level 2

Radix. The majority of the radix grafts are done with fascia. However, as radix hypoplasia increases, augmentation with "fascia only" is no longer sufficient (Fig. 3.26). One either adds diced cartilage below the fascia graft (DC+F) or wraps diced cartilage in the fascia (DC−F). The majority of DC+F grafts are done to raise the height of the radix area with the diced cartilage fusing to the bone and the fascia providing a smooth coverage. When one encounters a hypoplastic radix and upper half of dorsum, a DC−F graft is used to augment the more longitudinal deficiency.

Dorsum. As the height and cephalic extent of the dorsal reduction progresses upward, longer spreader grafts and more exotic osteotomies become necessary (Fig. 3.27a). Once the dorsal reduction reaches the level of the medial canthus, the open roof deformity is quite extended. Lateral osteotomies cannot mobilize the lateral walls sufficiently and spreader grafts must be used to avoid an inverted-V deformity.

1) The dorsal width can be quite wide at the junction level of the two vaults. In these cases, I will often do a medial oblique osteotomy prior to a low-to-low osteotomy as the combination produces a major narrowing of the dorsal width (Fig. 3.27b). I do not use this technique routinely as there is often a palpable bony step-off in the radix area.
2) The lateral walls can be very convex due to angulation at the nasal bone/frontal process of the maxilla suture line. Thus, one must achieve a true change in the intrinsic shape of the lateral walls rather than mere mobilization. A "double-level" osteotomy is required (Fig. 3.27c). The upper osteotomy fractures the lateral wall at the junction of the nasal bone and the frontal process of maxilla. The lower osteotomy goes across the frontal process of the maxilla as close to the maxilla as possible. Finally, a transverse osteotomy is done. Often three osteotomies per side are necessary with the sequence being high, transverse, and low-to-low.
3) Spreader grafts must be cut longer and placed more cephalically to insure closure of the bony vault following the osteotomies. One may have to do a three-layer suture fixation high-up within the bony vault area.

PRINCIPLES

● Radix augmentation is progressive with regard to height and length, beginning with F, then DC+F, and finally DC−F for combined radix and upper dorsal deficiencies.
● Selection of lateral osteotomies is based on the degree of movement with none, low-to-high, and low-to-low sufficient in 95% of the cases.
● Medial oblique osteotomies are useful for the very wide flared dorsum. Note: one should concentrate on narrowing dorsal width, not just base bony width.
● A double-level and transverse osteotomy can effectively change the most convex lateral wall.

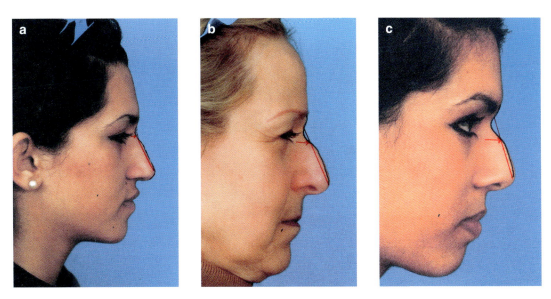

Fig. 3.26 Radix decisions. (**a**) Fascia, (**b**) DC+F, (**c**) DC−F

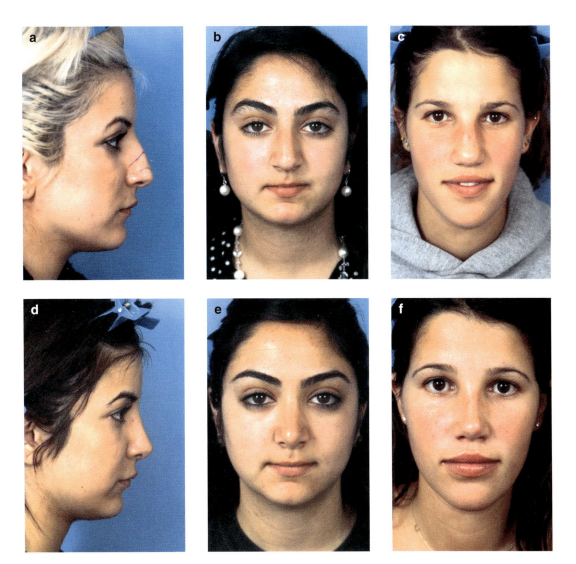

Fig. 3.27 Dorsal decisions. (**a,d**) High bony dorsum, (**b,e**) wide dorsum, (**c,f**) convex lateral walls

Case Study: Asymmetric Bony Vault

Analysis

A 27-year old presented with an asymmetric deviated nose and a vague history of nasal trauma which was not treated (Fig. 3.28). Functionally, she was obstructed at her left external valve. Aesthetically, the patient was bothered by the deviated nose, the prominent dorsum, and the overall size. The technical challenge was to straighten both the very asymmetric bony dorsum and the entire nose while creating a smaller more refined look. Relocation of the caudal septum was an absolute necessity for straightening the nose and opening the external valve. Different osteotomies on the two sides improved the inherent asymmetry of the bones. The spreader grafts were longer than usual (25 mm) and placed higher into the bony vault to insure stability. A fascia graft over the dorsum was done to insure smoothness.

Operative Technique Highlights

1) Harvest of deep temporal fascia
2) Exposure of dorsum and septum
3) Creation of 6 mm rim strips and extra mucosal tunnels
4) Incremental dorsal reduction: bone 0.5 mm, cartilage 3 mm
5) Caudal septal resection: 3 mm
6) Septal harvest followed by caudal septal relocation L to R
7) Asymmetric osteotomies: R double level, L low-to-low
8) Columellar strut and tip sutures: CS, DC, ID, DE
9) Insertion of dorsal fascia graft and tip fascia graft
10) Nostril sill excisions: R 1.7 mm, L 2.0 mm
11) Alar rim support grafts sutured into marginal incisions

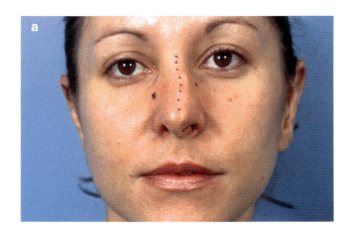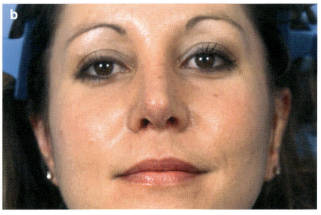

Fig. 3.28 (a–j)

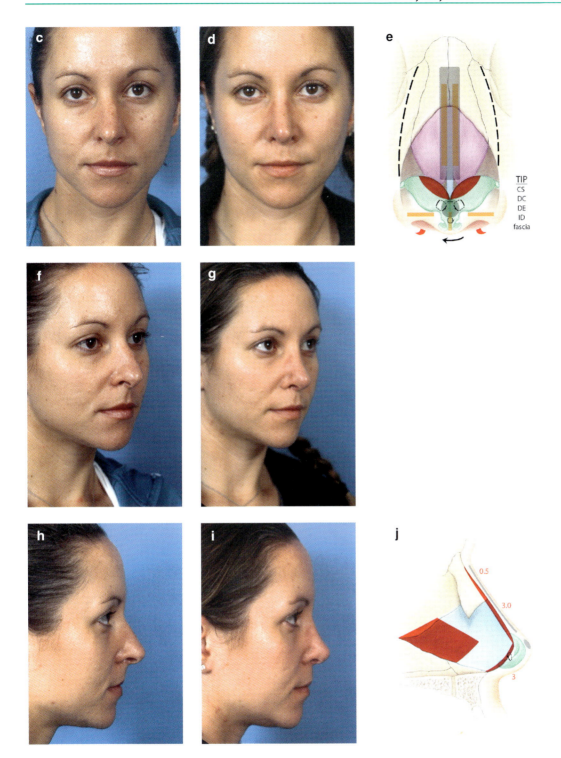

Fig. 3.28 (continued)

Radix. Radix reduction is not as easy or effective as one might wish (Fig. 3.29). Thus, one should be careful in thinking that a major reduction is possible – never design an "all or none" operative plan based on a major radix reduction. Do not over-reduce the dorsum to fit a new nasion which would be produced by a large radix reduction. In operative planning and execution it is important to separate the *radix area* from the dorsum. I will usually do an incremental dorsal reduction first using a rasp for the bony vault and scissors for the cartilage vault. This initial dorsal reduction is conservative. Then the double-guarded osteotome is inserted against the cephalic edge of the bony vault. The handle is levered upward towards 45° and then tapped with the hammer. After several taps, one should palpate the amount of bone being removed. If satisfied, the tapping is continued until the osteotome strikes the skull which is indicated by a dull thud. Rotating the osteotome causes the radix bone to disarticulate from the nasofrontal suture line. If the bone is not easily removed, a 2 mm osteotome can be driven transversely across the radix via a stab incision beneath the eyebrow.

Dorsum. As previously stated, dorsal augmentation has changed dramatically (Fig. 3.30). I no longer use solid grafts of septum or layered conchal grafts, but rather diced cartilage grafts in fascia (DC–F). Since the vast majority of dorsal augmentations have been done in Asian, secondary, or reconstructive cases, this technique will be discussed in-depth in those sections. As regards primary Caucasian noses, the need for augmentation is usually in the 1–3 mm range and can be achieved progressively with either a double layer of fascia (F) or a very small tapered DC-F graft with the thickest portion in the supratip area. In these patients, I make the dorsal graft *construct* on the back table. The fascia is pinned to a silicone block. The diced cartilage is placed on the fascia in the desired amount, the fascia folded over, and the edges sutured with 4–0 plain catgut. The graft is molded with the fingertips until the desired shape is achieved. These grafts are kept on the conservative side and can always be augmented with small amounts of diced cartilage placed underneath, usually in the supratip area. Most overresected secondaries will require maximum fullness over the bony vault, whereas most Asian noses require a graft of uniform thickness.

PRINCIPLES

- Be conservative in planning a radix reduction, but be relatively aggressive in how much bone you remove.
- A double-guarded osteotome is safer than a drill.
- DC-F grafts have replaced dorsal grafts of septum or concha.
- DC-F grafts can be customized to fit the dorsal defect, ranging from half-length to full-length, as well as thickness (2–8 mm).
- DC-F grafts are never made larger than required, there is no absorption.

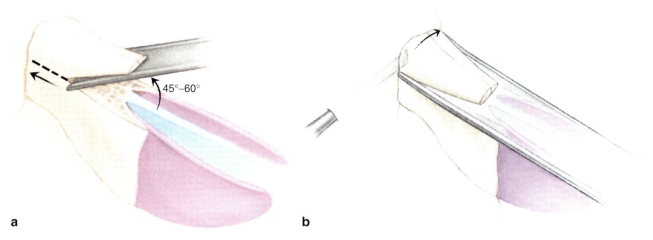

Fig. 3.29 (**a, b**) Bony excision of the radix

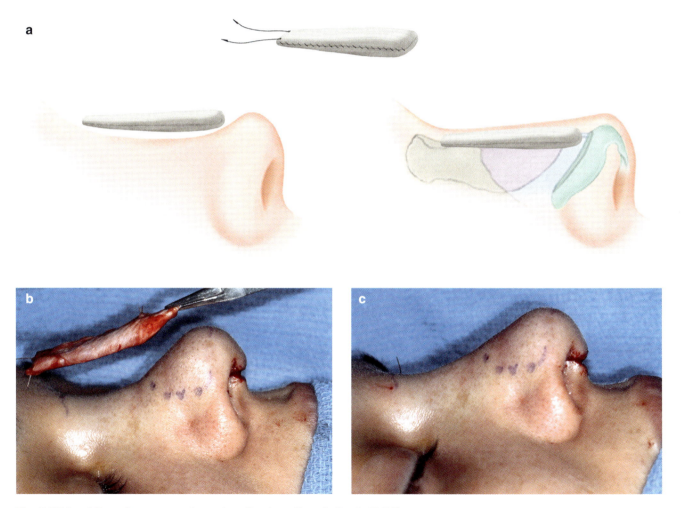

Fig. 3.30 (**a–c**) Dorsal augmentation using diced cartilage in fascia (DC-F)

Case Study: Radix Reduction

Analysis

A 19-year-old girl of Persian descent felt that her nose was too big, too wide, and too unattractive (Fig. 3.31). Compounding the problem of a heavy skin sleeve was the radix fullness which gave the impression that the nose started at the eyebrows. Palpation indicated that the radix fullness was soft tissue rather than bone. Muscle resection followed by elevation of the medial brow resulted in a more specific nasion point and also lowered the start of the nose from the medial brow to the lash line. The width of the bony vault was narrowed markedly, but required a total of eight osteotomies plus stabilization with long spreader grafts.

Operative Technique

1) Maximum soft tissue defatting over the tip and dorsum
2) Maximum muscle resection in the radix area
3) Incremental dorsal reduction: bone 2 mm, cartilage 4 mm
4) Caudal septal resection 5 mm and ANS resection
5) Septal harvest
6) Maximum narrowing of the bony vault: medial oblique, double-level and transverse osteotomies
7) Spreader grafts placed high into the bony vault
8) Insertion of columellar strut and tip sutures; CS, DC, and LCC
9) Open structure tip graft sutured to domes and columellar
10) Alar wedge resections and alar rim grafts
11) Central endoscopic forehead lift with no temporal sutures

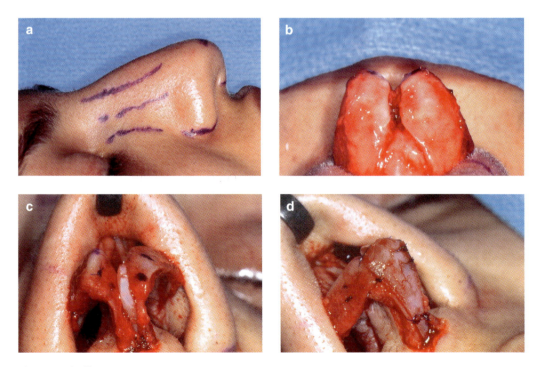

Fig. 3.31 (a–l)

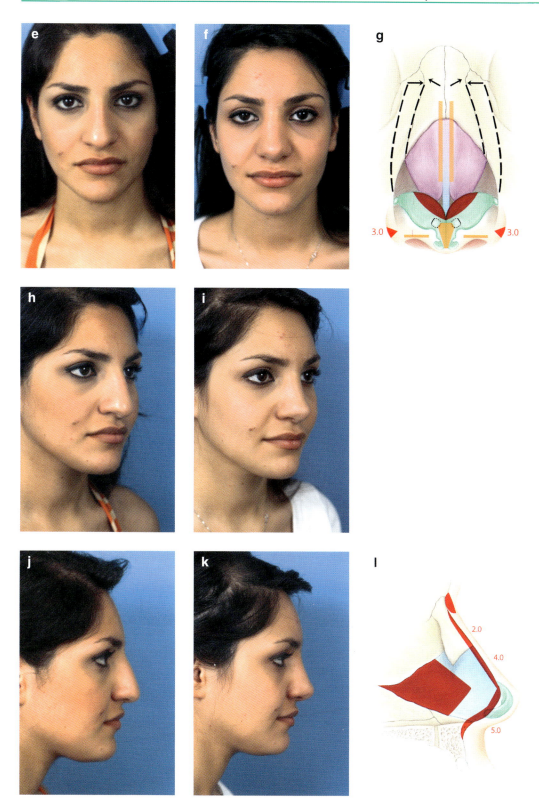

Fig. 3.31 (continued)

Reading List   Aiach G, Gomulinski L. Resection controlée de la bussé nasal osseuse au niveau de l'angle naso-frontal. Ann Chir Plast 27: 226, 1982

Byrd S, Hobar PC. Rhinoplasty: A practical guide for surgical planning. Plast Reconstr Surg 91: 642, 1993

Daniel RK. The radix. In: Daniel RK (ed) Aesthetic Plastic Surgery: Rhinoplasty. Boston: Little, Brown, 1993

Daniel RK, Lessard ML. Rhinoplasty: A graded aesthetic anatomical approach. Ann Plast Surg 13: 436, 1984

Daniel RK, Farkas LG. Rhinoplasty: Image and reality. Clin Plast Surg 15: 1, 1988

Daniel RK, Letourneau A. The superficial musculoaponeurotic system of the nose. Plast Reconstr Surg 82: 48, 1988a

Daniel RK, Letoumeau A. Rhinoplasty: Nasal anatomy. Ann Plast Surg 20: 5, 1988b

Gruber R, Chang TN, Kahn D et al Broad nasal bone reduction: An algorithm for osteotomies. Plast Reconstr Surg 119: 1044, 2007

Guerrosantos J. Nose and paranasal augmentation: Autogenous, fascia, and cartilage. Clin Plast Surg 18: 65, 1991

Guyuron B. Precision rhinoplasty. Part I: The role of life-size photographs and soft-tissue cephalometric analysis. Plast Reconstr Surg 81: 489, 1988

Guyuron B. Guarded burr for deepening of nasofrontal junction. Plast Reconstr Surg 84: 513–516, 1989. Updated, Plast Reconstr Surg 106: 1417, 2000

Lessard ML, Daniel RK. Surgical anatomy of the nose. Arch Otolaryngol Head Neck Surg 111:25,1985

Miller TA. Temporalis fascia graft for facial and nasal contour augmentation. Plast Reconstr Surg 81: 524–533, 1988

Nievert H. Reduction of nasofrontal angle in rhinoplasty. Arch Otolaryngol 53: 196, 1951

Parkes ML, Kamer, F, Morgan, WR. Double lateral osteotomy in rhinoplasty. Arch Otolaryngol 103: 344, 1977

Rohrich Rj, Hollier, LH. Versatility of spreader grafts in rhinoplasty. Clin Plast Surg 2: 225, 1996

Rorhrich RJ, Gunter JP, Deuber MA et al The deviated nose: Optimizing results using a simplified classification and algorithmic approach. Plast Reconstr Surg. 110: 1509, 2002

Rorhrich RJ, Muzaffar, AR, Janis, JE. Component dorsal hump reduction: The importance of maintaining dorsal aesthetic lines in rhinoplasty. Plast Reconstr Surg 114: 1298, 2004

Shah AR, Constantinides M. Aligning the bony nasal vault in rhinoplasty. Facial Plast Surg 22: 3, 2006

Sheen, JH. Aesthetic Rhinoplasty. St. Louis: Mosby, 1978

Sheen JH. The radix as a reference in rhinoplasty. Perspect Plast Surg 1: 33, 1987

Sheen JH. Rhinoplasty: Personal evolution and milestones. Plast Reconstr Surg 105: 1820, 2000

Skoog T. A method of hump reduction in rhinoplasty. Arch Otolaryngol Head Neck Surg 101: 207, 1975

Tardy MA Jr, Denneny, JC. Micro-osteotomies in rhinoplasty. Facial Plast Surg 1: 137, 1984

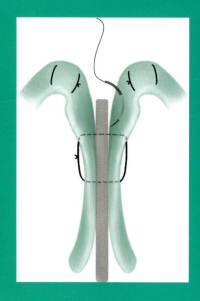

Tip Techniques 4

Introduction

Tip surgery remains the most discussed and least understood aspect of the rhinoplasty operation. The foundation of tip surgery is the interrelated "3 As" of anatomy, aesthetics, and analysis. The six tip characteristics of volume, width, definition, projection, rotation, and shape will be related to the underlying anatomy and overlying surface aesthetics. The surgeon will learn to distinguish the intrinsic tip from the lobule, as well as the influence of intrinsic and extrinsic factors on the tip itself. Then, in perhaps the most controversial aspect of this book, I will present only two tip operations, albeit with numerous variations. The operations are open tip suture and open tip graft. With these two operations, the surgeon can correct 95% of primary tip deformities. Each step in the procedure will be presented in great detail and must be mastered by the reader. Rather than try every tip operation available, the novice surgeon has the luxury of mastering only two interrelated procedures, thus achieving a greater understanding of surgical cause and effect. This chapter will serve as the foundation for all tip surgeries. Additional applications to a wide range of specific tip deformities are discussed throughout the book, especially in Chapter 8 and Chapter 9.

Overview   Tip surgery can appear extraordinarily complex due to the wide variation in tip anatomy, patient desires, and surgical options. To overcome this complexity, I favor the following progressive tip operation, which a surgeon can master and then expand to cases of increasing levels of difficulty (Fig. 4.1)

Level 1. A Five-Step Tip Suture Technique. The combination of an open approach and tip suturing has revolutionized tip surgery allowing the surgeon to control the individual tip characteristics of width, projection, definition, and supratip break. Suturing provides a graded controlled method of tip shaping. The five components are as follows: (1) create symmetrical rim strips, (2) insert and fix a columellar strut, (3) domal creation sutures for definition, (4) an interdomal suture for tip width control, and (5) a tip-positioning suture to create a supratip break (Fig. 4.2). This relatively simple approach using standard absorbable sutures will work for at least 60% of all primary tips. As long as the surgeon is conservative in suturing tension, all sutured tips will be more symmetrical and refined than when first exposed. Careful records must be kept as the surgeon must teach themself surgical cause and effect at each postoperative visit. Obviously, judgment comes from experience which can only be gained in the operating room.

Level 2. Advanced Suturing and Add-On Tip Grafts. Once the surgeon has a moderate experience with tip sutures, additional sutures can be employed in dealing with more challenging tips as regards asymmetry and excessive width. The domal equalization suture brings the domes into alignment while the lateral crural convexity suture reduces convexity of the lateral crura. Yet, it is the application of add-on Tip Refinement Grafts to the sutured tip that can give the requisite shape and definition which elevates and refines the final result.

Level 3. Structure Tip Grafts. In contrast to add-on grafts, which accentuate the sutured tip, a structure tip graft replaces the tip anatomy. The tip definition as seen through the skin is created by the tip graft and not the alar cartilages. The majority of structure tip grafts are simply golf-tee shaped shield grafts inserted *within* the alar architecture or positioned *above* the alar domes to achieve greater definition. These grafts reach their ultimate expression as isolated entities in secondary cases where the entire alar cartilages have been previously excised.

Simplifying Tip Surgery. It is only in the last 5 years that I have become convinced that *95% of all primary tips* are Level 1 and 2 cases. This fact means that the surgeon can get good results mastering one operation – *open tip suture techniques with optional add-on grafts*. The ability to master all the nuances of one progressive operation that can be individualized to each specific case is revolutionary. There is no need to struggle with ten different tip operations unless you want to do the remaining 5% of cases which are Level 3. Equally, I do not recommend a closed delivery approach for tip suturing as my experience indicates that it rarely achieves the symmetry or precision of an open approach.

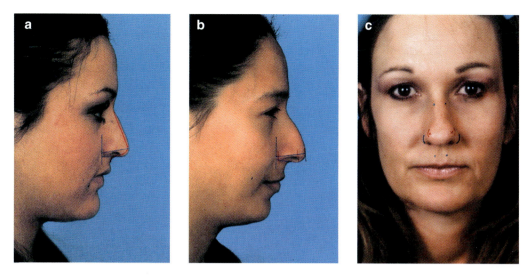

Fig. 4.1 Tip analysis. (**a**) Level 1, (**b**) Level 2, (**c**) Level 3, see case studies at end of chapter **DVD**

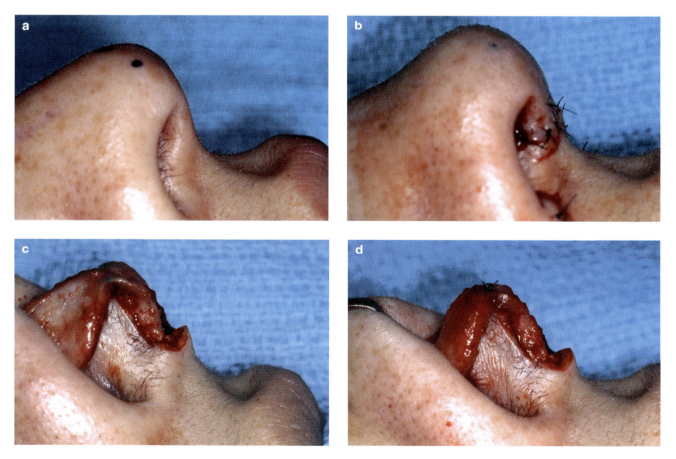

Fig. 4.2 (**a–d**) Intraop changes created by tip sutures

Case Study: Tip Suture

Analysis

A 20-year-old girl presented with the complaint that she felt her bridge was too convex and her tip too droopy (Fig. 4.3). She wanted a smaller, cuter nose. There were no functional issues. This patient demonstrates that a simple tip suture technique can dramatically change a tip. There were no destabilizing excisions or incisions of the lateral crura. Also, there is no need for either an open structure or multilayer tip graft underneath this thin skin. On anterior view, the tip change is quite dramatic. Tip suture techniques have revolutionized rhinoplasty surgery because they allow the surgeon to make significant yet controlled changes in the tip with minimal morbidity.

Operative Technique

1) Open approach with confirmation of pre-op tip analysis and op plan.
2) Creation of symmetrical rim strips – 12 mm wide reduced to 6 mm.
3) Incremental dorsal reduction: bone (1 mm), cartilage (3 mm).
4) Shortening of caudal septum (2.5 mm), the anterior nasal spine (ANS) was resected.
5) Septal harvest.
6) Low-to-less and transverse osteotomies.
7) Bilateral spreader grafts.
8) Insertion of columellar strut and tip sutures: CS, DC, ID, TP.
9) Nostril sill excisions (R:2, L:2)

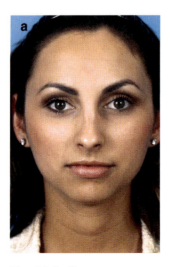
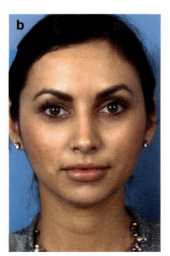
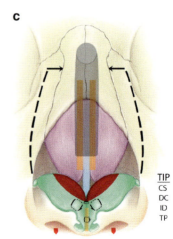

TIP
CS
DC
ID
TP

Fig. 4.3 (a–j)

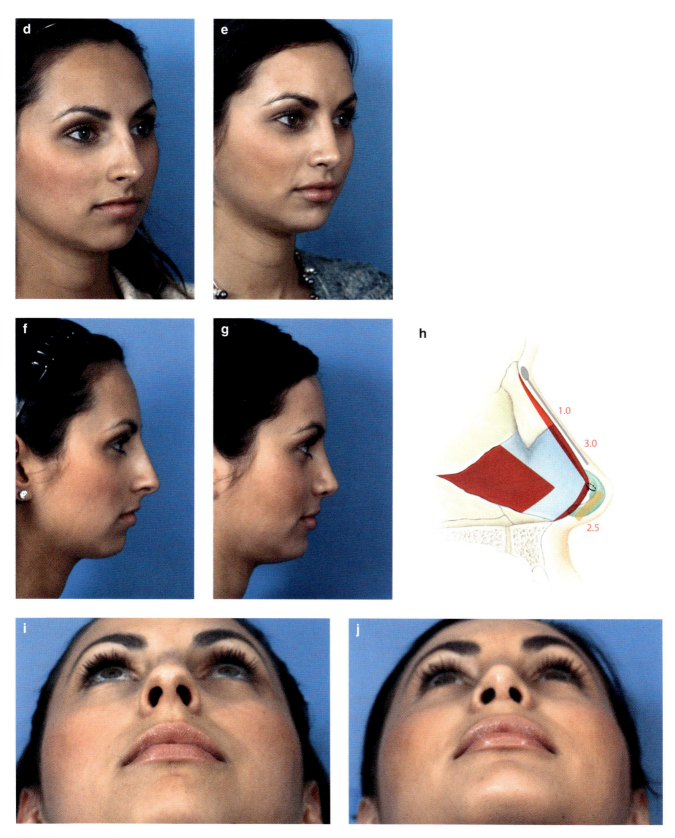

Fig. 4.3 (continued)

Tip Anatomy   Based on extensive fresh cadaver dissections and intraoperative observations during open rhinoplasty (Daniel 1992), I have divided the alar cartilages into three crura (medial, middle, and lateral), each composed of two segments with distinct junction points of aesthetic importance (Fig. 4.4).

Medial Crus. The medial crus is the primary component of the columella and can be subdivided into two portions: lower footplate segment and superior columellar segment. The footplates vary in size, shape, and angulation. The superior columella segment represents the narrow waist of the columellar and its overall length correlates with nostril length.

Columella-Lobular Junction. A distinct junction occurs between the paired vertically oriented medial crura and the divergent angular middle crura. It marks the transition from nasal base to the tip lobule and usually corresponds with the nostril apex ±1–2 mm. It is the breakpoint in the columella's "double break."

Middle Crus. As originally defined by Sheen (1987), the middle crus begins at the columellar-lobular junction and ends at the lateral crura. It can be subdivided into a lobular segment and a domal segment. The shape of the lobular segment varies in width and length, which can have a profound effect on tip shape, e.g., short segments produce snubbed tips. The lobular segments abut in the midline cephalically but diverge caudally similar to an open book standing on end. The *domal segment* extends from the medial genu, which marks its transition with the infralobular segment, to the lateral genu, which marks its junction with the lateral crura. and bracket the *domal notch*, which in turn determines the soft triangles or soft tissue facets of the lobule. The shape of the domal segment varies from concave to smooth to convex.

Domal Junction. The domal junction is the critical landmark of the refined tip and marks the transition from middle crura to lateral crura. The tip-defining points fall consistently on the domal junction line. Anatomically, the most aesthetic configuration is a convex domal segment adjacent to a concave lateral crura. It is this configuration that one is trying to produce with domal sutures.

Lateral Crura. The lateral crura may be subdivided into the lateral crus and the accessory cartilage ring. The lateral crus is the main component of the nasal lobule and influences its shape, size, and position. Each of its borders has surgical significance. Cephalically, a "scroll formation" exists between lateral crus and upper lateral cartilage with interspersed sesamoid cartilages. Laterally, the crus passes posterior away from the nostril rim and tapers in size. Three additional factors are critical: configuration, axis of orientation, and axis of curvature. The configuration has been subdivided into six shapes based upon relative concavity and convexities. For example, the severely concave lateral crura produces a pinched tip but is easily corrected by flipping rather than excising the excess cephalic lateral crura.

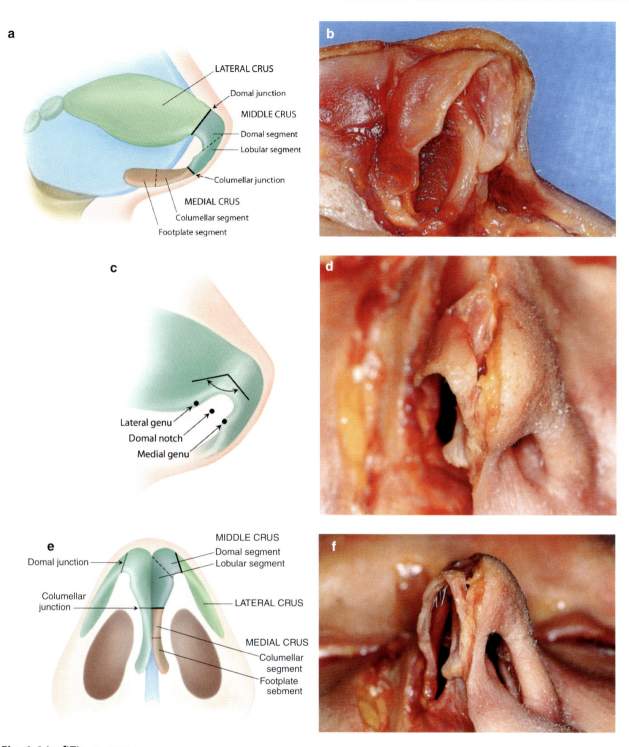

Fig. 4.4 (a–f) Tip anatomy

Aesthetics:
Intrinsic factors

Although tip analysis can be subjective, decisions must be made and an operative plan formulated. The goal of analysis is to determine what the tip characteristics are and how far they deviate from ideal. Over the years, I have evolved a set of six criteria which facilitate decision-making. These characteristics consist of three intrinsic tip factors (volume, definition, and width) and three additional factors (projection, rotation, and position) that can be intrinsic, extrinsic, or both (Fig. 4.5). Each criterion can be graded as normal or abnormal with progression from minor, moderate, to major. Although initially confusing, this system is rapidly applied and serves as a decision-making ladder for formulating the operative plan.

Volume. Tip volume refers to the size of the lateral crura. Essentially, one evaluates the size, shape, and axis of the lateral crura. In 90% of female rhinoplasties, some degree of cephalic lateral crura resection is done which reduces volume, minimizes overlap at the scroll formation, and reduces intrinsic convex curvature of the lateral crura. This excision produces three *aesthetic improvements*: (1) it makes the tip smaller, (2) it sets off the tip thereby improving definition, and (3) it rotates the tip slightly upward. It also makes tip suturing easier.

Definition. Definition is a true aesthetic concept which implies the degree of detail, refinement, and angularity of the tip. It is determined anatomically by the adjacent relationship between the *convexity* of the domal segment and the *concavity* of the lateral crura with its surface expression revealed or obscured by the overlying skin. The anatomical configuration which correlates with the best tip definition is a convex domal segment with an adjacent concave lateral crura. The critical importance of the skin envelope should never be forgotten (Fig. 4.6).

Width. Width refers to the interdomal distance and is easily measured on the skin surface between the two tip-defining points. The ideal interdomal width correlates often with the width of the philtral columns and the dorsal lines.

Shape. Virtually every clinician recognizes certain tip shapes including the 3 Bs (broad, ball, and boxy), the 3 Ps (Pinocchio, pinched, and parenthesis) plus a myriad of other shapes. Each of these shapes denotes a certain combination of anatomical deformities and, more important, a certain set of potential postoperative problems. For example, the boxy tip consists often of thick alar cartilages, but weak alar sidewalls which can easily collapse postoperatively unless supported with rim grafts.

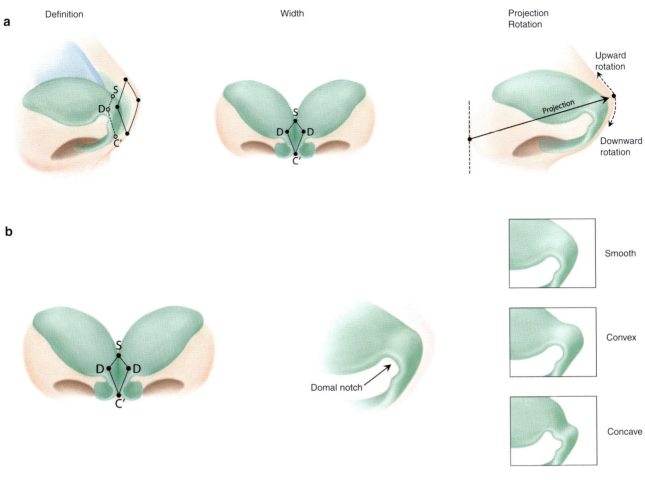

a Definition — Width — Projection / Rotation

Upward rotation

Projection

Downward rotation

b

Smooth

Convex

Concave

Domal notch

Fig. 4.5 (**a, b**) Aesthetics – intrinsic factors **DVD**

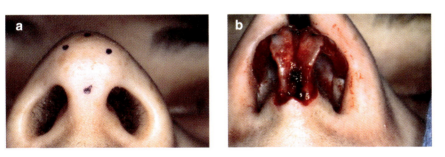
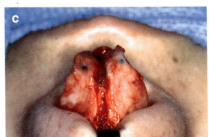

Fig. 4.6 (**a–c**) Intraopertive aesthetics

Aesthetics: Extrinsic factors

The *intrinsic* characteristics are dictated by the configuration of the alar cartilages. In contrast, the *extrinsic* factors are often determined by the abutting supporting structures (Fig. 4.7). A classic example is the high-arched tension nose. Total tip projection may be excessive, but once the large dorsal hump and long caudal septum are excised, the tip may even be intrinsically deficient due to small alar cartilages. Thus, one must learn to analyze the tip, both for its intrinsic and extrinsic factors (Fig. 4.8). Ultimately, one has to consider the total characteristic comprised of both intrinsic and extrinsic contributions.

Projection. Tip projection can be defined as the distance from a vertical facial plane passing through the alar crease to the nasal tip. According to Byrd (1993), ideal tip projection is considered to be two thirds the ideal dorsal length which in turn is two thirds the ideal midface height. It is determined by the intrinsic tip cartilage configuration, the extrinsic structural abutments, or both. One can measure intrinsic projection by a vertical from the columellar breakpoint to the tip projection line. For example, the true Pinocchio tip is due to extremely long alar cartilages, whereas the more common over-projecting tip is most frequently due to a large cartilaginous vault that pushes the tip outward. Surgically, the extrinsic factors are eliminated first and then the intrinsic tip modification is done if necessary.

Rotation. Tip rotation is most easily defined as the *tip angle*, which is measured from the vertical plane at the alar crease to the tip. This angle is set at 105° for females and 100° for males. Anatomically, it is determined by the intrinsic tip cartilage configuration, the extrinsic structural abutments, or both. For example, the tip can be pushed down by large lateral crura (intrinsic), a prominent caudal septum (extrinsic) or both. It is critical to determine the etiology in order to design the ideal operation. Essentially, the diagnosis can be made by evaluating each of the three crura and then by palpating the caudal septum/ANS.

Position. Tip position refers to the location of the tip along the dorsal line (N-T) and is of great concern in shortening the long nose. Essentially, one will often excise cephalic lateral crura (intrinsic) and caudal septum (extrinsic) to shorten the nose. Certainly, septocolumellar grafts demonstrate the concept of extending dorsal length without altering rotation. Another, critical relationship is to remember that the dorsal line (N-T) can be dramatically effected by changes at the nasion (N) which creates an illusion that tip position has been altered. For example, augmenting the radix will make the dorsum longer and create the illusion that the tip is more dependent.

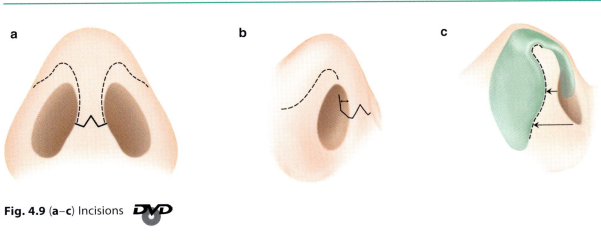

Fig. 4.9 (**a**–**c**) Incisions *DVD*

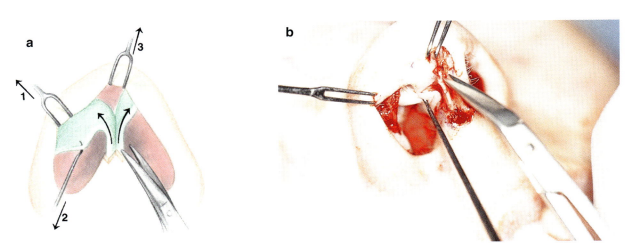

Fig. 4.10 (**a**, **b**) Exposure: columellar to tip *DVD*

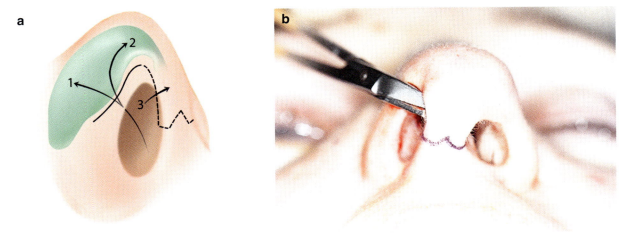

Fig. 4.11 (**a**, **b**) Exposure: bidirectional *DVD*

Open Tip Suture Technique: An Overview

Without question, tip surgery is the most complex, frustrating portion of a rhinoplasty due to the patient's expectations and anatomical variations. In my first Atlas, I fell into the trap of being encyclopedic and presenting a large number of tip techniques. Today, I find that I use tip sutures plus simple add-on grafts of excised alar cartilage in 85% of my primary cases (Tables 4.1 and 4.2). The other 15% consists of either a closed rhinoplasty with minimal tip change (10%) or an open structure tip graft for maximum change (5%).

I published my first paper on open tip sutures in 1987 and over the subsequent 20 years, I have reached certain conclusions (Daniel 1987, 1999). First, tip sutures are effective at achieving significant permanent tip refinement. Second, the technique need not be complex, but rather can be sequentially additive until the desired tip change is achieved. Third, each tip characteristic can be achieved using a specific suture; i.e., tip definition with domal creation sutures. Fourth, the suture material is always absorbable (polydioxanone suture [PDS]), which eliminates long-term extrusion or infection, is colored (violet) to improve visibility, is usually small (5–0 PDS), and is on a short-cord sharp needle (PS3). Five, asymmetry is minimized through out the tip suturing process with the final results always less asymmetrical than the original alar configuration. Six, one should use only as many sutures as needed to achieve the desired tip, there is no need to put eight sutures in every nose. Seven, I never hesitate to take out a suture that is not right – a pointy dome will show through the skin and too vertical a columellar will result in a long infralobule. Eight, sutures should be tied to the ideal tension point, neither too tight nor too loose. Avoid excess tension, if one must err always use less tension rather than too much. Nine, there is no need to undermine the mucosa prior to placing the suture; one simply penetrates the cartilage without going through the underlying mucosa. If necessary, the underlying mucosa can be injected with local anesthesia prior to suture placement to avoid penetrating it. Ten, one must learn surgical cause and effect, so keep a detail diagram of the sutures and refer to it at each postoperative visit. Better yet, take intraop photos from four different views and print them out – look at them at every post-op visit.

Recently, it became obvious to me that surgeons are teaching tip suture techniques the wrong way. Traditionally, the emphasis was placed on the direct and indirect consequences of each individual suture. In contrast, I now teach tip suture techniques from exactly the opposite view point – what tip characteristic do I want to achieve and which suture will produce it. Fortunately, the operation is sequential and a true "sew as you go" method. One simply stops when the desired refinement is obtained.

Be fore warned that numerous authors use different names for the same suture. I have always tried to respect the original name of the suture as its author intended. This same courtesy has not been extended by others and thus there is total confusion between various texts. Fortunately, the suture is more important and longer lasting than its name.

Table 4.1 Tip factors and tip sutures

Volume	Excision lateral crura
Projection	Columellar strut
Definition	Domal creation suture
Tip width	Interdomal suture
Tip position	Tip position suture
Asymmetry	Domal equalization suture
Crural convexity	Lateral crural convexity sutures
Extra definition projection	Add-on grafts (TRG)

Table 4.2 Open Tip Suture Technique: Step-by-Step

Step	Surgical technique	Effect	Frequency
Step #1	Symmetrical rim strips	Decreases volume	99%
	Cephalic lateral crura excision	More suturable	Leave 6 mm
Step #2	Columellar strut with strut suture	Increases projection	99%
		Prevents drooping	
Step #3	Domal creation suture R & L	Increases definition	95%
Step #4	Interdomal suture	Decreases tip width	90%
		Creates tip diamond	
Step #5	Domal equalization suture	Increase symmetry	75%
Step #6	Lateral crural convexity suture	Decreases convexity of lateral crura	20%
		Crua straight	
Step #7	Tip position suture	Increase projection	75%
		Increases rotation	No excess
Step #8	Add-on grafts (TRG)	Increases definition	40%
		Increases projection	
Step #9	Alar rim grafts	Supports alar rims	10–15%

Step #1 Symmetrical Rim Strips (Tip Volume Reduction)

Purpose

The cephalic portion of the lateral crura is excised in virtually all cases to reduce the volume of the nasal tip and to increase the malleability of the cartilages for suturing. The excision also produces a significant change in the convexity of the cartilages. The lateral crura is not excised when major concavities of the lateral crura exist that can be treated by folding or flipping the crura.

Technique

The skin is elevated over the nasal tip using the open approach. The alar cartilages are analyzed as to configuration, size, and symmetry. The operative plan is reevaluated to see if any changes are warranted based on anatomical findings. An example of changing the operative plan would be if a significant concavity was found in the alar cartilage which one decides to treat with a lateral crural "fold" rather than excision. The line of planned excision is marked on the alar cartilage using a caliper and a marking pen. The excision line is marked 6 mm from the caudal edge (Fig. 4.12). Preservation of a 6 mm rim strip allows insertion of any requisite shaping sutures as well as retaining sufficient support for the nostril rim and preventing any alar retraction. However, three points are important in drawing the excision line: (1) the initial 6 mm width is drawn at the widest point of the lateral crura, (2) the line is then tapered to preserve the natural width of the domal notch, and (3) the line follows the caudal border of the lateral crura laterally preserving a 6 mm width (Fig. 4.13). Once the line is drawn, the underlying mucosal surface of the alar cartilage is injected with local anesthesia to facilitate dissection. The cartilage is then held with forceps and a #15 blade is used in incise the lateral crura along the marked excision line. The actual excision of the cartilage begins at the domal notch and then progresses laterally. The excision follows the scroll junction with the upper lateral cartilages cephalically. Every effort is made to remove the cartilage intact as it is often used for add-on tip refinement grafts (TRG).

PRINCIPLES

- Volume reduction of the tip is achieved by excising the lateral crura.
- Removing the lateral crura creates symmetrical rim strips which will be sutured.
- Keep a 6 mm wide rim strip for support and suturing.
- Follow the caudal border of the lateral crura, tapering your excision at either end.
- It is rarely necessary to narrow the domal notch area.

Symmetrical Rim Strips

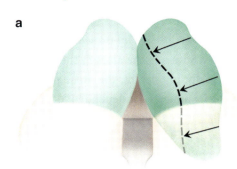

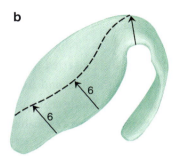

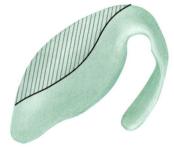

Fig. 4.12 (a, b) Symmetrical rim strips *DVD*

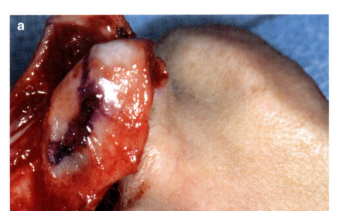

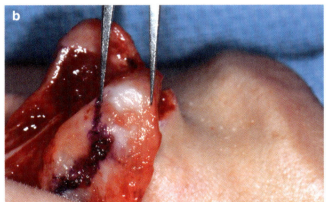

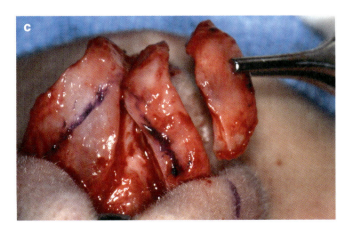

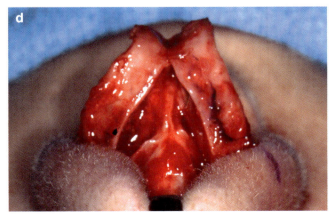

Fig. 4.13 (a–d)

Step #3 Domal Creation Suture (Tip Definition)

Purpose

The domal creation suture produces tip definition by creating the ideal aesthetic tip anatomy even from flat or concave cartilages (Fig. 4.16). Essentially, one inserts a horizontal mattress suture at the domal notch and cinches it down to create a convex domal segment next to a concave lateral crura. This anatomical configuration produces a very attractive tip when the skin is redraped. Rather than being an abnormal shape, this configuration is a normal anatomical finding in attractive tips when viewed during an open rhinoplasty. Our desire is to replicate the most attractive normal domal configuration.

Technique

Although conceptually simple, the surgeon must become facile with insertion of the domal configuration suture. I prefer to use a short-cord needle (P3) with highly visible violet-colored absorbable suture material (Fig. 4.17). The *domal notch* is located. The domal segment is gently squeezed using an Addson-Brown forceps to determine the exact location for the suture and the amount of convexity. The desired dome-defining point is marked. Then a horizontal mattress suture is placed from medial to lateral with the knot tied medially. The tension is gradually tightened until the desired domal convexity is achieved. The goal is the *juxtaposition* of gradually increasing domal *convexity* next to gradually increasing lateral crura *concavity*. One should concentrate on these two areas and not worry about any persistent convexity of the lateral crura which can be controlled with another suture. The following five suture errors are to be avoided: (1) too tight can result in a sharp point under thin skin, (2) too loose fails to achieve the desired definition, (3) too medial a placement snubs off the tip, (4) too lateral a placement lengths the infralobule, and (5) do not try to modify the entire lateral crura, just the portion immediately adjacent to the dome. Unlike incision and excision techniques which weaken the rim strip and often lead to bossa, the domal suture is initially reversible and can be replaced several times depending upon the rigidity of the cartilage. In contrast to grafts, tip sutures achieve definition without visibility, cartilage atrophy, or thinning of the skin.

PRINCIPLES

- Learn to recognize the *domal notch* – it is the key reference point for locating the domal creation suture.
- Gently squeeze the domal notch with an Adson-Brown forceps and determine the desired convexity and ideal location of the dome-defining point.
- Place the suture from medial to lateral with the knot tied medially.
- As you tighten, the domal segment will become convex. Try to avoid too concave an adjacent lateral crura or alar rim grafts will be necessary.
- Do not tighten excessively. Consider adding a second domal creation suture.
- Stand at the head of the table to assess symmetry.

Domal Creation Suture

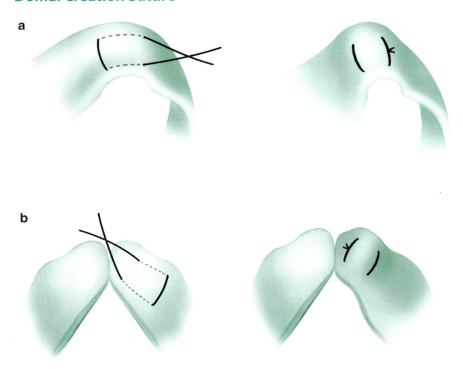

Fig. 4.16 (**a**, **b**) Domal creation suture 🅳🆅🅳

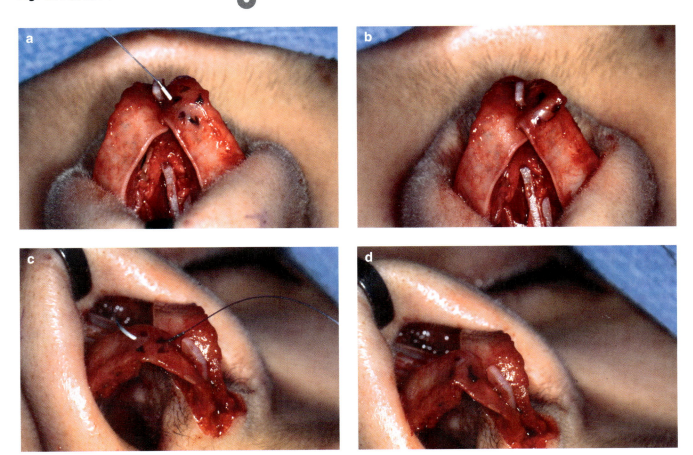

Fig. 4.17 (**a–d**)

Step #4
Interdomal
Suture
(Tip Width)

Purpose

The interdomal suture controls tip width both at the domes and in the infralobule. It is a simple vertical suture that begins on one crura adjacent to the domal creation suture, exits above the columellar suture, crosses over to the opposite crura at the same level, and then exits adjacent to the domal creation suture. The knot is gradually tightened until the ideal width is achieved. One must avoid producing either a single pointy tip or close the infralobule too much. One must maintain a normal angle of domal divergence. It is wise to remember the usual anatomical variations of the middle crura (Fig. 4.18).

Technique

The simplicity of inserting this stitch is due to its occurrence in the tip suturing sequence (Figs. 4.19 and 4.20). Since the columellar strut suture and domal creation sutures are already in place, the location of the interdomal suture is virtually predetermined. The suture enters just below the domal creation knot on the left and exits just above the strut suture on the middle crura. Then, the needle enters the right crura directly across on the middle crura and exits just below the domal creation knot. The only decisions are how far back from the caudal border to insert the suture and how tight to tie the knot. In general, the suture is placed 2–3 mm back from the caudal border of the crura. If placed too close to the edge then excessive narrowing of the columellar occurs. Too far back a placement is almost impossible because of the columellar strut. The suture is gradually tightened to reduce the interdomal width, not to create a single pointy tip. Remember the "tip diamond" concept. Also, the columellar flares at its base, narrows at its mid point, and gradually widens in the infralobule. Thus, one must avoid narrowing the infralobular columellar excessively.

PRINCIPLES

- Too tight a knot produces a pointy tip while too loose causes a wide tip.
- The normal angle of domal divergence is approximately 30°.
- Very rarely a tip will present as too narrow. Interdomal width can be increased using a wider columellar strut and no interdomal suture.
- As with all sutures, if the tip shape is good to begin with then there is no obligation to insert this suture.

Fig. 4.18
Middle crura variations

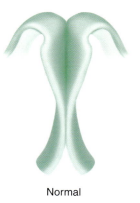 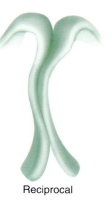 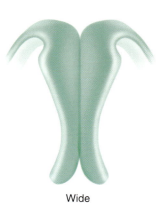

Normal   Reciprocal   Wide

Interdomal Suture

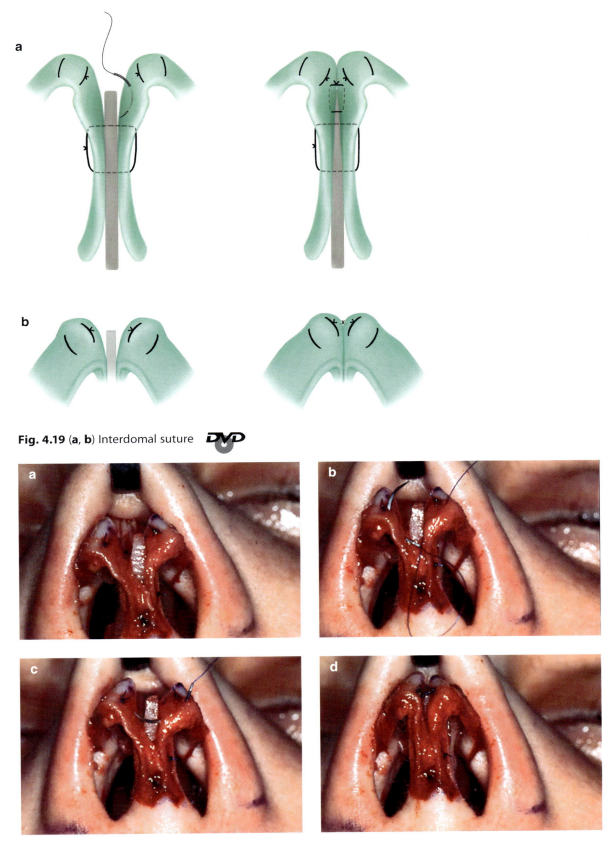

Fig. 4.19 (**a, b**) Interdomal suture

Fig. 4.20 (**a–d**)

Step #5 Domal Equalization Suture (Tip Symmetry)

Purpose

The domal equalization suture helps to insure symmetry of the tip. It is inserted through the cephalic border of the domal segments and tightened until the cartilages touch (Fig. 4.21). Conceptually, the suture insures tip symmetry, creates the cephalic point of the tip diamond, and lowers the cephalic portion of the rim strip below the tip-defining points. Although the domal equalization suture is a primary insurer of tip symmetry, every step in the tip suturing process improves symmetry; i.e., fixation of crura on the columellar strut and domal creation sutures.

Technique

Of all the tip sutures, the domal equalization stitch is probably the easiest to insert and the most difficult to do wrong. The needle enters the right dome beneath its cephalic edge, exits 1.5–2.5 mm on to the domal segment, then enters at a comparable point on the left domal segment, and exits beneath the cephalic edge of the left (Fig. 4.22). The knot is then tied until the cartilages touch. The suture brings the cephalic edge of the two convex domal segments together, thus creating the apex of the tip diamond. The knot is cut short and it becomes buried beneath the cephalic edge of the rim strips. Equally, it depresses the cephalic border of the rim below that of the caudal border, thus moving the tip-defining point toward the caudal border of the domal segment.

PRINCIPLES

- This suture is used frequently, but it is not always required.
- Small differences in placement point are done on either alar to fine tune symmetry.
- This suture is surprisingly effective with minimal risk.

Domal Equalization Suture

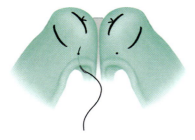 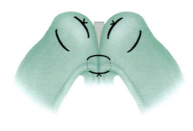

Fig. 4.21 Domal equalization suture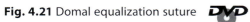

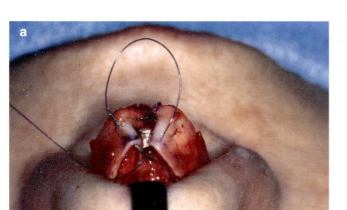 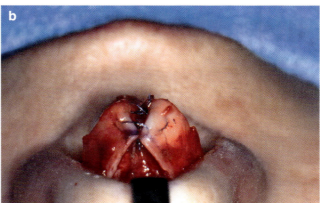

Fig. 4.22 (**a**, **b**)

Step #6 Lateral Crural Mattress Suture (Crural Convexities)

Purpose

The lateral crural mattress suture (LCMS) pioneered by Gruber (2005) has revolutionized our treatment of the wide tip as well as broad, boxy, and ball tips. It is a simple transverse mattress suture that is placed at the point of maximum convexity on the lateral crura (Fig. 4.23). The point of convexity is marked with a pen and then a mattress suture straddles it perpendicular to the rim strip beginning from the caudal border. The needle enters about 1 mm from the caudal edge and exits 1 mm from the cephalic edge, then a similar bite is taken 6–8 mm laterally, coming from the cephalic to the caudal border. The suture is gradually tightened until the convexity is flattened.

Technique

The lateral crural mattress suture solves one of the greatest challenges in tip rhinoplasty – how to eliminate convexity and width in the alar rim strip without incising or excising the alar cartilage. For years, the only solution was some variation of interdigitating cuts or segmental excisions that ultimately led to bossa formation or lateral crura collapse. Thus, this suture must be mastered. Fortunately, it is rather straightforward. Since the rim strip has been cut at 6 mm, there is sufficient cartilage to work with. When first using this suture, mark the convexity and then measure 3 mm on either side (Fig. 4.24). The needle is inserted about 1 mm from the caudal edge and exits 1 mm from the cephalic edge. One then moves laterally an equal distance from the marked point of maximum convexity. The needle enters 1 mm from the cephalic edge and exits 1 mm from the caudal edge. The knot is gradually tightened until the convexity disappears. The lateral crura should be straight or slightly concave. One wants to avoid too much tightening as it can cause marked concavity. If insufficient change has occurred which is often the case with rigid cartilages, an additional suture can be added, usually lateral to the original. Why insert the suture from the caudal border? Gruber prefers this method as it makes the knot less visible. In contrast, I feel that the cephalic location somehow depresses and can bunch up the cephalic border, both problems are avoided with a caudal placement.

PRINCIPLES

- Creation of 6 mm wide symmetrical alar rim strip facilitates future insertion of the lateral crural mattress suture.
- With experience, one can insert the suture in 3–4 mm wide rim strips that are often encountered in secondary cases.
- One wants to avoid penetrating the mucosa and exposing the suture, One can add local anesthesia beneath the convexity prior to suturing.

Lateral Crural Mattress Suture

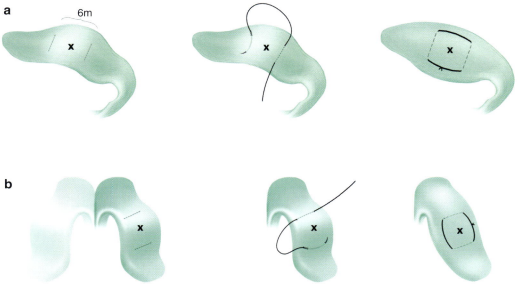

Fig. 4.23 (a–d) Lateral Crural Mattress Suture

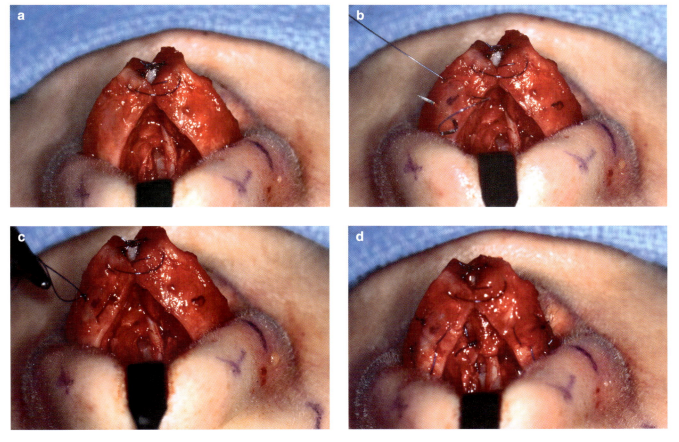

Fig. 4.24 (a–d)

Step #7 Tip Position Suture (Tip Rotation and Projection)

Purpose

The tip position suture achieves both tip rotation and increased projection which in turn creates the supratip break that most patients want (Fig. 4.25). It is a simple transverse suture between the infralobular mucosa and the anterior dorsal septum. It is placed from the top through an open approach using 4–0 PDS on a medium-size needle (FS2). As the knot is tightened, the tip rotates upward and projects above the dorsal line creating a supratip set-off. Early on, one should do a single throw, redrape the skin, and assess its effect – be careful, over rotation is a disaster.

Technique

Despite the disasters it can produce if over-tightened, the tip position suture achieves two very much desired tip characteristics – tip rotation and sufficient tip projection to produce a supratip break. It is not inserted until the ideal intrinsic tip has been created. Once satisfied with tip width and definition, then the final position becomes critical. A 4–0 PDS suture on an FS2 needle is used. The surgeon stands at the top of the table. The suture is transverse beginning with a pass through the mucosa of the infralobule with optional inclusion of the columellar strut (Fig. 4.26). The next pass is through the dorsal septum about 3–4 mm back from the anterior septal angle usually avoiding the spreader grafts. In general, I will do a double throw, redrape the skin, and asses the changes before adding additional sutures. It is never tied tightly. Rather, the suture serves as a loop bringing the tip above the anterior septal angle. The goal is to rotate the tip slightly while giving additional support to the tip which in turn creates the desired super tip break. I find this method of suturing more effective and with less risk of columellar distortion than Gruber's columellar-septal suture. Equally, I am not a fan of the tongue-in-groove technique where the alar cartilages are rotated on either side of the caudal septum and then fixed with sutures. The problem is that fine-graded adjustments in rotation and projection cannot be made once the alars are sutured to the septum. In contrast, the tip position suture is inserted after the ideal tip is created and tension can be added incrementally.

PRINCIPLES

- The tip position suture is the *most powerful* of all the tip sutures and must never be tied too tight!
- The needle passes through the mucosa of the columellar just behind the upper middle crura. There is no need to include the columellar strut.
- Judging the effect of the suture is best done by placing a single throw on the knot, redraping the skin, and evaluating. Too loose is much better than too tight.

Tip Position Suture

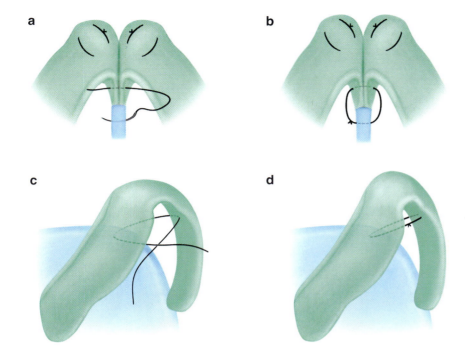

Fig. 4.25 (a, b) Tip position suture **DVD**

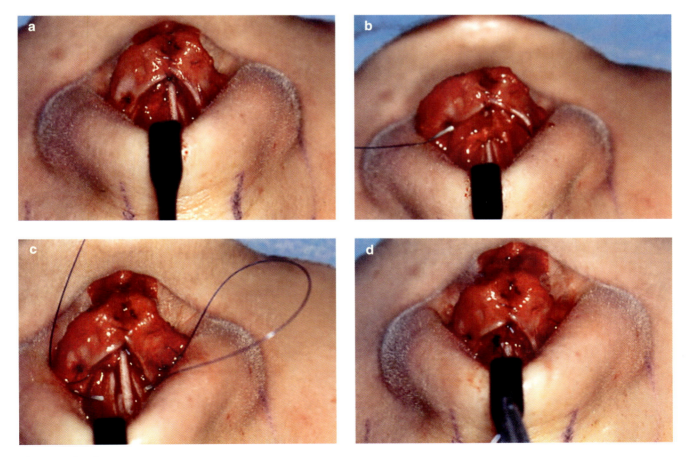

Fig. 4.26 (a–d)

Step #8 Add-on Grafts (Tip Refinement)

Purpose

Once suturing is completed, small tip grafts of excised alar cartilage can be added to provide additional refinement (Fig. 4-27). They are truly "Tip Refinement Grafts – TRG" which are added to the final sutured tip as an "enhancement" rather than incorporated into the structure of the tip (Daniel 2009).

Technique

Whenever possible, excised alar cartilage is used as it is quite pliable, easily shaped, and can be layered. These grafts have minimal risk of showing through the skin in contrast to rigid grafts of septal or conchal cartilages. There are 5 types:

1) *Domal TRG*. These grafts accentuate the dome defining points and are relatively small (8x4mm). They are sutured over the domes covering the domal creation sutures. Single or double layers are employed depending upon the desired definition.
2) *Shield TRG*. These are shield shape with a distinct dorsal edge to produce dome defining points. The shoulder of the graft is sutured to the domal notch. A second "booster" graft can be placed behind the shield to force the tip more caudal.
3) *Diamond TRG*. These grafts are diamond in shape and cover the entire tip diamond to set the tip off from the rest of the tip lobule. They are sutured at each domal notch, the columellar breakpoint, and the midline junction of the cephalic lateral crura.
4) *Folded TRG*. These grafts have the same shape as a long diamond, but are folded at their widest point with the shorter end folded behind. The graft is projected 1-2mm above the domes. Essentially, one is pushing the dome defining points caudally while achieving both increased definition and projection.
5) *Combination TRG*. Any combination of these 4 grafts can be used to achieve a specific goal. One variation is to insert multiple shields and diamonds to increase volume. Another grouping is to add a domal graft first, then bend a diamond over it which accentuates the tip diamond under thicker skin.

Inherently, these grafts are also concealing any asymmetries. If the grafts are too visible, the first choice is to remove them. If the grafts are absolutely essential as in an asymmetric tip with thin skin, then one can consider over laying a fascia graft.

PRINCIPLES

- Whenever possible use excised alar cartilage for add-on TRGs.
- These grafts accentuate changes produced by suturing.
- If in doubt, remove the graft.
- Fascia grafts can cover concealer grafts under a thin skin envelope.

Final Photos

Always take 4 close-up (macro view) photographs of the tip before closing the skin. These should be top-down, lateral, basilar oblique, and basilar. Print the 4 photos on one page and place it next to the operative diagram in the patient's chart. Review the operative diagram and tip photos at every potop visit- it is how you teach yourself surgical cause and effect.

Add-On Grafts

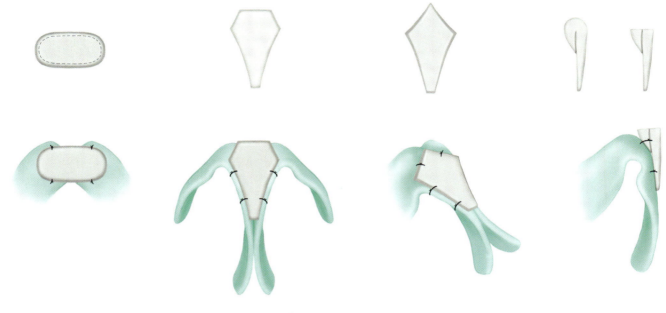

Fig. 4.27 Add-on tip refinement grafts (TRG) DVD

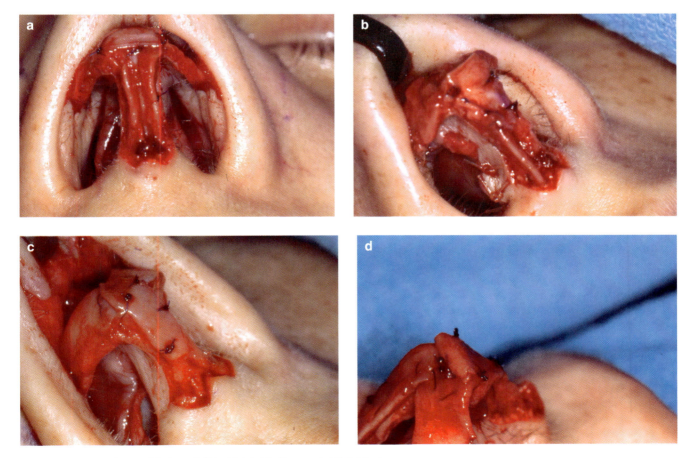

Fig. 4.28 Types of TRG. (**a**) domal, (**b**) shield, (**c**) diamond, (**d**) folded

Step #9 Alar Rim Grafts (Nostril Rim Shape)

Purpose

Alar rim grafts were developed to correct alar rim retraction in secondary cases. However, their use has increased dramatically as tip suture techniques have gained in popularity. Alar rim grafts counteract the subtle effects of tip suturing on alar rim shape, both rim retraction and rim depression. Small tapered pieces of rigid cartilage (8–10 mm long, 2–3 mm wide) are placed either subcutaneously along the alar rim (alar rim graft – ARG) or are sutured into a true rim incision (alar rim structure graft – ARS) depending upon the severity of the rim changes (Fig. 4.29).

Technique

The grafts are usually carved from septal or excised cartilaginous vault material. In general, I find excised alar cartilage too weak. The dimensions are 8–12 mm long and 2–3 mm wide with tapering cephalically both in width and thickness.

ARG. Insertion of an alar rim graft can be made either medially from the infracartilaginous incision or laterally from a stab incision on the mucosal surface of the alar base (Fig. 4.30a, b). Then a subcutaneous pocket is made 2–3 mm back and paralleling the alar rim. *One should never dissect into, or unfurl, the alar rim as it will cause irreparable rim distortion.* The graft is slipped into the pocket and one should see an immediate improvement in both alar rim retraction and depression. The cephalic end of the graft toward the tip is always checked to avoid future bossa formation or distortion of the soft tissue facet. The infracartilaginous incision is closed in the standard fashion. One should expect that patients will inquire about these grafts, especially those with inquisitive fingers. One can tell the patient that the grafts will soften with time and reduce in volume by 50%. In reality, most patients adjust to the grafts once they are reassured.

ARS. When the alar rim is extremely weak with preexisting external valve collapse, then the graft is sutured into a true marginal rim incision irrespective of the original open incision (Fig. 4.30c, d). The pocket is dissected away from the rim – never unfurl the alar rim. The graft is placed in the pocket. The graft is incorporated into the closure using 4–0 chormic. On occasion, the cephalic end can be too rigid and placed too far toward the tip resulting in either a tip bossa or distortion of the soft tissue facet. Treatment is excision. Avoidance is achieved by careful palpation and inspection followed by appropriate excision prior to closure. Too long a graft laterally can cause a wide nostril base, again excision is the treatment.

PRINCIPLES

- When indicated, alar rim grafts are a necessity, not an option.
- Detail inspection from the head of the table will reveal alar rim retraction, whereas inspection from the foot of the bed shows alar rim depression (think boxy tip).
- Careful carving of the graft is as important as careful placement of the graft.
- Too small a graft is much preferred to too long a graft.
- Nostril changes are very three-dimensional, so inspect the nostrils carefully.

ARG and ARS Grafts

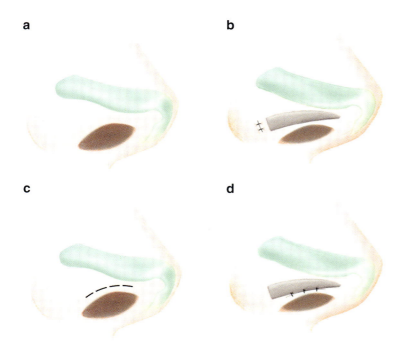

a

b

c

d

Fig. 4.29 (**a,b**) Alar rim grafts (ARG) and (**c,d**) alar rim structure grafts (ARS)

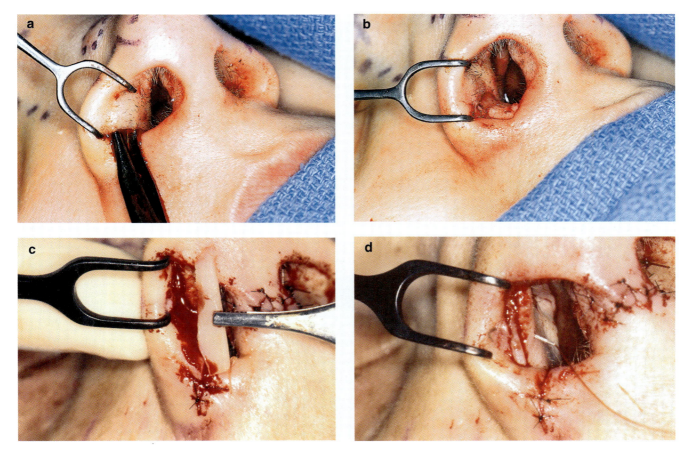

a

b

c

d

Fig. 4.30 (**a,b**) Alar rim grafts (ARG), (**c,d**) alar rim structure grafts (ARS)

Open Structure Tip Graft

At its simplest, an open structure tip procedure consists of a columellar strut and a shield shape tip graft sutured to the middle crura via an open approach. It originated with Johnson (1990) as a stunning solution for the "problem noses" of the endonasal era. During the past decade, I have modified the operation as follows: (1) domal sutures rather than domal excision to modify the anatomical domes whenever possible, (2) altering the shape and size of the crural strut as necessary, (3) columellar-septal sutures to effect adjustments in projection and rotation rather than relying solely on the tip graft, and (4) recognition of the limitations for the procedure.

Indications. I divide the indications into three groups: (1) severe deformities where excision of a domal segment is necessary followed by a concealing tip graft, (2) major deformities where domal sutures would be inadequate thus necessitating a tip graft, and (3) moderate deformities where tip sutures were tried, but the addition of a tip graft was an intraoperative decision. This "reverse" approach from severe to moderate parallels my preference to use a destructive (domal/excision), reconstructive (tip graft), tip technique only for the most difficult of cases. I do an open structure tip for the following cases: (1) asymmetric and abnormal shapes, (2) major deformities of width or definition, (3) major inadequacies of projection or rotation, and (4) most ethnic and cleft lip noses.

Technique. Although one's initial impression is that it is a fixed rigid procedure, the reality is that the open structure tip graft can be varied widely to accommodate a diversity of tips.

Step #1 Cephalic Rim Strips. Following exposure of the alar cartilages, I reassess my preoperative analysis and operative plan. I tend to excise cephalic lateral crura early to improve dorsal exposure and septal access (Fig. 4.31a, b). The goal is to establish symmetrical rim strips rather than symmetrical excisions.

Step #2 Columellar Strut. Shape, insertion, and fixation of the columella strut are all critical. In most cases, I favor the standard straight 20 × 3 mm crural strut made from septal cartilage (Fig. 4.31c, d). I prefer a longer wider columellar strut when the columella is retracted or the columella labial angle is acute. The insertion pocket is created by passing the Stevens scissors vertically between the crura down toward, but at least 2 mm short of, the anterior nasal spine thereby avoiding clicking of the strut. The graft is temporarily held in place with a #25 needle. A single mattress suture of 5–0 PDS is inserted across the columella at the columellar breakpoint. Next, the domes are modified either with sutures or excision.

Step #3A Domal Modification (Sutures). I have found that domal creation sutures are an excellent nondestructive method of achieving the desired changes in domal angle prior to insertion of the tip graft (Fig. 4.31e, f). I use domal sutures for the majority of cases and reserve domal excision for severe deformities. These are the same domal creation sutures used in open suture tips (4.31c, d). Domal equalization and interdomal sutures are contraindicated as interdomal width will be controlled by the width of the tip graft.

Open Structure Tip Graft

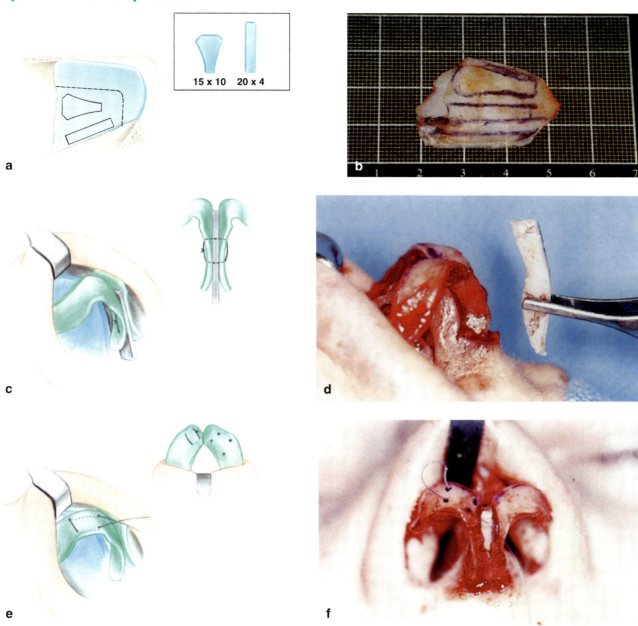

Fig. 4.31 Open Structure Tip Graft (OST) **DVD** (**a**, **b**) Symmetrical rim strips (**c**, **d**) columellar strut **DVD** (**e**, **f**) domal suture

Step #3B Domal Modification (Excision). Excision of a domal segment is done as a tapered full-width domal segment excision (Fig. 4.32a, b). I excise a domal segment to make major tip changes. Once the crural strut is sutured in place, I measure up from the columella breakpoint 6–8 mm and mark a transverse cut in the lobular segment of the middle crura (a point that often corresponds with the medial genu of the domal notch). Then the cut is made without going through the underlying mucosa, a move simplified by injecting it first with local anesthesia. The domal segment and lateral crura are then elevated off the mucosa, overlapped at the transverse cut, and then the redundancy is excised, ranging from 4-8mm. The cut edges are then repaired with interrupted 5–0 PDS.

Step #4 Graft Shaping. A three-stage sequence is used for shaping the tip graft. The shape has shifted from shield shape to a more tapered golf-tee shape graft integrated between the divergent middle crura. The initial triangular "block" is cut with a superior edge 10 mm wide and tapered sides to a 4 mm wide inferior edge with a total length of 15–18 mm (Shaping #1). Then, the dorsal edge is beveled and shoulders cut on either side. The sides are beveled creating a narrow waist (Shaping #2). The final shaping occurs in situ once the graft is sutured in place (Shaping #3).

Step #5 Graft Placement. I now conceive of graft placement as being either integrated or projected (Fig. 4.32c, d). Usually, I integrate the graft into the divergent middle crura allowing the tip of the graft to rise slightly above the domes. The goal is to create ideal tip definition and width by accentuating the preexisting tip, but without any visibility of the graft. When the skin is thick or major changes are required, then the tip graft is placed to project above the domes and create a new tip. As one begins to project the graft 2–3 mm above the domes, it becomes necessary to add a cap graft behind the tip graft to give support and fill the dead space.

Step #6 Graft Suturing. In most cases, I use four stitches of 5–0 PDS to hold the graft in place: two at the level of the middle crura and two just above the columella incision (Fig. 4.33). I do not hesitate to add sutures at the level of the domes to integrate the graft into the domal architecture. If the graft is angulated or asymmetrical, then I will insert small "door stop"-shaped booster or leveling grafts behind the main tip graft.

Open Structure Tip Graft

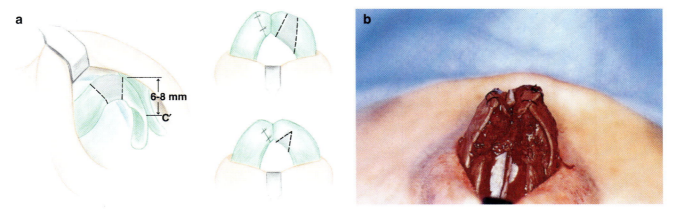

Fig. 4.32 (**a**, **b**) Open structure tip graft (domal excision) *DVD*

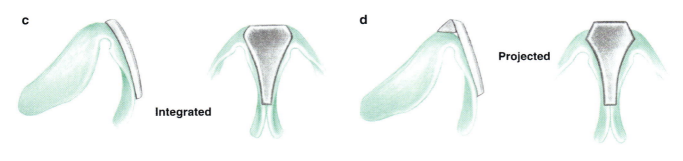

Fig. 4.32 (**c**) Tip graft integrated *DVD* (**d**) tip graft projected *DVD*

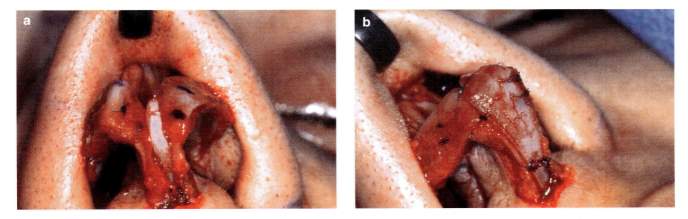

Fig. 4.33 (**a**, **b**) Domal sutures with open structure tip graft

Decision Making: Level 1

The Problem

In these cases, the tip is simply unattractive. The goal is to eliminate the negatives thereby producing a much more refined tip. Open *tip suture* techniques are highly effective in correcting these problems. The operative sequence is a variation of the following (Fig. 4.34).

Technique

Step #1. The overall volume of the tip is reduced by creating the symmetrical rim strips. The excision of cephalic lateral crura parallels the caudal border and never encroaches on the domal notch medially. A 6 mm wide strip is left.

Step #2. The columellar strut insures stability and projection of the tip. A pocket is made between the middle crura down toward the ANS. The alar cartilages are elevated, rotated medially, and then temporarily fixed with a #25 needle in the infralobule. A vertical suture of 5–0 PDS fixes the crura to the strut.

Step #3. Definition is created at each tip point with a domal creation suture that crosses the domal notch. This horizontal mattress suture of 5–0 PDS begins and ends on the medial side of the domal notch. As the suture is tied, the dome becomes convex while the adjacent lateral crura becomes slightly concave.

Step #4. Tip width is controlled with an interdomal suture. Suture placement is easily determined. Tension is increased until the domes approach each other cephalically, while the caudal border is often separated by 4–6 mm. One has the option of adding a domal equalization suture to improve symmetry if necessary.

Step #5. Frequently, a supratip break is desired with a "set-off" of the tip above the dorsal line. A tip position suture is inserted between the mucosa of the infralobular columella and the septal angle. Tension is increased to achieve rotation and finalize projection. Note: do not tie this suture too tight – err on the side of conservatism.

Lessons Learned

After 20 years and a few thousand sutured tips, experience has taught me the following:

1) Always use a columellar strut. It promotes stability, symmetry, and projection, while minimizing tip droop. It prevents a plunging tip – so much to gain for so little effort.
2) Use absorbable sutures to minimize infection. Dyed sutures are easier to see.
3) Most problems occur from too much tension, not too little.
4) The "domal notch" is the location for the domal creation suture – learn to recognize it.
5) The middle crura should be "open" – do not tie the interdomal suture too tight.
6) The domal equalization suture improves symmetry and lowers the cephalic rim.
7) The tip position suture creates supratip break, but be very careful – do not tie too tight.
8) Be prepared to do alar rim grafts – they are often necessary.
9) If the strut is too long and pushes down the columellar base, then shorten it.
10) Record your tip operation with intraop photos and drawings on the op diagram. Refer to them at every post-op visit. Only you can teach yourself surgical cause and effect.

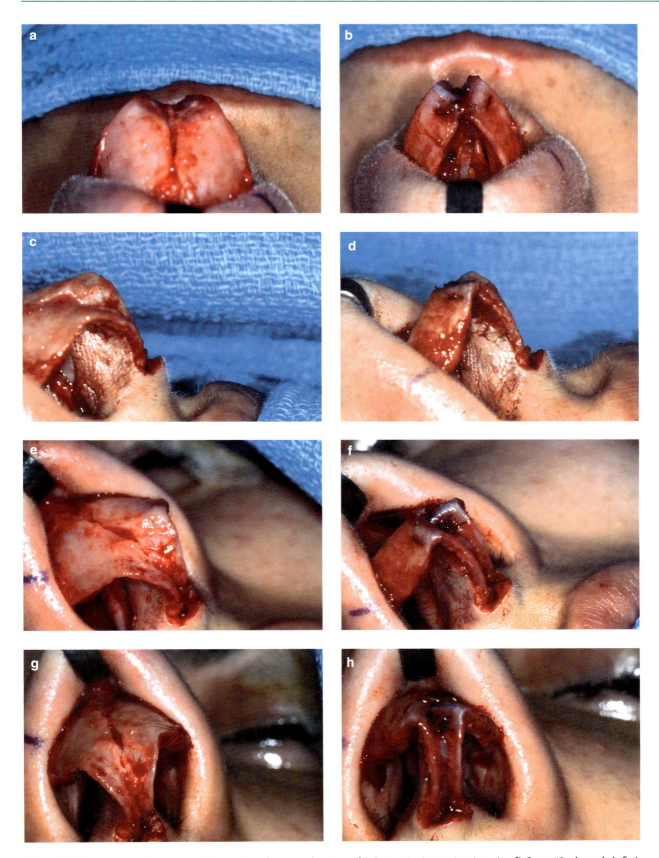

Fig. 4.34 Tip suture technique: (**a**) Step #1: volume reduction, (**b**) Step #2: tip projection, (**c**, **d**) Step #3: domal definition, (**e**, **f**) Step #4: interdomal width, (**g**, **h**) Step #5: supratip break

Case Study: An Unattractive Tip

Analysis

A 21-year-old patient of Middle Eastern descent presented with a wide unattractive tip (Fig 4.35). She wanted a significant change in the nose, but especially a cuter tip. She agreed to having a chin implant done at the same time. This is truly a Level 1 case as all the surgeon has to do is rasp down the small bump, narrow the base bony width, and refine the tip. A balanced approach was done to establish the profile including a fascia graft to the radix. The tip change was achieved with just five steps: (1) volume was reduced by excising cephalic lateral crura, (2) projection was increased with a columellar strut (CS), (3) definition was created with domal creation suture (DC), (4) symmetry was improved with a domal equalization suture (DE), and (5) supratip break was insured with a tip position suture (TP).

Operative Technique

1) Harvest of deep temporal fascia
2) Open approach and confirmation of tip analysis and operative plan
3) Incremental reduction – bony 0.5 mm, cartilage 3 mm
4) Caudal septal resection (3 mm)
5) Low-to-high osteotomies. Bilateral spreader graft placement
6) Columellar strut insertion followed by tip sutures: CS, DC, DE, TP
7) Radix graft of fascia

A large chin implant was inserted at the beginning of the case.

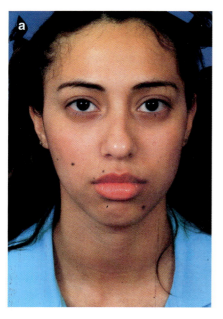
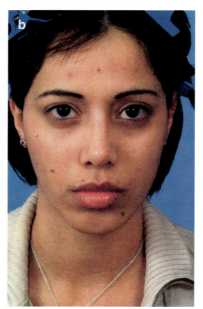
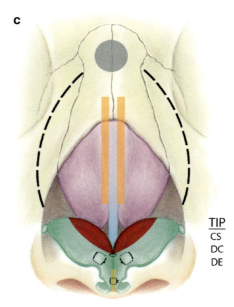

TIP
CS
DC
DE

Fig. 4.35 (a–j)

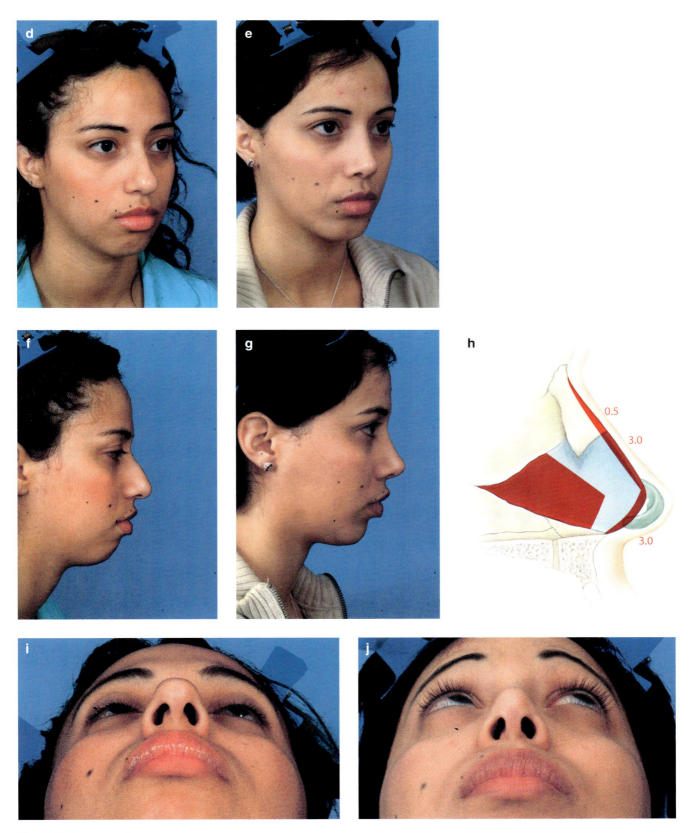

Fig. 4.35 (continued)

Decision Making: Level 2

The Problem. Most Level 2 patients consider their tip to be *the major reason* for having a rhinoplasty and they want a significant tip improvement. Technically, a fundamental change in the underlying tip anatomy is required to achieve the desired aesthetic goal. It is at this point that *add-on* and *structure* tip grafts have to be considered. These are intermediate cases between the refinement of Level 1 and the total change of Level 3. The surgeon should feel confident with their tip suturing skills before progressing to these more challenging cases.

Techniques. Several sutures can be added to the standard five-step technique with the most common being the lateral crural mattress suture (LCC). The broad tip is characterized by lateral crura convexity which is easily corrected with the LCC thereby avoiding destabilizing incisions or excisions. Once suturing is completed and there is a need for more tip definition, then add-on grafts are used. If one has totally misdiagnosed skin thickness or compliance such that add-on grafts are ineffective, then a structured tip graft is the only solution.

Specialized Sutures. After creating an attractive tip, the most common challenge is excessive convexity of the lateral crura which is often seen as a broad tip. The point of lateral convexity is marked with a pen and then the lateral crura mattress suture straddles it (Fig. 4.36a). The tension is increased until the convexity disappears and the crura is straight – one should avoid producing a concave lateral crura. When the skin is closed it may be necessary to add an alar rim graft, especially in a boxy tip.

Add-On Tip Grafts. The use of add-on Tip Refinement Grafts (TRG) made from excised alar cartilage has revolutionized the finesse aspect of tip suturing. Grafts can be placed in the infralobule to conceal asymmetries or to create fullness (Fig. 4.36b). Alternatively, a domal graft can be placed over the domes to improve definition and in double layer to increase projection by 1 mm. Both shield shape and domal shape grafts can be placed in combination to increase refinement and produce additional volume. Due to their pliability and thinness, visibility or absorption of the grafts is rarely a problem (Daniel 2009).

Structure Tip Grafts. Following completion of tip suturing, definition and projection may be inadequate especially in thicker skin patients. The solution is a rigid shield shape graft of septal cartilage (Fig. 4.36c). These grafts are highly tapered and designed to fit within the crural framework. Therefore, it is *critical* to remove any interdomal or domal equalization sutures before suturing the graft into place. In most cases, the top two fixation sutures pass through the caudal border of the domal notch and are fixed to the shoulders of the tip graft. This maneuver insures that the graft fits between the crural edges and provides greater tip definition. In Level 3 cases, a structure tip graft is planned from the beginning, the domes often require excision, and the tip graft is placed higher with a cap graft backing to maximize tip projection

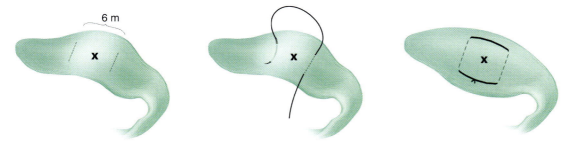

Fig. 4.36 (**a**) Lateral crural convexity sutures

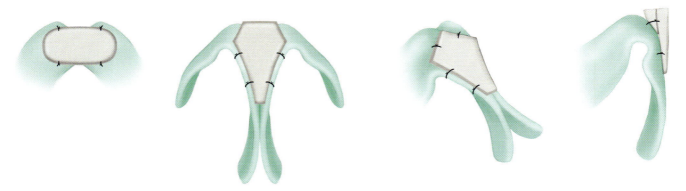

Fig. 4.36 (**b**) Tip Refinement Grafts (TRG)

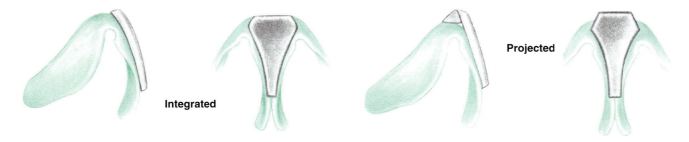

Fig. 4.36 (**c**) Open structure tip grafts

Case Study: Intrinsic Tip Deficiency

Analysis

This 31-year-old woman disliked the beaky appearance of her nose (Fig. 4.37). The tip had a flat dependent look – there was simply no intrinsic tip. On lateral view, a large nostril/small tip disproportion was obvious (Fig. 4.37). Success in this case depended on being able to increase the volume and definition of the intrinsic tip. The critical steps of her tip surgery consisted of columellar strut insertion, tip projection, and add-on grafts. Following tip suturing, the entire tip complex was rotated and projected above the septal angle using the tip position suture. Redraping of the skin indicated that more tip definition was required and thus a double layer add-on graft of excised alar was placed across the domes. This patient has the world's fastest blink response.

Operative Technique

1) Open approach and confirmation of tip analysis and op plan
2) Creation of symmetrical rim strips and extramucosal tunnels
3) Incremental dorsal reduction – bony 1.5 mm, cartilage 5 mm
4) Excision of caudal septum (3 mm)
5) Fascia harvest. Septal harvest and caudal septal relocation, R to L
6) Low-to-high osteotomies then placement of spreader grafts
7) Insertion of columellar strut and tip sutures: CS, DC, ID, DE, TP
8) Add-on domal tip graft using a double layer of excised alar
9) A "ball and apron" fascia graft to augment the radix and smooth the dorsum
10) Nostril sill excisions (2.5 mm)

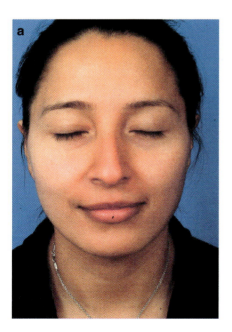 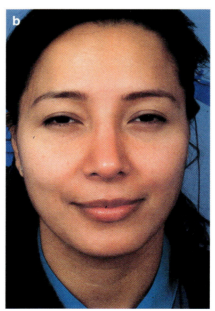 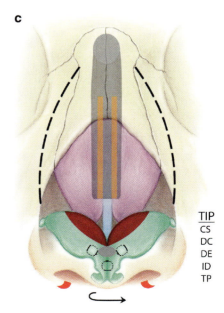

TIP
CS
DC
DE
ID
TP

Fig. 4.37 (a–j)

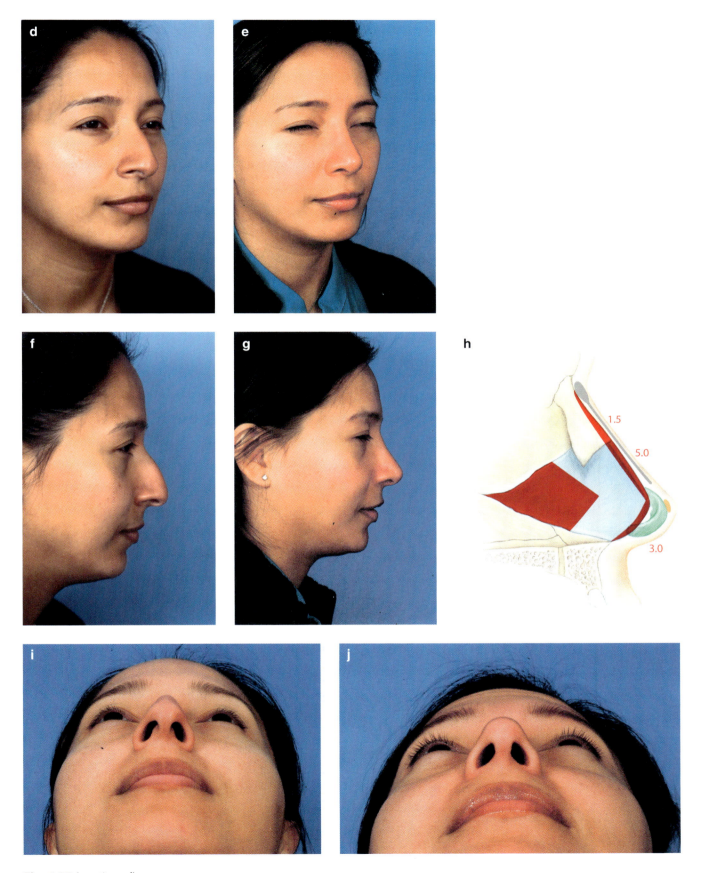

Fig. 4.37 (continued)

Decision Making: Level 3

The Problem. Put simply, these patients hate their tip and want a new one. Success or failure rests on the surgeon's ability to create a new tip. These tips are often "extreme" deformities where the surgeon needs to deconstruct the existing tip followed by reconstruction of an attractive tip. Further complicating the challenge is collapse of the external valve on deep inspiration. The actual etiology is most often abnormal or extreme variations of alar anatomy ensheathed in thin or thick skin. A typical comparison is that a Level 2 case would have a broad tip while a Level 3 patient would have a severe alar malposition requiring alar transposition. A true Pinocchio tip is a Level 3 deformity as the intrinsic anatomy of the alar cartilage is deformed thereby requiring excision of the domes and replacement with a structure tip graft. Due to the severity of the problem and the minimal margin of error, these cases should be approached with caution.

Structure Tip Graft with Domal Excision. The ball tip ensheathed in thick skin is a classic example where sutures may prove inadequate, especially if there is over-projection (Fig. 4.38a–d). Following the open approach, the alars are analyzed, symmetrical rim strips created, and the definitive dorum established. A columellar strut is inserted and sutured. Then, a mark is made about 6 mm above the columellar breakpoint and the alars divided. The lateral portion is undermined and a domal segment is excised (2–6 mm). Depending upon its location, the domal excision can reduce tip projection or tip width or a combination of the two. The excised edges are repaired with 5–0 PDS. A tip graft is then sutured to the repaired alars with the leading edge of the tip graft 1–2 mm above the repaired domes. The skin is redraped, tip projection and definition assessed, and the graft shaped as necessary. Then a transverse cap graft is sutured over the domes and behind the tip graft to prevent flattening of the tip graft.

Alar Transposition. In cases of significant alar malposition, it is often necessary to mobilize the lateral crura and reposition them toward the nostril rim (Fig. 4.38e–h). These cases frequently have nostril rim weakness that may lead to total collapse on deep inspiration preoperatively. Alar transposition plus lateral crura strut grafts have revolutionized our treatment of the unstable boxy tip. If the alars are too vertically oriented (malposition), then alar transposition is indicated. The lateral crura are dissected laterally and transected at their juncture with the accessory cartilages. The domal notches are marked. A columellar strut is sutured between the middle crura. With the lateral crura mobilized, domal creation and interdomal sutures are inserted. The skin is redraped. Lateral crura strut grafts are often necessary to stabilize and contour the nostrils. Most of these cases have thin skin and a fascial blanket graft is added over the tip.

Secondary Cases. As will be discussed in Chapter 10, a wide variation of tip grafts may be needed as the alar cartilages have often been excised or severely compromised. In certain cases, an isolated tip graft is inserted and alar rim support grafts added along the rims without any replacement of the lateral crura. Secondary cases are truly demanding and one must be comfortable with complex primary cases before attempting them.

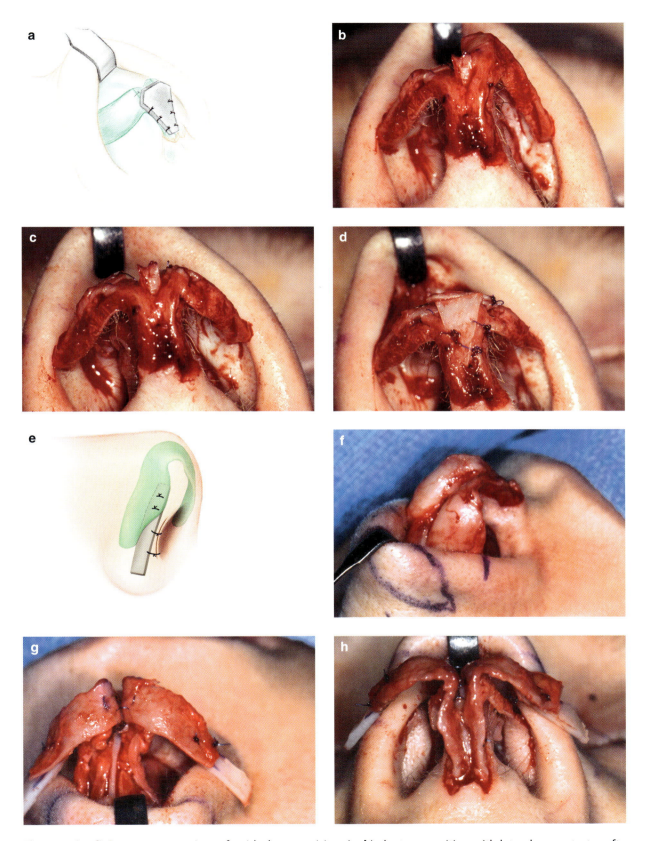

Fig. 4.38 (**a–d**) Open structure tip graft with dome excision, (**e–h**) alar transposition with lateral crura strut grafts

**Case Study:
Open Structure
Tip Graft**

Analysis

A 38-year-old patient felt that her nose and upper eyelids made her look older. The nasal challenge was obvious – a ball tip sheathed in thick skin (Fig. 4.39). The goal was not to make the tip better, but rather to create an entirely new tip, both smaller and with more definition. Compounding the problem was a profile that needed minimal change thus emphasizing the dorsal/base disproportion. At 4 years post-op, the patient's nasal tip looks much more refined and narrower. When major changes are needed, an open structure tip graft with domal excision is the answer. Note: A short DVD of this case is available (Fig 4.39 **DVD**).

Operative Technique

1) Upper lid blepharoplasty and harvest of fascia
2) Open approach with tip analysis and symmetrical rim strips
3) Minimal dorsal modification – bony smoothing, cartilage <1 mm
4) Septal harvest
5) Low-to-high osteotomies and asymmetric spreader grafts: R 2.5 mm, L 1 mm
6) Insertion and suture fixation of columellar strut
7) Excision of a 4 mm domal segment
8) Open structure tip graft
9) Alar wedge excision (4 mm) and insertion of alar rim grafts

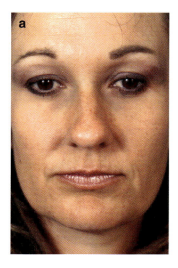 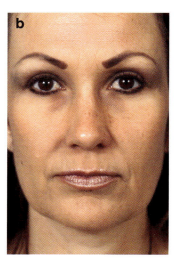 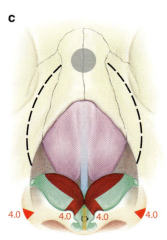

Fig. 4.39 (a–j) Open Structure Tip Graft

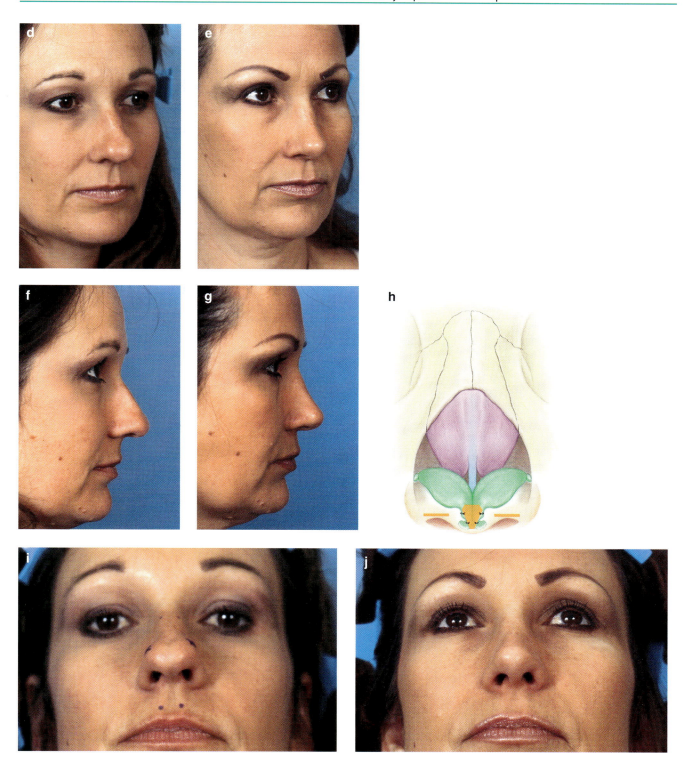

Fig. 4.39 (continued)

Tip Sutures That Do Not Work for Me

Over the years, I have found that a variety of specialized sutures do no not work for me. Since I also find them in secondary cases, it appears that they do not work for others. The explanation may be that these sutures are technically demanding and unforgiving for surgeons who do not use them frequently. Obviously, the proponents of these sutures can make them work, but I find them challenging. The latter three sutures illustrated come from the case study that follows (Fig. 4.41).

Lateral Crural Spanning Sutures (LCSS). As originally conceived by Tebbetts (1994), the LCSS is designed to shape and reposition the lateral crura, especially reducing their convexity (Fig. 4.40a, b). The key steps are the following: (1) place a needle across both lateral crura at their point of maximum convexity, (2) insert a horizontal mattress suture, and (3) tighten incrementally to reduce convexity and narrow the tip. The problem with the LCSS is its tendency to cause true alar rim retraction. The LCSS has been supplanted by Gruber's LCMS which is more effective in fixing a convexity in a single lateral crura and has minimal risk of causing alar retraction as a by product.

Midline Sutures. I have no idea who proposed multiple midline sutures between the caudal border of the two crura, but it can have devastating consequences (Fig. 4.40c, d). These sutures produce real distortion in the columellar resulting in a narrow hanging columella. As the midline suturing progresses toward the tip, a unified *single point tip* is produced followed by retraction of the alar rims resulting in a snarl tip. Do not even think about using midline sutures.

Lower lateral cartilage (LLC) to Upper lateral cartilage (ULC) Suture. Several surgeons have suggested suturing the cephalic border of the lateral crura to the caudal border of the upper lateral cartilages to achieve upward tip rotation and stabilization (Fig. 4.40e, f). A significant degree of sophistication and experience is required to make this suture work. Unfortunately, these sutures are difficult to execute and can produce bulging in the area similar to excessive scroll formation. I do not recommend it.

Columellar to Caudal Septum Overlap. The concept of suturing the columellar to the caudal septum has been used by surgeons ever since rhinoplasties were first done and it can be effective. However, other surgeons have extended this concept to the *tongue-in-groove technique*. In this procedure, the medial crura are sutured to the caudal septum in a more upwardly rotated position thereby using the caudal septum as a columellar strut (Fig. 4.40 g, h). For the surgeon who performs this technique rarely, it can be difficult to position the crura correctly. Once fixed in position, the surgeon cannot make the fine adjustments in tip projection as the tip has been fixed caudally, i.e., a tip position suture will not be effective in creating the supratip break. I do not recommend this suture for occasional use as too much judgment is required and there is too little flexibility for finesse.

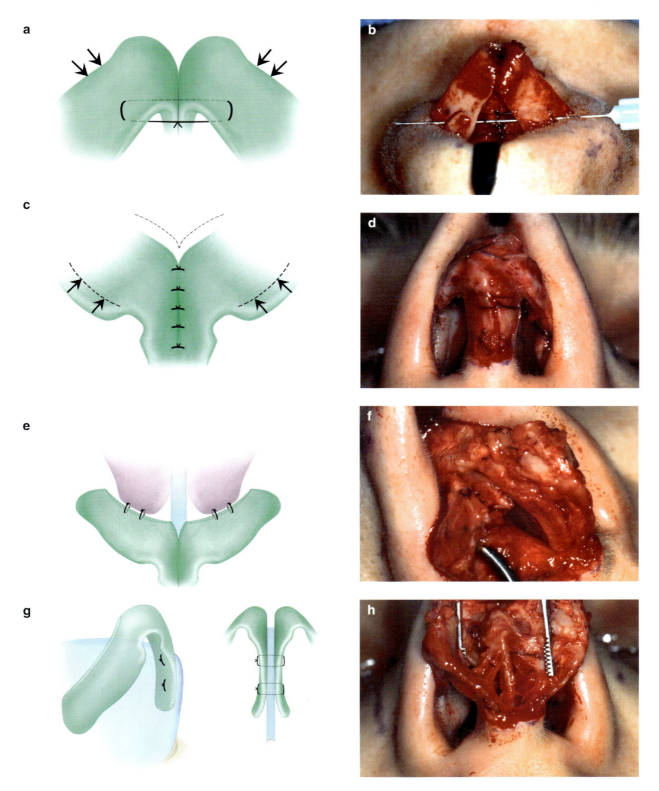

Fig. 4.40 (**a**, **b**) Lateral crural spanning suture, (**c**, **d**) midline sutures. (**e**, **f**) LLC to ULC suture, (**g**, **h**) tongue-in-groove

Case Study: An Over-Sutured Nose

Analysis

A 28-year-old woman had a rhinoplasty at age 18. Ten years later, her primary complaints were that her nose looked "done" and stuck out too far (Fig. 4.41). This case illustrates why a surgeon has to be prepared for any and all surprises during a secondary rhinoplasty. It was hard to decide which surprise was greater – the extent of previous tip suturing or the Skoog dorsal graft. Certainly, removal of the dorsal graft meant that the tip was grossly over-projected. The alar cartilages were encased in scar tissue and the prior suturing was certainly not "reversible." Also, the vestibular valve collapse meant that the alars had to be transposed and lateral crural strut grafts added. This case illustrates why secondaries can be extraordinarily difficult – there is always a moment when you wish that you had never agreed to do the case.

Operative Technique

1) Transfixion incision revealed tongue-in-groove sutures (Fig 4.40b).
2) Open approach using the previous transcolumellar incision. Thin skin encountered.
3) Visible midline sutures explaining alar retraction and pointy tip (Fig 4.40d).
4) Dorsal dissection revealed "Skoog" graft of reinserted dorsum.
5) Incremental dorsal reduction – cartilage only, tapered 3 mm.
6) Caudal septal resection (3 mm). Septal and fascial harvest.
7) Medial oblique, transverse, and low-to-low osteotomies.
8) Insertion of bilateral spreader grafts.
9) Transposition of the alars revealed LLC to ULC sutures (Fig 4.40f).
10) Insertion of columellar strut and 5 mm domal excision to drop projection.
11) Concealer tip graft of excised cartilage with fascia graft coverage.
12) Dorsal fascia graft.

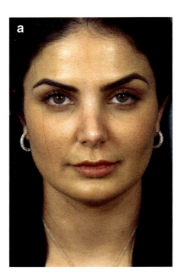 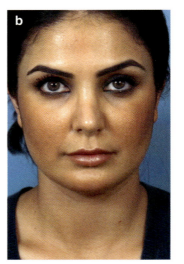 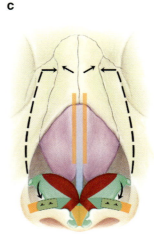

Fig. 4.41 (a–j)

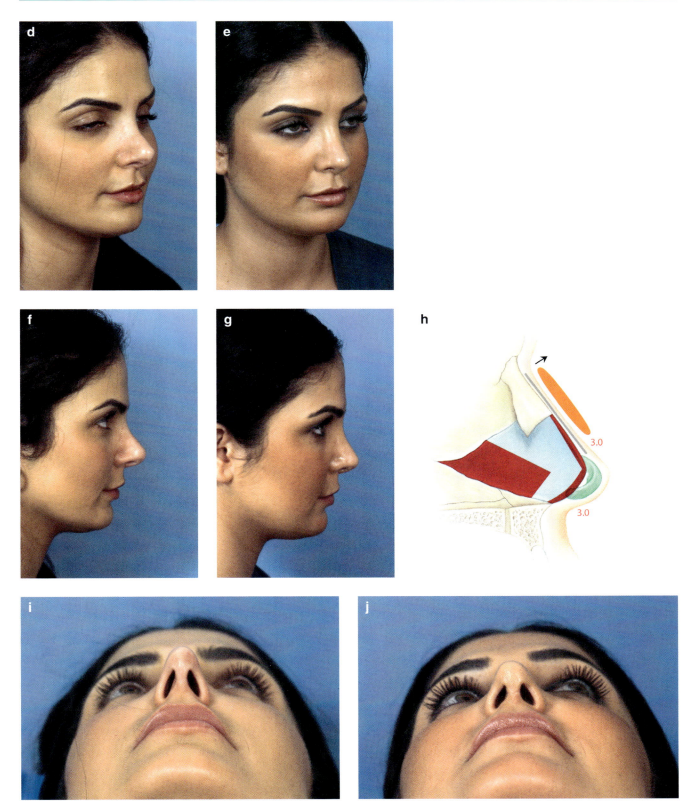

Fig. 4.41 (continued)

Reading List   Byrd HS, Hobar PC. Rhinoplasty: A practical guide for surgical planning. Plast Reconstr Surg 91: 642, 1993

Byrd HS, Andochick S, Copit S, and Walton KG. Septal extension grafts: A method of controlling tip projection shape. Plast Reconstr Surg 100: 999, 1997

Daniel RK. Rhinoplasty: Creating an aesthetic tip. Plast Reconstr Surg 80: 775, 1987

Daniel RK. Anatomy and aesthetics of the nasal tip. Plast Reconstr Surg 89: 216, 1992

Daniel RK. The nasal tip. In: Daniel RK (ed) Aesthetic Plastic Surgery: Rhinoplasty. Boston: Little, Brown, 1993

Daniel RK. Open tip suture techniques. Part I: Primary rhinoplasty, Part II: Secondary rhinoplasty. Plast Reconstr Surg 103: 1491, 1999

Daniel RK. Broad, boxy, and ball tips. Open Tech Plast Surg 4: 7, 2000

Daniel RK. Tip refinement grafts: the designer tip. Aesth Surg J 29: 528, 2009

Gruber RP, Nahai F, Bogdan MA, et al Changing the convexity and concavity of nasal cartilages and cartilage grafts with horizontal mattress sutures. Part I. Experimetnal results. Plast Reconstr Surg 115: 589, 2005. Part II: Clinical results. Plast Reconstr Surg 115: 595, 2005

Gruber RP, Bates SJ, Le JL. Advanced suture techniques in rhinoplasty. In Gunter, JP, Rohrich RJ, Adams WP Dallas Rhinoplasty: Nasal Surgery by the Masters. (2nd ed.), St. Louis: QMP Publishing, 411–446, 2007

Guyuron B, Behmand RA. Nasal tip sutures. Part II: The interplays. Plast Recon Surg 112: 1130, 2003. Part I: The evolution. Plast Reconstr Surg, 112: 125, 2003

Johnson CM, and Toriumi DM. Open Structure Rhinoplasty. Philadelphia: Saunders, 1990

Kridel RWH, Scott BA, Fonda HMT. The tongue-in-groove technique in septorhinoplasty: a 10 year experience. Arch Facial Plast Surg 1: 246–256, 1995

McCollough EG. Nasal Plastic Surgery. Philadelphia: Saunders, 1994

Natvig P, Setler LA, and Dingman RO. Skin abuts skin at the alar margin of the nose. Ann Plast Surg 2: 248, 1979

Rees TD, and La Trenta OS. Aesthetic Plastic Surgery (2nd ed.) Philadelphia: Saunders, 1994

Rohrich RJ, Adams WP Jr. The boxy nasal tip: classification and management based of alar cartilage suture techniques. Plast Reconstr Surg 107: 1849, 2001

Sheen JH. Middle crus: The missing link in alar cartilage anatomy. Perspect Plast Surg 5:3 1, 1991a

Sheen JH. Tip graft: A 20-year retrospective. Plast Reconstr Surg 91: 48, 1991b

Sheen JH. Rhinoplasty: personal evolution and milestones. Plast Reconstr Surg 105: 1820, 2000

Sheen JH, Sheen AP. Aesthetic Rhinoplasty (2nd ed.) St. Louis: Mosby, 1987

Tardy ME. Rhinoplasty: The Art and the Science. Philadelphia: Saunders, 1997

Tardy ME, and Cheng E. Transdomal suture refinement of the nasal tip. Facial Plast Surg 4: 317, 1987

Tebbetts JB. Shaping and positioning the nasal tip without structural disruption: A new, systematic approach. Plast Reconstr Surg 1994;94:61. Additional information in Tebbetts JB. Primary Rhinoplasty: A New Approach to the Logic arid Techniques. St. Louis: Mosby, 1998

Toriumi, DM. New concepts in nasal tip contouring. Arch Facial Plast Surg 8: 156, 2006

Toriumi DM, Johnson CM. Open structure rhinoplasty. Featured technical points and long-term follow-up in Facial Plast Clin 1: 1, 1993

Zelnik J, Gingrass RP. Anatomy of the alar cartilage. Plast Reconstr Surg 64: 650, 1979

Nasal Base 5

The nasal base is probably the least understood and most complex area of the nose. Surgical errors of omission lead to less than optimal results, while errors of commission can produce irreparable deformities. Errors occur because surgeons assume that these are "ancillary techniques" rather than an integral part of a rhinoplasty. Or perhaps not enough time is taken to study the aesthetic and anatomical subtleties of the area. Unfortunately, analysis can be complex and the etiology of a problem multifactorial. Anatomically, the nasal base is not a distinct anatomical entity. The impact of adjacent structures is of critical importance. One must always assess the influence of the caudal septum on the columella which can result in deviation, retraction, or a hanging deformity. Despite the analytical complexity, most of the surgical solutions are straightforward once the correct diagnosis is made. The procedure must be done meticulously or permanent deformities can occur. Although challenging, it is my belief that a properly planned and executed alar base modification can have as great an impact on a rhinoplasty result as a tip graft.

Overview   Patients frequently complain about the width of their nasal base, the size of their nostrils, or their plunging tip. Many surgeons try to ignore these complaints as they do not feel confident that they can correct them. Yet these deformities can be improved quite easily provided the surgeon analyzes their etiology and design an effective operative plan (Fig. 5.1). The key is to think of the *ABCs* of the nasal base – *A*lar Rim, *B*ase, and *C*olumellar.

Level 1

Alar Rim. The most effective way of supporting the alar rim is the alar rim graft (ARG). A small tapered piece of cartilage (3 × 10 mm) is placed in a subcutaneous pocket paralleling the alar rim. It corrects most preexisting rim weaknesses or any that might occur following tip suturing.

Base. The surgeon must master the *nostril sill excision* which reduces nostril show on anterior view, and the *alar wedge excision* which reduces alar flare. These excisions are extraordinarily effective with minimal risk when properly executed.

Columellar. Excisions of the caudal septum and anterior nasal spine (ANS) are tailored to upwardly rotate or shorten the long nose. Their effect on tip position is perhaps as important as alar anatomy.

Level 2

Alar Rim. As alar rim retraction and abnormal nostril shape become greater, the surgical solution becomes the direct suturing of the alar rim graft into a marginal rim incision – the *alar rim support graft* (ARS). Essentially, one is using the same graft but suturing it directly along the nostril rim for greater support and shaping.

Base. As alar flare and nostril width both increase, the surgical solution becomes a *combined* nostril sill/alar wedge resection.

Columellar. The insertion of a columellar strut between the crura is extremely effective in pushing down the columellar inclination. In most cases, straightening a deviated columellar requires both correction of the deviated caudal septum and insertion of a major columellar strut.

Level 3

Alar Rim. As rim retraction becomes severe, one adds composite grafts of conchal cartilage and skin to correct the deficiency. When alar rim support is totally absent, rigid alar battens of rib cartilage may be necessary.

Base. In certain ethnic and cleft cases, cinch procedures are used to maximally narrow the nostril sill width. A great deal of imagination is needed to revise secondary nostril deformities.

Columellar. Retraction of the columellar can be due to telescoping of the septum or prior resection of either the caudal septum or membranous septum. Reconstruction can be demanding.

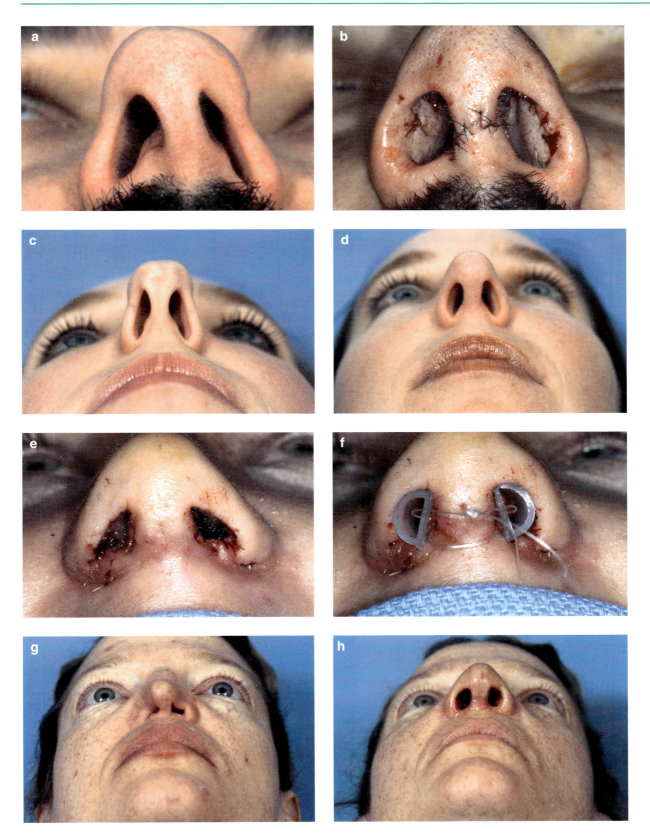

Fig. 5.1 Overview – illustrations, (**a**, **b**) correcting deviation and assymetry, (**c**, **d**) supporting and changing intrinsic nostril shape, (**e**, **f**) external valve splinting, (**g**, **h**) total collapse of the nostril treated with alar battens

Anatomy

Anatomical Components. From both an anatomical and an aesthetic perspective, the nasal base is subdivided into eight components: (1) columella base, (2) central columellar pillar, (3) infralobular triangle, (4) soft triangle, (5) lateral wall, (6) alar base, (7) nostril sill, and (8) nostril (Fig. 5.2). This component approach is best appreciated on basilar view. The transverse width of the columella base is related to the separation of the footplates and the quantity of the intervening soft tissue. The caudal septum/ANS is the critical factor in determining the columellar labial angle as seen on lateral view. The central columellar pillar is created by medial crura apposition and their termination at the columellar lobular junction. The infralobular triangle and soft triangle are the capstone of the basilar pyramid. The length of the columella segment of the middle crura determines the height of the triangle and the width of its divergence. The soft triangle is a reflection of the width of the domal notch and consists of a web of surface and vestibular skin devoid of cartilage. The lateral wall reflects the support and proximity of the lateral crura to the alar rim. It is the cephalic sweep of the lateral cartilage away from the rim that creates the alar rim breakpoint and marks the junction between lobule and alar base. The alar base is composed of subcutaneous tissue and muscles. It serves as an external baffle for the nose as influenced by the facial musculature. It is an area of surgical importance as it determines the amount of alar flare and interalar width. The nostril sill varies widely in its vestibular and cutaneous surfaces. The alar base can end abruptly creating a flat nostril sill or it can have a rolled continuous border. Equally, the footplates can extend laterally leaving an ill-defined nostril sill. The nostril is obviously the void whose shape is determined by the surrounding structures.

Extrinsic Influences. It is on lateral view that one begins to appreciate the important interrelationship between the nasal base and its abutting structures. The *columellar labial angle* is a critical aesthetic landmark. As seen on cadaver dissection, the key anatomical finding is that the distance from the maxilla's A-point to the tip of the nose is often 4 cm. It breaks down into four 1 cm segments: anterior nasal spine, caudal septum, medial crura, and middle crura. The ANS determines the projection from the maxilla and may have a webbed bony ridge beneath it. The caudal septum determines the columellar limb as it is covered by soft tissue centrally, but no cartilage for 1 cm before the medial crura meets in the midline. The labial limb is determined by the shape of the maxilla and its relationship with the soft tissues that comprise the upper lip. On anterior view, the key anatomical factor is the alar flare (AL) and the width of the alar bases (AC).

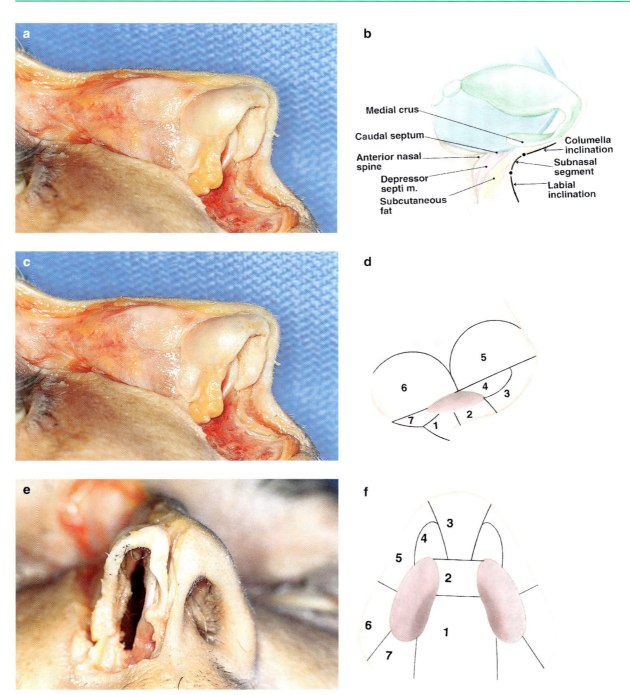

Fig. 5.2 (**a–f**) Basilar anatomy

Aesthetics/
Analysis

The aesthetics of the four nasal base components are carefully analyzed: alar flare/width, columella, columella labial angle, and nostril (Figs. 5.3 and 5.4).

Alar flare (AL-AL) refers to the widest point between the alar bases which usually occurs several millimeters above the alar crease. In contrast, *interalar width* (AC-AC) denotes the distance between the alar creases which is usually less than alar flare. The distinction is important in that alar flare can be easily reduced by alar wedge excision, whereas interalar width requires combined excision of the alar base and the nostril sill. Aesthetically, the alar bases should be narrower than the intercanthal width (EN-EN). These values are easily measured with a ruler or caliper on anterior or basilar view.

The *columella* relationship to the tip and the presence of a hanging columellar can be assessed by the "seagull-in-flight" concept on anterior view. Essentially, the columella breakpoint and each alar rim breakpoint are connected in such a way that it represents a seagull in flight. The more vertical the wings are, the more the columellar hangs (see Fig. 10.15 p377).

As previously noted, the *columella labial angle* (CLA) is created by the intersection of the columella tangent and the lip tangent at the subnasale (SN). Each component must be analyzed separately. The columella limb is a very powerful indicator of upward nasal rotation. A true *columellar angle* is measured by extending the columellar tangent line back to the vertical axis passing through the alar base. It should parallel the tip angle and be approximately 105° in females and 100° in males. The columella should have a slight convexity rather than a retruding concavity or a hanging prominence. The labial limb relates to the upper lip with the ideal at −6° from the upper lip vertical while avoiding either retrussion or prominence. One must consider the obvious influences of maxilla, occlusal relationship, teeth inclination, and upper lip composition. The subnasal segment should be a gradual curve interconnecting the two limbs, not a sharp acute point nor a blunted convex web which shortens the upper lip. Next, careful assessment of the caudal septum and ANS is mandatory. The examination is done mainly by palpation which often indicates either bony or soft tissue etiologies. Note: the term nasolabial angle is no longer used as CLA is of greater accuracy and surgical relevance.

Analysis of the *alar rim–nostril–columellar complex* (ARNC) requires careful scrutiny of multiple factors. The first step is to assess four inclinations on lateral view: (1) tip angle, (2) tangent of alar rim, (3) nostril inclination, and (4) columellar inclination. Second, tip angle and columellar inclination will be critical factors in determining the overall result of the rhinoplasty and must be addressed before the nostril. Third, one assesses the size, shape, and inclination of the nostril itself. Fourth, the alar rim configuration becomes a primary determinant of nostril show and its retraction is a common post-rhinoplasty stigmata.

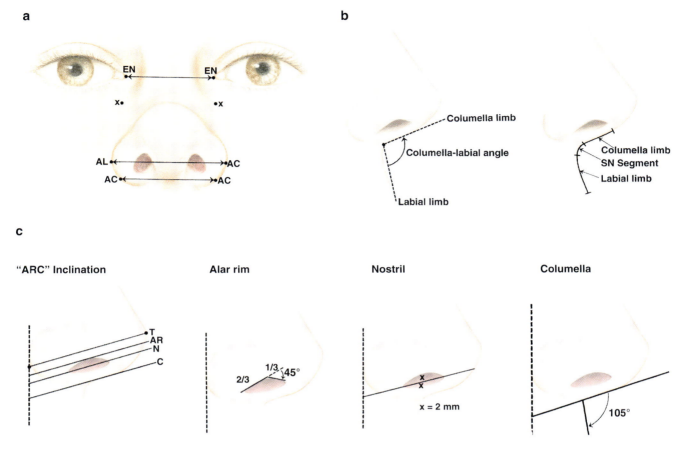

Fig. 5.3 (a–c) Aesthetics/analysis

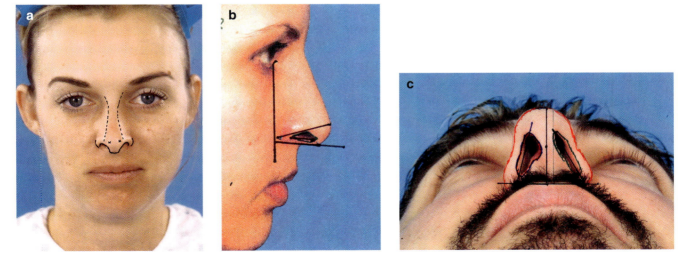

Fig. 5.4 (a–c) Case analysis **DVD**

Base Modification

Although many excisional configurations exist for narrowing the alar bases, I have simplified them into three types of excisions: nostril sill, alar wedge, and combined (Fig. 5.5). A few technical points: (1) the decision as to the indication and type is made preoperatively, (2) the alar crease is marked preoperatively and all alar incisions are made in the crease, (3) all excisions are carefully measured with a caliper prior to injection of local anesthesia, (4) 98% of the time, similar procedures are done on each side with only the size of the excision varied to accommodate asymmetries, (5) a fresh #15 blade is used and all cuts are made with the area under skin hook traction, (6) the sill is closed with a horizontal mattress suture of 4–0 plain catgut to insure eversion and thus avoid a depressed scar (Q sign), (7) the skin is closed with interrupted 6–0 nylon and no deep sutures, and (8) the sutures are kept clean until removal at 1 week.

Nostril Sill Excision

This excision is designed to reduce "nostril show" on anterior or oblique view. The wedge is centered in the floor vertically and is not angulated laterally nor does it have a comma shape (Fig. 5.6a, b). It is essentially a vertical trapezoidal wedge excision measuring 2–4 mm in width at the nostril sill with vertical side walls of 2–4 mm height that taper downward. Closure is begun with a horizontal mattress suture of 4–0 plain catgut in the vestibule followed by one or two 6–0 nylon sutures. The goal is a smooth scar not a depressed scar that distorts the floor of the nostril (Q sign).

Alar Wedge Excision

The alar wedge excision is an elliptical excision with an inferior border placed in the alar crease and a width 2–5 mm that may approach 7–9 mm in certain Black noses (Fig. 5.6c, d). The alar wedge is designed to reduce alar flare. Using a #15 blade, a V-excision is done down to the mid-muscle level, but without penetrating the underlying vestibular skin. Cauterization is necessary. The ellipse is closed from either end toward the middle with the knots tied on the lower side. With rare exception, I have not found the scars to be a problem and disagree with those who limit their alar base modification.

Combined Sill/Base Excision

This combined excision is designed to narrow the alar base maximally while reducing flare at the same time (Fig. 5.6e, f). Essentially, one draws the lower portion of the alar wedge excision around to the medial vertical wall of the nostril sill excision. Then using the calipers, one determines the sill width component and then the height of the alar wedge component. Under skin hook traction, the vertical sills are cut first, then the lower alar incision, and last the superior wedge incision. Following cauterization, the sill is closed first with 4–0 plain catgut and then the rest with 6–0 nylon. Note: throughout the text, I will denote the sill component first and alar component second so that a 3/4 excision is 3 mm of sill and 4 mm of alar wedge.

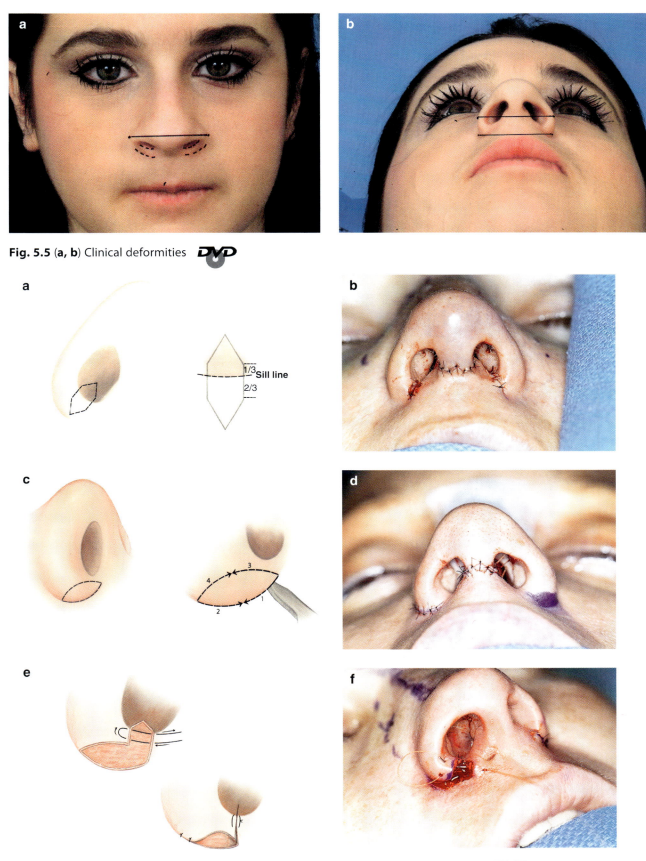

Fig. 5.5 (**a, b**) Clinical deformities *DVD*

Fig. 5.6 Base modifications, (**a, b**) nostril sill excision *DVD* (**c, d**) alar wedge excision *DVD* (**e, f**) combined sill/alar wedge excision *DVD*

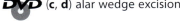

Columellar Labial Angle

Careful visual and tactile analysis of the columella labial angle (CLA) in repose and smiling is essential in determining whether the etiology of a deformity is isolated or combined. Surgical modification consists of preservation, resection, or augmentation of either the columellar or the anterior nasal spine (ANS).

Columella

The vast majority of columellar problems are deviations due to the caudal septum which require caudal septal relocation. The next most common deformity is the hanging columellar due to a prominent caudal septum which can be resected to affect either shortening and/or rotation (Fig. 5.7). In most cosmetic rhinoplasties, only the *upper half* of the caudal septum is resected to achieve tip rotation without altering the columellar limb. Resection of the *lower half* of the caudal septum affects the columella limb of CLA. Straight excisions of the entire caudal septum effectively shorten the nose. Clinical retraction of the columella limb is corrected by insertion of a long wide columellar strut graft (30 × 4), which extends below the medial crura footplates. The graft pushes down both the columellar limb and the CLA segment. One must avoid excessive length to prevent the graft from rocking across the ANS. "Plumping grafts" of excised cartilage are placed in the CLA to fine tune and correct the acute CLA.

Anterior Nasal Spine

The prominent ANS can be either shortened or its underlying bony webb deepened using a double-action rongeur. Shortening reduces the prominence of the SN point while resection lets the upper lip inclination become negative. The retracted ANS can be an isolated entity or part of a hypoplastic premaxilla which will often be expressed as an acute CLA. In most cases, I correct the retro position of the SN point with a large columella strut graft and additional small cartilage grafts placed subcutaneously in the columellar base beneath the CLA (Fig. 5.8). Others have tried a pyriform graft of either preformed Proplast or rolled GoreTex. The idea is to bring both the alar bases and the CLA forward. Unfortunately, I have had to remove several alloplastic grafts for the following reasons: (1) visibility in thin patients especially on smiling, (2) restricted movement of the upper lip, and (3) general dissatisfaction. For this reason, I use 2–3 ccs of diced cartilage (DC) when peripyriform augmentation is required, especially in the cocaine nose. In very asymmetric primary cases, I may build up the hypoplastic maxilla with hypdroxyapatite granules, if sufficient cartilage is not available. I do not recommend routine peripyriform grafts. Note: in many secondary cases, the caudal septum has been overly resected and one must reestablish both the columellar segment and the columellar inclination. In these cases, a large columellar strut can create the illusion of significant tip rotation without direct tip surgery. It is important to understand the columellar labial angle both as an isolated entity and as an integral part of rhinoplasty.

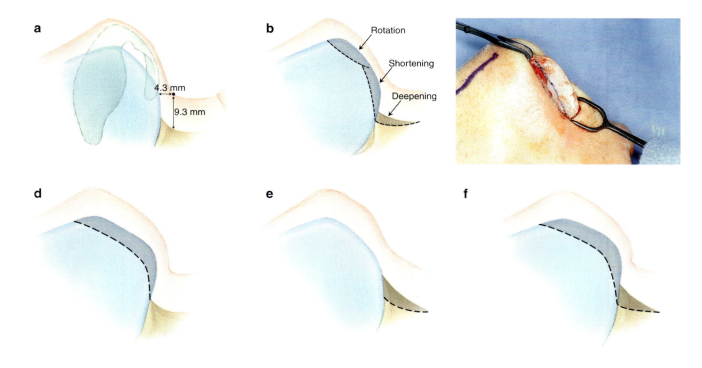

Fig. 5.7 (**a–f**) Caudal septum/ANS resection

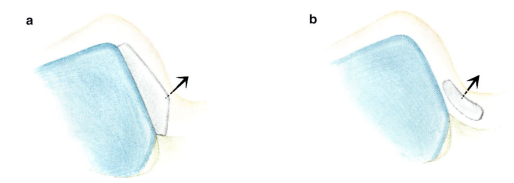

Fig. 5.8 (**a, b**) Grafting CLA

**The Alar Rim–
Nostril–
Columellar
Complex**

Analysis of the alar rim–nostril–columellar complex (ARNC) begins with drawing four inclinations on lateral view: (1) tip angle, (2) tangent of alar rim, (3) nostril inclination, and (4) columella inclination (Fig. 5.9). It is critical that the requisite tip angle and columellar inclination be achieved before modifying the nostrils. The breakpoint of the alar rim is marked as well as the proximal limb which should be twice the distal limb and the angle of intersection should be approximately 45°. The nostril circumference is drawn, which incorporates the alar rim cephallically and the posterior portion of the columellar caudally. A line is drawn through the terminal points of the nostril and the resulting bisection classified as follows: (1) ideal with 2 mm on either side, (2) excesses greater than 2 mm indicating a retracted alar, hanging columella or both, and (3) reductions of 1 mm or less denoting a hanging alar or retracted columellar. Alar rim surgery can be divided into those for the hanging or retracted alar rims.

Lowering the Alar Rim

Level 1. The easiest method for lowering the alar rim by 2 mm or blunting a notched alar rim is the simple alar rim graft (ARG) (Fig. 5.10). A straight piece of cartilage measuring 10 × 2.5 mm is cut. A small transverse incision is made in the lateral vesitibule 3–4 mm behind the rim and a subcutaneous pocket is dissected paralleling the rim. The graft should fit snugly in the pocket and correct the visible deformity. The usual errors are a thick cephalic end which can be visible in the soft tissue facet or create a bossa over the dome. Rigid support can be achieved by suturing the graft into the alar rim as an ARS.

Level 2. For cases with 2–4 mm of alar rim retraction, I prefer to use a composite graft from the cymba concha (Fig. 5.11). Several technical points: (1) mark the alar rim border and its apex on the patient; (2) make the incision 2 mm behind the rim; (3) spread perpendicular to the rim and never dissect toward the rim; (4) have equal amounts of cartilage and skin in the graft; and (5) know that the graft works by filling the defect. The major problem has been the three-dimensional challenge of getting rim descent without widening the nostril horizontally or creating excess fullness cephalically.

Level 3. Any alar retraction greater than 5 mm is a severe problem and composite grafts in the alar rim position tend to be inadequate. In severe cases with associated vestibular steosis, I have used a large conchal cartilage graft (20 × 8 mm) placed in the vestibule.

Elevation of the Alar Rim. Elevating the hanging alar rim is of limited effectiveness as only 2–3 mm can be achieved at the maximum. An ellipse is drawn 3 mm above the alar rim and centered at the desired point of maximum elevation. The width is twice the desired elevation. This pattern is then transferred to the vestibular lining and a full thickness ellipse of soft tissue is excised. The wound is closed with 5–0 plain catgut which should elevate the alar rim. A more aggressive method is direct excision along the alar rim which I do not recommend as the scarring is unpredictable.

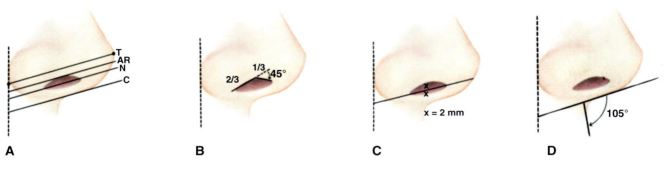

Fig. 5.9 (**a–d**) Alar rim–nostril–columellar complex analysis

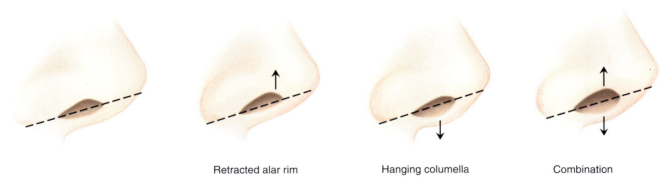

Retracted alar rim   Hanging columella   Combination

Fig. 5.10 Nostril analysis

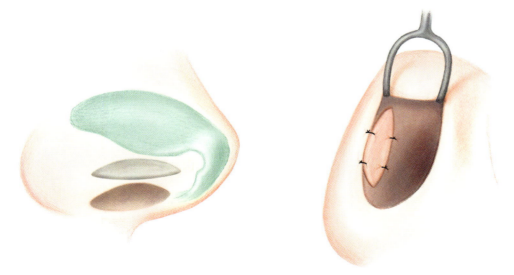

Fig. 5.11 Composite grafts

Changing Nostril Size and Shape

Many surgeons tell patients that the inherent size and shape of the nostrils cannot be changed – nothing could be further from surgical reality. Both the size and shape of the nostrils can be altered significantly, but it requires Level 2 and Level 3 techniques.

Changing Nostril Size. Large nostrils are similar to "stretchy doughnuts." The aperture is affected by the convexity and projection of the cartilaginous vault as well as the downward rotation of the caudal septum. These extrinsic forces must be eliminated before true nostril size can be determined (Fig. 5.12a–c). The combination of dorsal reduction and caudal septal resection plus the appropriate nostril base excision, usually a combined nostril sill/alar wedge, will adequately reduce 90% of large nostrils. In the truly massive alar nostril (1–2% of my cases), it is necessary to either excise a portion of the lateral crural segment or do a domal excision plus open structure tip graft to reduce the nostrils. Note: increasing nostril size is a nightmare and virtually never required in primary aesthetic cases. This subject will be dealt with under cleft and secondary rhinoplasties later in the text.

Nostril/Tip Disproportion. Many patients complain of large nostrils and an under projecting poorly defined tip. On lateral analysis, it is a small tip which is accentuating normal or large nostrils (Fig. 5.13a–c). One must increase intrinsic tip projection to achieve balance in the ideal 2:1 nostril to tip ratio. The most common method is to suture the middle crura to a columellar strut followed by tip suturing. Add-on grafts are used to increase infralobular tip volume and domal definition.

Changing Nostril Shape. Virtually nothing has been written about changing *intrinsic nostril shape*. After using a large number of ARS grafts, I realize how dramatically nostril shape could be altered. However, it requires careful analysis, surgical skill, and checking of the most minute details (Fig. 5.14a–c). The boxy tip with its weak alar rims is the most common deformity requiring a change in nostril shape. The steps are as follows: (1) eliminate the deforming forces of the dorsum and caudal septum, (2) achieve the desired tip which may involve domal excision or even alar transposition, (3) reduce the nostril base with the appropriate excision technique, and (4) control nostril shape with an ARS graft. The key is to suture an ARS graft into a true marginal rim incision. For the ARS graft, the steps are as follows: (1) make a true rim incision 2 mm back from the rim extending into the alar base, (2) undermine cephalically, never caudally into the nostril rim, (3) one should see a distinct change in nostril shape with release of the mucosa, (4) the ARS graft must be shaped meticulously – a length of 10–14 mm with a width of 2–3 mm but tapered medially and thinned to 1–2 mm, (5) the graft is inserted along the marginal incision and sutured at its central point with 4-0 plain sutures, and (6) the medial portion must not overlap the domal segment or a visible "bossa" will appear postoperatively.

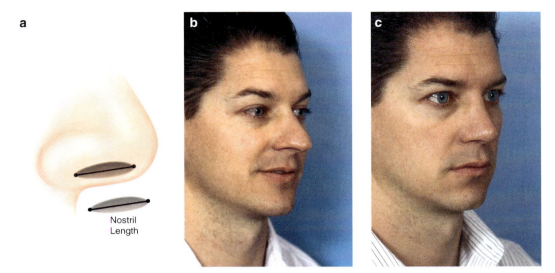

Fig. 5.12 (a–c) Changing nostril size

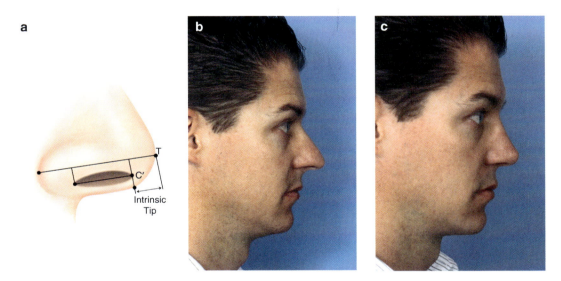

Fig. 5.13 (a–c) Correcting nostril: tip disproportion

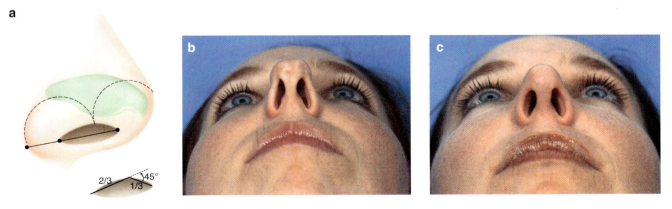

Fig. 5.14 (a–c) Changing nostril shape

Decision Making Level 1

Operative Planning. The truth is that in the majority of Level 1 cases, there is no surgery indicated for the nasal base. The exceptions are those patients who complain of wide nostrils or have a significant caudal septum deviation that influences the columellar. When first starting out, the surgeon should be forced into doing a particular operative step, either by patient request (nostrils too wide) or presenting deformity (crooked columellar). Intraoperatively, a base excision might become necessary if a major dorsal reduction is done which results in a secondary widening of the base. In contrast, alar rim grafts following tip suturing may be necessary to minimize loss of alar rim support. To correctly analyze the problem, the surgeon should answer the following questions.

Base. Do I need to narrow the base of the nose? One should look on anterior and basilar views to determine alar flare and alar width as compared to intercanthal width. One can either do this on photos or by measurements with a caliper directly on the patient (my preferred method). How much nostril sill do I see on anterior view or with the head slightly back? Will a simple nostril sill excision solve the problem or is the alar flare so severe that I need to do a wedge resection? A nostril sill excision has less risk of a visible scar, but does little for alar flare. Always choose the simplest procedure.

Columellar/Caudal Septum. Is the nose too long? Is the tip rotated downward? Is the upper lip crowded? Is the columellar deviated because of a caudal septal deflection? In addition to direct inspection, one must answer these questions by palpating the columellar and caudal septum as well as observing their changes on maximum smiling. The most common deformity is that the nose is too long and the tip is somewhat downwardly rotated. Both problems are minimized by excising 2–3 mm off the upper two thirds of the caudal septum. The ANS is rarely excised unless the upper lip is very crowded. One must correct caudal septal deviations both for functional and aesthetic reasons. A columellar strut between the alars can reduce the impact of a deviated caudal septum.

Nostril Rim. Is the alar rim retracted on anterior view or weak on basilar view? After suturing the tip, did the alar rims loose support? In the vast majority of primary cosmetic rhinoplasties, the alar rim is rarely a problem preoperatively. However, tip suturing can cause a subtle change in alar rim contour requiring alar rim grafts to restore rim contour. These are important grafts and if in doubt, insert them.

PRINCIPLES

- Surface measurements with a caliper allow direct comparison of EN-EN, AL-AL, and AC-AC. It insures a complete pre-op analysis.
- Base modification is a critical step in the operative plan, not an optional ancillary minor detail.
- Meticulous closure of the excision is essential, especially eversion of the nostril sill.

Analysis

Pre-op, the patient has a long downwardly rotated nose and a convex profile. The nostrils are quite visible on all views, but especially the oblique, which would only be accentuated postoperatively. For this reason, 2 mm nostril sill excisions were done on both sides. Note how much smaller the nostrils look on the post-op oblique view. There were no ARG or ARS grafts – just bilateral nostril sill excisions (Fig. 5.15).

Nostril Sill Excisions

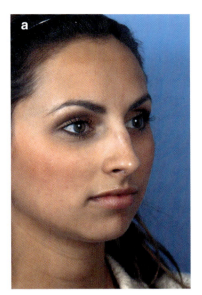
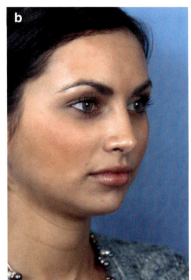
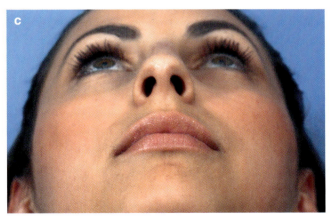
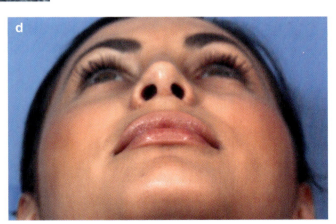

Fig. 5.15 (a–d)

Alar Wedge Excisions

This patient presented with the complaint of a large nose crowned by a bulbous tip. The skin envelope was relatively thick. At surgery, her cartilaginous dorsum was reduced 5 mm and tip projection dropped using bilateral transfixion incisions. The tip went from an over-projecting narrow isosceles triangle to a wider equilateral triangle. Alar wedge excisions, 4 mm wide, were an intraoperative necessity which is a fairly rare occurrence (Fig. 5.16).

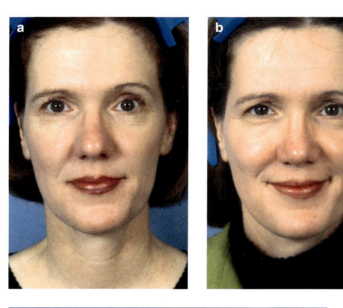

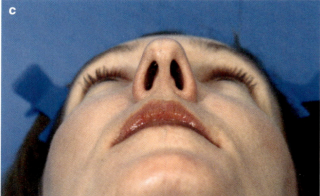

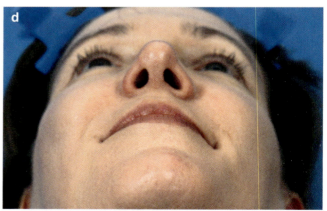

Fig. 5.16 (a–d)

Analysis

Pre-op, the patient's surface measurements were as follows: EN 28, AC 30, and AL 35. The alar flare (AL) was +7 mm relative to the intercanthal distance (EN) thus leading to the combined nostril sill/alar base excision (R & L: 2.5/2.5). Post-op on basilar view, the nasal base is significantly narrower while the nostrils are smaller. The nostril sills no longer hang down below the alar rims on anterior view. There were no osteotomies (Fig. 5.17).

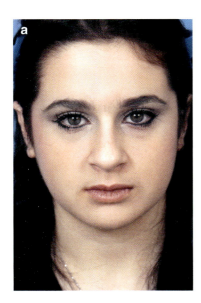
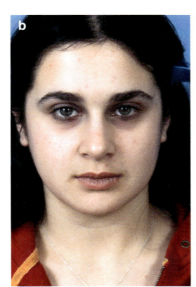
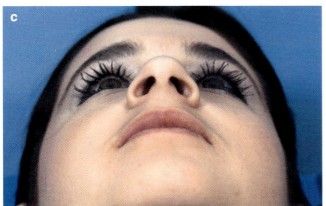
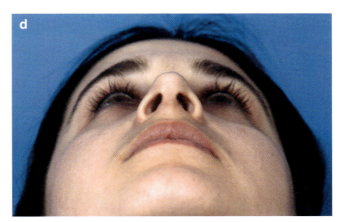

Fig. 5.17 (a–d)

Decision Making Level 2

In the majority of Level 2 cases, the problems are both aesthetic and functional with correction a necessity rather than an option (Fig. 5.18). One has to be prepared to deal effectively with both a wider range and greater severity of problems. A classic example is the combination of a boxy tip and a deviated caudal septum. One wants to reduce the rigid alar tip cartilages, but the flimsy nostril rims are already weakened. On deep inspiration, the external valve collapses on the side of the caudal septal deviation.

Base. A combined nostril sill/alar wedge resection is necessary when a major reduction in the base width is planned. Asymmetry is common and asymmetrical excisions of each component are often required. I mark the nostril sill component first in the standard fashion. Then the lower alar wedge incision is placed in the alar crease. The amount of excision varies from the usual 2–3.5 mm to the exceptional 6–7 mm in Black patients. The nostril sill component is incised first using parallel vertical cuts. Then the alar wedge component is incised from lateral to medial, with tapering on the upper border into the nostril sill. Closure of the nostril sill with an everting horizontal mattress suture of 4–0 plain catgut is critical to avoid an inverted scar (Q sign). Due to the alar rim notching that follows major excisions, ARS grafts are inserted after the alar base excision in most cases.

Columellar/Caudal Septum. The columellar is frequently deviated due to a caudal septal deflection. The septum must be relocated to, and fixed in, the midline. Simple positioning without rigid fixation is insufficient. Thus, the septum is fixed to the ANS in the correct position. Next, a columellar strut is placed between the alar cartilages. The tip cartilages are appropriately modified and supported on the columellar strut.

Nostril Rim. Support of the nostril rim becomes critical in these cases and a simple alar rim graft (ARG) is rarely adequate. Rather, one must use alar rim support grafts (ARS) where the graft is sutured into a true *marginal rim incision*. The rim incision is made rather than the infracartilaginous incision to allow the graft to support the rim. Then a tapered 12 × 2.5 mm piece of septal cartilage is sutured into the rim incision. These grafts offer both rim support and the ability to change nostril shape significantly. The suturing is first at the midpoint and then laterally. The medial extent of the graft must be carefully checked to avoid overlap above the dome which can result in a bossa or distortion of the soft tissue facets. When in doubt, a shorter graft is better.

PRINCIPLES

- One must straighten the foundation first (caudal septum), then reduce asymmetry in the columellar using a strut, and then the tip.
- Any major combined nostril sill/alar wedge resection will require either an ARG or ARS graft.

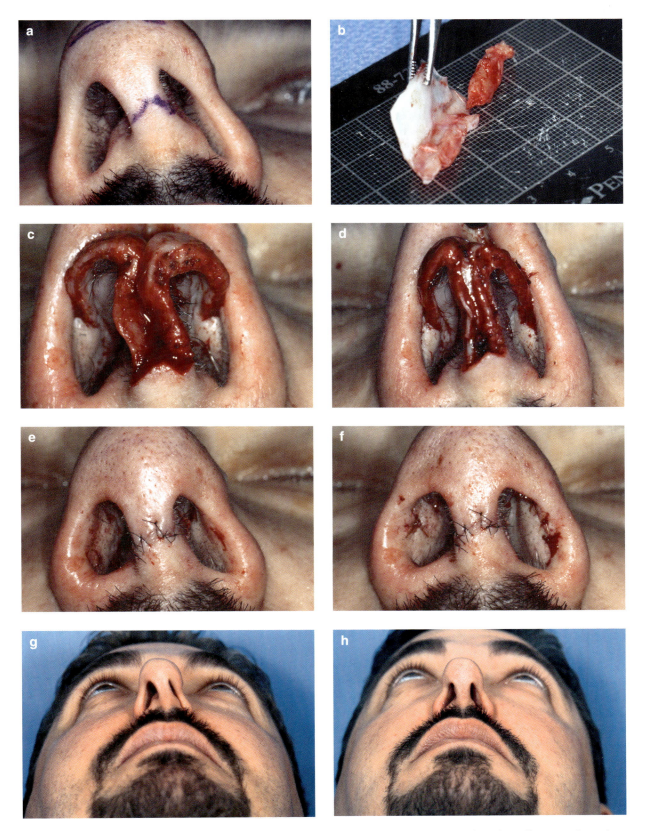

Fig. 5.18 (**a**) Pre-op base, (**b**) septal deviation, (**c**) post-caudal sepal relocation, (**d**) columellar strut insertion, (**e**) closure, (**f**) ARG (R), ARS (L), (**g**) pre-op/deep inspiration, (**h**) post-op/deep inspiration

Case Study: Base Collapse

Analysis

A 41-year-old male presented with a history of severe nasal obstruction, but no prior nasal trauma (Fig. 5.19). Literally, everything that could cause nasal obstruction was present including the following: (1) caudal septal deviation to the left, (2) alar rim weakness with collapse on deep inspiration, (3) a severe S-shape deviation of the septal body, and (4) midvault narrowing. The latter would be treated by detaching the upper laterals, inserting spreader grafts, and no osteotomies. As shown on the previous page, straightening the caudal septum improved the columellar while the nostrils were supported with an ARG on the right and an ARS on the left. Aesthetically, the patient wanted a nose that was more compatible with his life style.

Operative Technique

1) Exposure of alar cartilages and dorsum
2) Septal exposure through right transfixion incision
3) Detachment of upper laterals for bidirectional septal access
4) Inferior tunnel for bony septal exposure
5) Major septoplasty, but maintaining a 12 mm L-shape strut
6) Caudal septal relocation L to R with suture fixation
7) Columellar strut plus tip sutures: CS, DC, ID, LCC × 2
8) ARG on R, ARS on L
9) Out fracture of turbinates
10) No lateral osteotomies, no nostril sill excisions

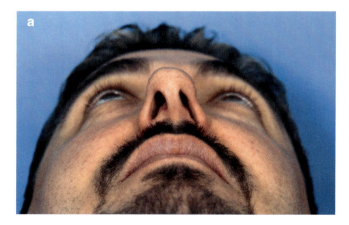
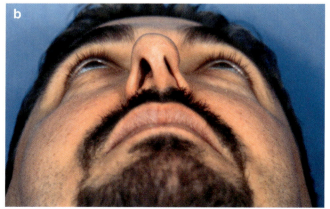

Fig. 5.19 (a–j)

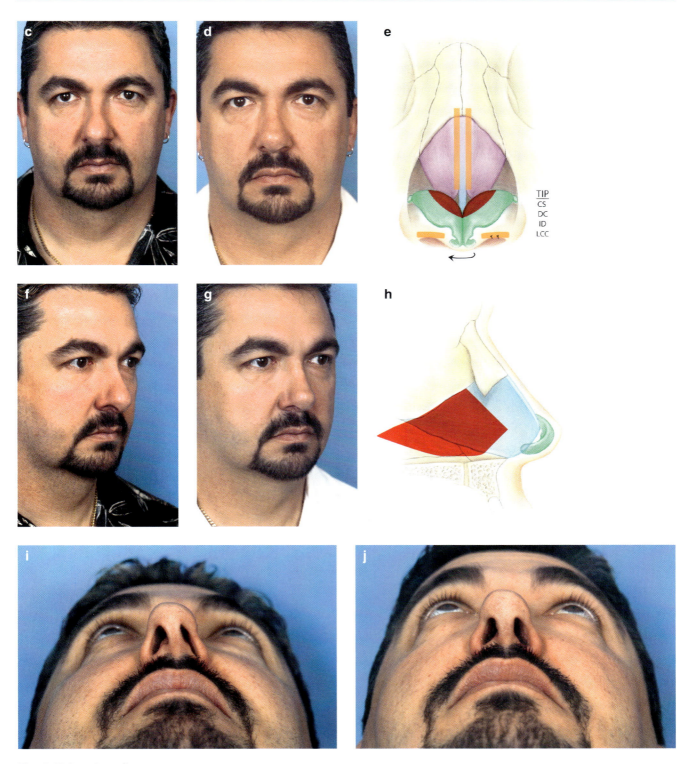

Fig. 5.19 (continued)

Decision Making Level 3

These cases often demand both creativity and surgical humility. In primary cases, the progression is from unusual nostrils to ethnic challenges to cleft lip asymmetries. The critical requirement is to combine base excisions with rigid alar rim support using either cartilage or composite grafts. Nostril retainer splints are used at night for 2-3 weeks (Fig.5.20).

Composite Grafts. Although frequently used in secondary and cleft lip rhinoplasty, I rarely use composite grafts in primary cases (<3%). These unusual cases involve significant isolated alar rim retraction where the caudal septum cannot be excised. ARG or ARS grafts would not solve the problem because true hypoplasia of the lateral crura is present. The solution is to fill the defect with both cartilage support and skin lining. These grafts are custom tailored to the defect and are usually "composite strips" (12 × 2–3 mm) in contrast to the 4–6 mm wide composite grafts required in cleft or secondary cases. It is important to shave down the cartilage surface until it has the thickness and pliability of alar cartilages.

Cartilage Grafts. A decade ago, the choice of cartilage grafts for the alar rim was simple – an alar batten graft. These large grafts provided support, but often obscured the alar crease or altered symmetry. ARG and ARS grafts work well for the nostril rim, but are probably insufficient for most major external valve collapses. Thus, *the lateral crural strut graft* has become the graft of choice because its size and position can be tailored to fit the problem (Fig. 5.21). As discussed in Chapter 7, the three positions for the lateral crural strut graft are pyriform (Type I), alar base (Type II), and nostril rim (Type III). The critical factor is that the graft is placed beneath and sutured to the lateral crura which in turn can be in its normal position or transposed. Simplistically, transposition of the lateral crura is a tip decision, whereas the position of the lateral crural strut graft is a functional decision. The Type I pyriform location supports the alar crease, the Type II alar base location supports the vestibule, and the Type III nostril rim location supports and reshapes the nostril. Lateral crural strut grafts are ideally made from rigid septal or rib cartilage and are highly tapered. This complex subject is discussed extensively in Chapters 7 and 8.

PRINCIPLES

- Composite "strip" grafts are effective in lowering the alar rims in primary rhinoplasty cases.
- Lateral crural strut grafts have replaced alar batten grafts in the majority of primary cases.
- Lateral crural strut grafts provide support, but should never be visible. Hiding the graft beneath the lateral crura is essential.
- A true marginal rim incision is used when the Type III lateral crural strut graft is placed into and sutured along the nostril rim.

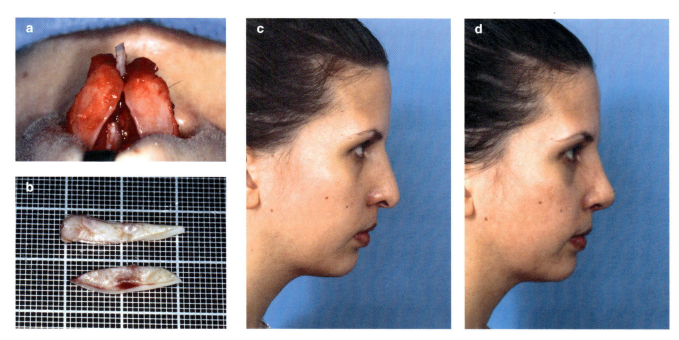

Fig. 5.20 (**a–d**) Composite grafts and the use of nostril splints ***DVD***

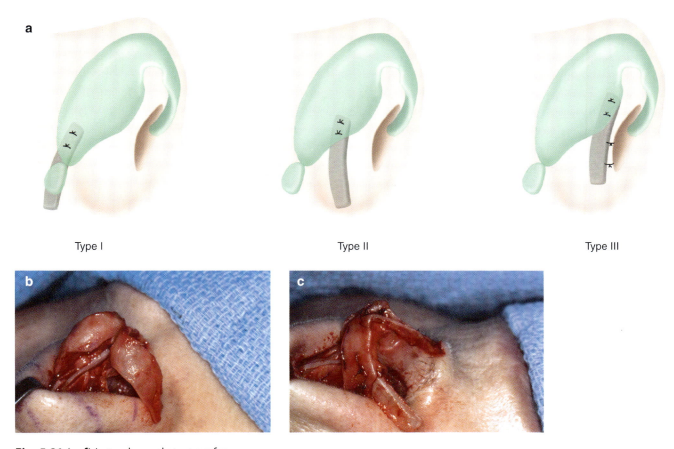

Type I   Type II   Type III

Fig. 5.21 (**a–f**) Lateral crural strut grafts

Case Study: Alar Retraction

Analysis

A 28 year old who works in the beauty industry requested a rhinoplasty (Fig. 5.22). Her three complaints were the following: "(1) beaky on profile, (2) nostrils too big, and (3) tip plunges." I agreed with her diagnosis. In addition, there was a significant large nostril/small tip disproportion. Technically, the major problem would be the preexisting retracted alars which would require composite grafts, especially if a major tip change was accomplished. Since analysis of the intrinsic tip was virtually impossible until the deforming extrinsic forces were removed, it was elected to use a "closed/open" approach. The composite grafts lowered the alar rim and provided support for the nostril contour. The result is shown at 2 years post-op.

Operative Technique Highlights

1) Intercartilaginous and transfixion incisions plus septal exposure.
2) Dorsal reduction (bone 0.5 mm, cartilage 2.0 mm).
3) Caudal septal (4 mm) and ANS resection followed by septal harvest.
4) Open approach. Minimal "scroll only" cephalic resection.
5) Low-to-high osteotomies. Insertion of spreader grafts.
6) Insertion of crural strut plus tip sutures: CS, DC, DE, TP.
7) Combined nostril sill/alar base excision R: 2.5/1.5, L: 3.5/2.0.
8) Composite conchal grafts to each nostril rim.

Note: patient had a chin implant (small) and submental liposuction.

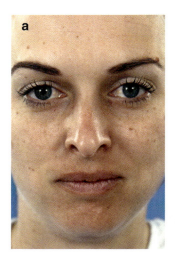 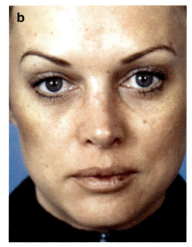 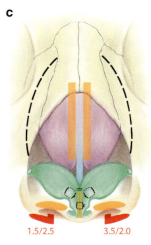

Fig. 5.22 (a–j)

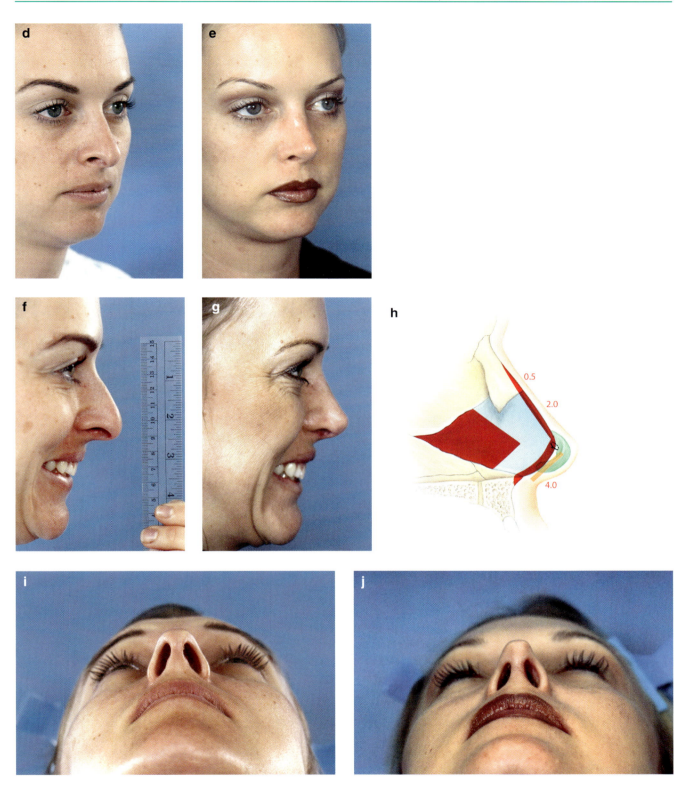

Fig. 5.22 (continued)

Reading List   Bennett GH, Lessow A, Song P, et al The long-term effects of alar base reduction. Arch Facial Plast Surg 7: 94, 2005

Byrd HS, Hobar C, Shewmake K. Augmentation of the craniofacial skeleton with porous hydroxyapatite granules. Plast Reconstr Surg 91:15, 1993

Daniel RK. The nasal base. In Daniel, RK (ed) Aesthetic Plastic Surgery: Rhinoplasty. Boston: Little, Brown, 1993

Daniel RK. Rhinoplasty: Nostril/tip disproportion. Plast Reconstr Surg 107:1454, 2001

Davis RE. Diagnosis and surgical management of the caudal excess nasal deformity. Arch Facial Plast Surg 7:100, 2005

Ellenbogen R. Alar rim lowering. Plast Reconstr Surg 79:50, 1987

Farkas LG, and Munro JR. Anthropometric Facial Proportions in Medicine. Springfield: Thomas, 1987

Farkas LG, Hreczko TA, Deutsch CC. Objective assessment of standard nostril types – A morphometric study. Ann Plast Surg 11:381,1983

Farkas LG, Kolar JC, Munro JR. Geography of the nose: A morphometric study. Aesthetic Plast Surg 10:191, 1986

Gruber RP, Freeman MB, Hsu C, et al Nasal base reduction; a treatment algorithim including alar release with medialization. Plast Reconstr Surg 123: 716, 2009

Gruber RP, French MB, Hsu C, et al Nasal base reduction by alar release: A laboratory evaluation. Plast Reconstr Surg 123: 709, 2009

Gryskiewicz JM. The "inatrogenic-hanging columellar": preserving columellar contour after tip retroprojection. Plast Reconstr Surg 110:272, 2002

Gunter JP, Rohrich RJ, Friedman RM. Classification and correction of alar-columellar discrepancies in rhinoplasty. Plast Reconstr Surg 97:643, 1996

Guyuron B. Alar rim deformities. Plast Reconstr Surg 107:856, 2001

Guyuron B. Footplates of the medial crura. Plast Recosntr Surg 101: 1359, 1998

Guyruron B. Alar base surgery. In Gunter, JP, Rohrich, RJ, and Adams, WP (eds) Dallas Rhinoplasty: Nasal Surgery by the Masters. 2nd ed. St. Louis: QMP, 2007

Guyuron B, Behmand, RA. Caudal nasal deviation. Plast Reconstr Surg 111: 2449, 2003

Kridel RW, Castellano RD. A simplified approach to alar base reduction; a review of 124 patients over 20 years. Arch Facial Plast surg 7: 81, 2005

Lessard ML, Daniel RK. Surgical anatomy of the nose. Arch Otolaryngol Head Neck Surg 111:25, 1985

Letourneau A, Daniel RK. The superficial musculoaponecrotic system of the nose. Plast Reconstr Surg 82:48, 1988

Meyer R, Kessering WK. Secondary rhinoplasty. In: Regnault P and Daniel RK (eds) Aesthetic Plastic Surgery. Boston: Little, Brown, 1984

Millard DR. Alar margin sculpturing. Plast Reconstr Surg 40:337, 1967

Millard DR. The alar cinch in the flat, flaring nose. Plast Reconstr Surg 65:669, 1980

Natvig P, Setler LA, Dingman RO. Skin abutts skin at the alar margin of the nose. Ann Plast Surg 2:428, 1979

Ortiz-Monasterio F, Olmedo A, Oscoy LO. The use of cartilage grafts in primary aesthetic rhinoplasty. Plast Reconstr Surg 67:597, 1981

Peck GC. Techniques in Aesthetic Rhinoplasty, 2nd ed. Philadelphia: JB Lippincott, 1990

Powell N, and Humphreys B. Proportions of the Aesthetic Face. New York: Thieme Stratton, 1984

Randall P. The direct approach to the "hanging columella". Plast Reconstr Surg 53:544, 1974

Rohrich, Rj, Raniere J Jr, Ha, RY. The alar contour graft: correction and prevention of alar rim deformities in rhinoplasty. Plast Reconstr Surg 109: 2495, 2002

Rohrich RJ, Hoxworth RE, Thorton JF, et al The pyriform ligament. Plast Reconstr Surg 121:277, 2008

Functional Factors 6

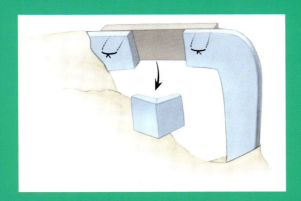

Introduction

As a plastic surgeon specializing in rhinoplasty, I deal with two patient populations: the cosmetic patient who wants a more attractive nose with the preservation of what they perceive to be normal respiration, and the secondary patient whose nasal function is often impaired. These problems are usually due to fixed anatomical deformities, which require surgical solutions rather than the more common form of nasal obstruction due to vasomotor rhinitis requiring medical management. This chapter provides a foundation for the younger surgeon to analyze, diagnose, and manage the rhinoplasty patient. The goal is to preserve normal respiratory function, recognize those who would be compromised by surgery, and treat those with fixed anatomical deformities. During the last decade, two radical changes have occurred in septo-rhinoplasty surgery as regards functional surgery. First, septal surgery has become far simpler and consists of four areas: body resection, caudal septal relocation, dorsal straightening, and total septoplasty. In contrast, a greater emphasis on valvular surgery requires attention to the external and internal valves. Second, the primary cause of post-rhinoplasty nasal obstruction has evolved from inadequate septal surgery (1980s)through untreated turbinate hypertrophy (1990s) to collapse of the nasal valves (2000). Currently, I am convinced that the major cause of post-rhinoplasty nasal obstruction is a failure to adequately diagnose and treat a preoperative problem. Careful preoperative history, examination, and planning for the functional portion of the internal nose are as important as the aesthetic improvement of the external nose. Compromise of nasal respiration severely downgrades even the most beautiful result.

Overview   Surgeons frequently want rhinoplasty to be simple. One of their favorite fantasies is that cosmetic rhinoplasty does not really require correction of functional nasal obstruction. They often ask the following questions. Can you do a rhinoplasty without fixing septal deviations? No. Do you really need to do spreader grafts? Yes, and frequently for both functional and aesthetic reasons. Can the operation be split into two parts with one surgeon doing the functional part and another surgeon the cosmetic portion? No, it is an integrated operation. I schedule all of my aesthetic cases as a "cosmetic septorhinoplasty with possible inferior turbincetomy and multiple grafts," which reflects the dual nature of the operation. Now that the delusion of a pure cosmetic operation has been put to rest, we can talk about functional factors that must be evaluated in every rhinoplasty.

Level 1. The surgeon should be able to deal with the following four functional factors: septal body deviation, caudal septal deviation, internal valve collapse, and inferior turbinate hypertrophy (Fig. 6.1a, b). The surgical solutions are straightforward: resect septal body deviations, relocate caudal septal deviations, insert spreader grafts to open the internal valve, and partially resect hypertrophic inferior turbinates.

Level 2. Additional surgical sophistication is required to deal with severe deviations of the septum due to either trauma or developmental causes. Caudal septal problems go beyond dislocation to instability or collapse, which may require either reinforcement or replacement using grafts of septal cartilage. Dorsal deviations are a reality and are corrected with the following sequence: (1) place spreader grafts on the nondeviated side, which is sutured above and below the deviation, (2) excise the deviated portion of the septum, and (3) place a spreader graft on the deviated side with five-layer suture fixation (Fig. 6.1 c, d). Problems in the external valve will require the use of alar rim grafts (ARG) or alar rim support grafts (ARS) in the nostril valve and lateral crura strut grafts for the vestibular valve. Problems can be found in the middle turbinate or synechiae between the turbinates and the adjacent tissues.

Level 3. Whenever one deals with severe primary cases (clefts, cocaine, and posttraumatic deformities) and virtually all secondary rhinoplasties, the surgeon must be prepared for a major challenge. One will need to fix the unstable septum and even do a total septoplasty (Fig. 6.1 e, f). These cases require a significant step-up in technical sophistication and I consider these cases to be "nasal reconstruction of the internal nose." In the septum a wide range of prior destabilizing incisions and extensive resections can be present. One must be prepared to establish septal support and to harvest grafts from alternative sites, including rib grafts for stability. Valvular surgery can range from opening up constricted stenotic areas with composite grafts to widening the bony valve. Turbinate surgery can be complicated by scar fusion with the septum or an over abundance of polyps.

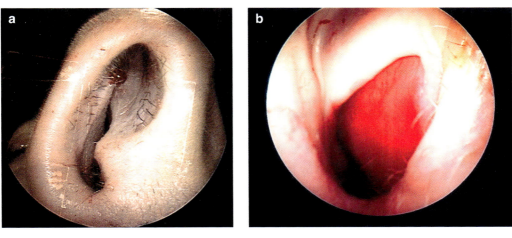

Fig. 6.1 (a,b) Septal and valvular obstructions **DVD**

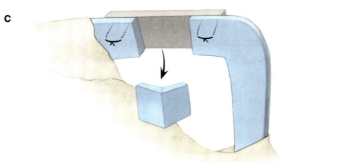

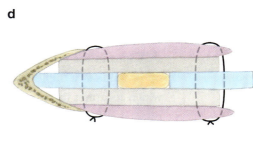

Fig. 6.1 (c,d) Dorsal septal deviation

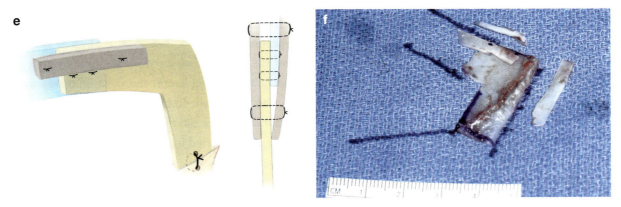

Fig. 6.1 (e, f) Total septoplasty

Septal Surgery

Anesthesia. After prepping the internal nose with Betadine swabs, the subperichondrial mucosal space is injected using 1% xylocaine with epinephrine 1:100,000. The goal is to achieve a hydrostatic dissection, which will facilitate subsequent elevation of the septal mucosa. Injections allow evaluation of mucosal quality and septal structure. Next, the mucosal lining is vasoconstricted using topical agents. Most surgeons use either a solution of 4% cocaine, local anesthesia, or Afrin. I find that two 18-in. strips of ½-in. gauze allows more accurate packing with better contact. In complex secondary cases, an endoscopic evaluation is often helpful.

Septal Exposure. Routinely, I use a full unilateral right transfixion incision combined with dorsal access to expose the septum. The caudal septum is exposed by retraction of columellar to the left side and then a full-length transfixion incision is made 2–3 mm back from the caudal border. Using the angled Converse scissors, the mucosa is elevated and the subperichondrial space is entered. To insure a clean dissection, I routinely crosshatch the lining with a #15 blade and then scrape through to the cartilage using a dental amalgam. Once the perichondrium is elevated, the dissection continues posteriorly over the cartilage and onto the ethmoid and vomer bones, In contrast to this uninterrupted passage, the dissection inferiorly is blocked at the junction of cartilage with premaxilla due to the joint fascia where perichondrium and periosteum meet. Any attempt to pass inferiorly will result in tears of the mucosa. For most cases, this degree of exposure via an "anterior tunnel" is sufficient. However, in complex cases with significant deformities involving the premaxilla, it is necessary to create an "inferior tunnel" for complete access to the premaxilla.

Access Alternatives. The classic septal access via the open approach was obtained through a top-down *dorsal split* technique in which the upper lateral cartilages are detached from the septum (Fig. 6.3 a, b). This dorsal split can be combined with a *tip split* separating the alar cartilages in the tip/columella, which adds exposure of the caudal septum and permits its correction (Fig. 6.3 c, d). However, the combination of a unilateral transfixion with the dorsal split, *dual exposure*, is used most frequently; especially in secondary cases (Fig. 6.3e, f). The elevator is passed from the transfixion incision up to the septal angle and into the gap between septal angle and attachment of upper lateral cartilages. In secondary cases, this subperichondrial dissection from the known (caudal septum) to the unknown (the dorsum with its heavily scarred disrupted anatomical planes) is much easier than a top-down dissection. The *tip flip* method is a combination of the intercartilaginous incisions extended into bilateral transfixion incisions plus the open approach with its transcolumellar and infracartilaginous incisions (Fig. 6.3g, i). Once the soft-tissue elevation is completed, then the entire tip lobule can be rotated downward onto the upper lip. One is starting directly at the septum end on.

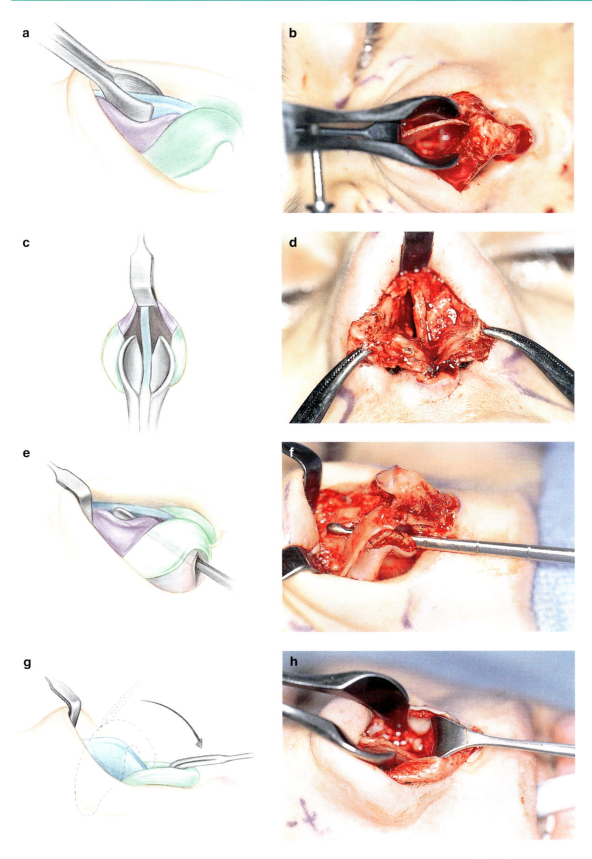

Fig. 6.3 Septal exposure. (**a, b**) Dorsal split **DVD** (**c, d**) combined dorsal/tip split **DVD** (**e, f**) transfixion **DVD** (**g, h**) tip flip **DVD**

Septal Body   In prior decades, septal body surgery ranged from complex to fantasy. Each surgeon devised a special operation, which was beautifully illustrated, but impossible for other surgeon to do. Fortunately, everything changed with the adoption of cartilage grafts and the need for harvesting large portions of septum. The concept of leaving a 10-mm L-shaped strut for septal support meant that there was essentially no difference between a septal harvest for acquiring graft material and excision of a severely deviated septal body. Suddenly, the technical complexity of parallel cuts and crosshatching became passé. The simplistic, but effective rule has become "when in doubt take it out." The obligatory corollary is to first assess the overall rigidity of the septal cartilage and be conservative when the cartilage is flimsy. One should take out only the necessary amount needed to correct the deflection or to obtain sufficient graft material.

Cartilaginous Correction. Conceptually, the "surgical septal body" is that portion of the septum beneath and behind the critical 10-mm L-shaped strut. Once the definitive dorsum and caudal septum have been established, one measures down and back 10 mm from the anterior septal angle (Fig. 6.4a–d). At this point, the septum is incised with a #15 blade paralleling the dorsum and staying 10 mm below the dorsum all the way back to the bony septum. Then the vertical caudal component is extended downward to the vomerine groove using a #15 blade parallel to the caudal septum while the mucosal leaflets are retracted with a nasal speculum. It is not a vertical cut but rather is angled posteriorly to insure a caudal 1-cm strut at the level of the caudal septum/ANS junction. Next, the inferior border of the cartilaginous septum is freed up along the vomerine groove. Then, the dissection comes downward from the dorsal cut, "popping through" the junction between cartilaginous septum and perpendicular plate of ethmoid. Next, the dissection continues posterior to free the *vomerine extension* of the cartilaginous septum. This extension overlaps the bony septum on one side, which is signaled by the "spur side" of the posterior septum; i.e., most spurs are cartilage on the convex side overlapped by bone. Thus, in a septoplasty one can dissect the cartilage in its entirety or plan to excise the bony spurs with their overlapped cartilage. The harvested cartilage is placed in a large basin of saline with antibiotics.

Bony Resection. With the mucosa elevated on both sides, it is possible to resect any fixed bony deformities using a small Takahashi forceps (Fig. 6.4e, f). These "bony spurs" are sharply "bitten off" with the forceps and not twisted out as the latter will risk disruption of the cribiform plate resulting in a cerebrospinal fluid leak. Correction of the bony septum should emphasize gentle relocation with limited resection. The exception to this rule is the posttraumatic nose where bony resection is obligatory. I am not convinced that trying to straighten the bony septum with a "speculum spread" is a good idea. It may work when the septum is essentially intact, but it risks septal disruption when a septal harvest has been done.

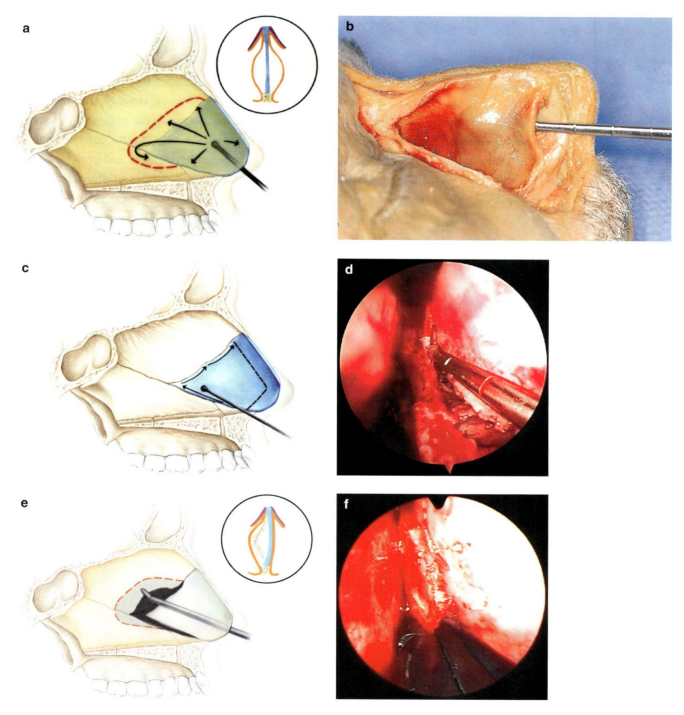

Fig. 6.4 (**a, b**) Septal exposure **DVD** (**c, d**) cartilaginous resection **DVD** (**e, f**) bony resection

Bony Septum/ Premaxilla: The Inferior Tunnel

Routine bony deviations are resected using a small Takahashi forceps (Fig. 6.5 a, b). Whenever possible, straight deflections are fractured back to the midline under direct vision using a Cottle elevator. When the bony deviation involves the premaxillary area, then an "inferior

Dorsal Septum

Dorsal problems are either deviations or asymmetries with the solution often being straightening, bracing, or concealing. Solving these problems requires one to assign specific causes to the various components of the entire osseocartilaginus vault and septum.

Level 1. Dorsal deviations are corrected via an open approach. The upper lateral cartilages are released from the septum to allow adequate septal mobilization, and then asymmetrical spreader grafts are inserted with the wider graft placed on the concave side. Differences in width may range from 0.5 to 3.5 mm with asymmetries of the middle vault often requiring onlay grafts over the upper lateral cartilages.

Level 2. These problems consist of linear or transverse deviations of the dorsal component of the L-shaped strut (Fig. 6.7). Again, any dorsal reduction must be done first followed by septal correction in the body and caudal septum. For transverse deviations or angulations, the upper lateral cartilages are detached from the septum allowing evaluation of the location and severity of the dorsal angulation (Fig. 6.7a). A spreader graft is placed on the concave side to serve as a brace and maintain structural relationships (Fig. 6.7b). It is sutured to the septum above and below the deviation. Then, the angulation in the septum is incised if possible and excised only if necessary (Fig. 6.7c). With the dorsum now straight, a spreader graft is placed on the previously deviated side and sutured as a five-layer "sandwich" incorporating upper lateral cartilages, spreader grafts, and septum (Fig. 6.7d).

For linear deviations/angulations, which result in "dorsal curling," total exposure on both sides is critical. One must carefully analyze the point at which the upper septum begins to curl and whether or not there is sufficient straight septum to fix a brace onto. If possible, a higher (6 mm) spreader graft of minimal width (1 mm) is sutured to the lower straight septum on the convex side extending longitudinally beyond the area of deviation. Then a longitudinal v-incision is made on the concave side of the septum at the point of maximum angulation. Next, the dorsal septum is sutured to the spreader graft and rigid support is provided. A similar spreader graft is placed on the opposite side as a brace across the cut.

Level 3. These cases require a "total septoplasty" and will be discussed in the next section.

Concealment/Camouflage. Although one can camouflage a deviated dorsum with crushed cartilage or a solid dorsal graft, they are rarely effective in the long term. The crushed cartilage will often melt away over time while the solid graft becomes visible as the skin shrink wraps around it. However, the greater problem is that although the dorsum may appear straighter the nose itself remains visibly deviated and the patient dissatisfied. Thus, one falls into a trap of doing a simpler procedure, which is ineffective rather than the more aggressive but more effective one.

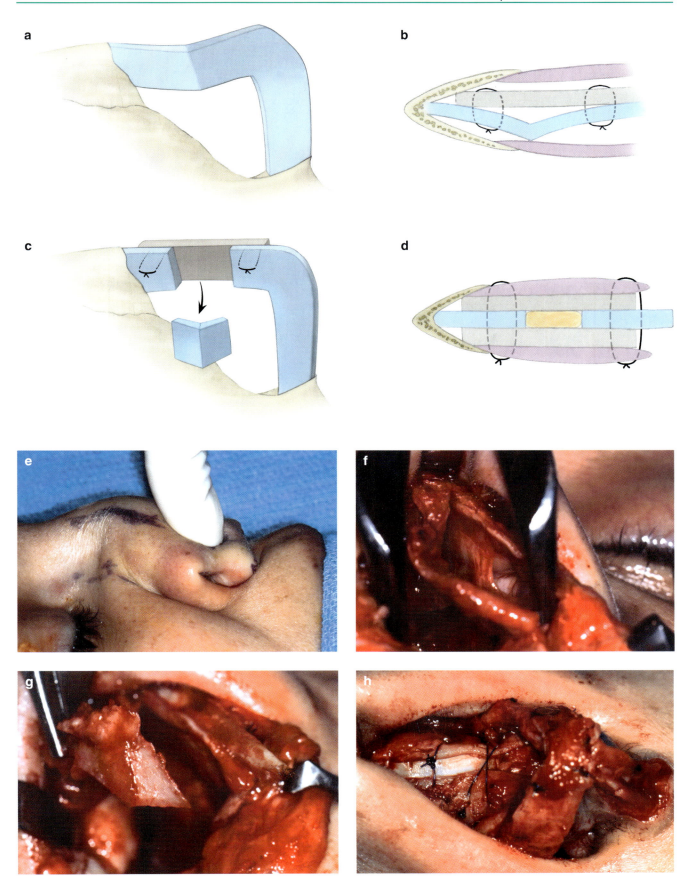

Fig. 6.7 (a–h) Dorsal straightening

Total Septoplasty

At first glance, complete removal of the cartilaginous septum with reinsertion of an L-shaped strut seems excessive and fraught with risk. Yet, the long-term results are excellent and the complications are few. Both Gubisch (2006) and Jugo (1995) have summarized their 20-year experience with total septoplasty in stunning step-by-step publications. The L-shaped strut replacement graft is a direct replica of the dorsal/caudal septum that is always preserved during a septorhinoplasty.

Operative Technique. The following operation is used for severe panseptal deformities (Figs. 6.8 and 6.9).

Step #1 Exposure. A top-down approach allows septal exposure while leaving the membranous septum intact. Extramucosal tunnels are completed and the upper lateral cartilages are detached from the dorsal septum. A top-down dissection is done beginning on the concave side to expose the body of the septum followed by a posterior-to-anterior elevation along the vomerine junction and across the caudal septum. The entire caudal septum–ANS complex must be exposed and any ANS deformity treated. If exposure is inadequate, I do not hesitate to add a "tip split" caudally. In sever cases, bilateral transfixion incisions can be done, which permits a "tip flip" for total access.

Step #2 Excision. Once the septum is completely exposed, I reassess the deformity and operative plan. Assuming total replacement is indicated, the point of deviation along the dorsal cartilaginous septum is defined, and then a vertical cut 10 mm in height is made just above the deviation point. Then, the cut is extended cephalically paralleling the dorsum back to the ethmoid plate. I then release the inferior septum from the ANS back along the premaxillary and vomerine grooves as far posterior as possible. Last, the separation extends upward from the vomer along the ethmoid plate juncture to the cephalic cut. The entire cartilaginous septum is removed.

Step #3 Shaping the Graft. The cartilage is then placed on a towel and its outline traced. In many cases, a pattern can be cut from this diagram; but with the dorsal component elongated for overlap. Then, the specimen is evaluated and a straight L-shaped replacement graft is designed using the previously drawn pattern.

Step #4 Graft Reinsertion. Reinsertion consists of the following steps: (1) the strut is placed in position and assessed, (2) the graft is placed on the side opposite to the preoperative dorsal deviation, (3) the graft overlaps dorsally with the cephalic septal cartilage stump and is held in place with #25 percutaneous needles, (4) fixation to the ANS is done with a 4–0 PDS placed through a drill hole in the ANS and the caudal septum positioned on the side opposite to the preoperative deviation, (5) the graft is sutured to the dorsal septum at two points with 4–0 PDS, (6) a contralateral spreader graft is usually added followed by "sandwich sutures' incorporating the upper laterals and graft, and (7) Doyle splints lubricated with polysporin ointment are sutured into place and left for 10 days.

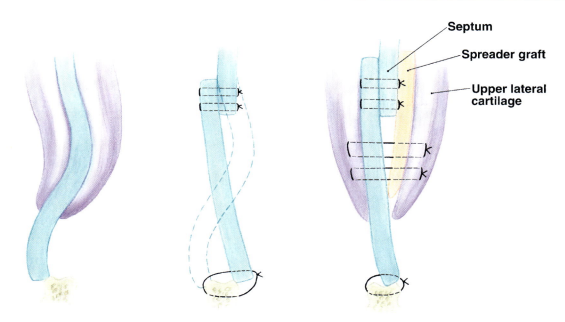

Fig. 6.8 Double shift of septum

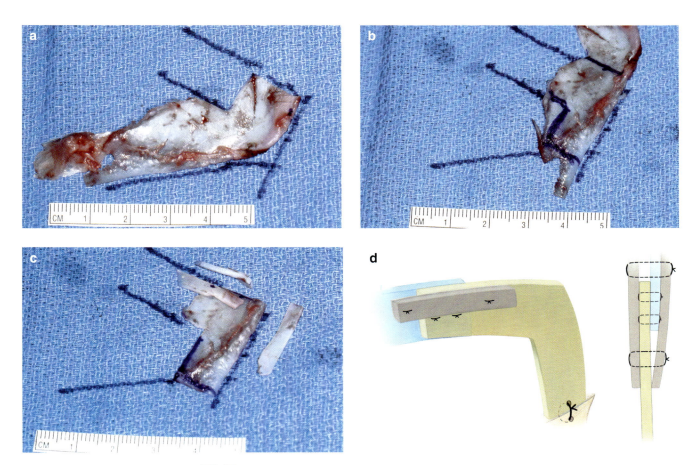

Fig. 6.9 (a–d) Total septoplasty

Nostril Valve   The nostril valve is composed of those structures that form and project into the nostril aperture. The three most common causes of nostril valve collapse in primary cases are caudal septal deviation, alar rim collapse, and nostril narrowing (Fig. 6.10a–c).

Caudal Septal Deviation. As previously discussed, the critical steps for correcting a caudal septal deviation are the following: (1) bilateral submucosal exposure and release of restricting mucosa, (2) analysis of the deformity and structural integrity of caudal septum/ANS, (3) selection of appropriate technique with repositioning being the first choice, (4) complete mobilization of caudal septum, and (5) suture fixation through the ANS in a corrected position.

Alar Rim Collapse. Instability of the alar rim with dynamic collapse may be either isolated or combined. Certain alar cartilage configurations contribute to lateral collapse including boxy and parenthesis tips with their strong cartilages medially and weak alar lobules laterally. In Level 1 cases, alar rim grafts (ARG) of septal cartilage will correct the problem. The grafts measure 3 mm in width, 8–14 mm in length, and are tapered in all dimensions. A small transverse incision is made in the vestibule behind the alar rim and then the recipient pocket is dissected parallel to the rim with blunt tip scissors. The tapered end of the graft is inserted first to provide minimal volume near the dome while the blunt end is hidden within the alar base. In Level 2 cases, alar rim support grafts (ARS) are sutured into true marginal rim incisions. In Level 3 cases, larger grafts of conchal cartilage or even bony septum are inserted. These grafts extend from the alar base and parallel the entire alar rim. In aesthetic cases, it is critical that the graft should not be so wide that it blunts the alar crease separating the alar base from the lobule.

Narrow Nostrils/Wide Columella. Although narrow nostrils may be multifactorial, the wide columellar base is a common causal factor. It is most often produced by divergent footplates of the medial crura and excess intervening soft tissue. A frequent form is the "comma nostril." The technique I currently favor is excision of the intervening soft tissue and suturing the divergent footplates (Fig. 6.10e, f). The technique is as follows: (1) incise the mucosa just above the cephalic border of the footplates, (2) dissect subcutaneously transverse across the columellar base, (3) deliver the intervening muscle (depressor nasalis), (4) resect the muscle using a cautery, (5) place a vertical mattress suture of 5–0 Prolene (yes a permanent suture) between the footplates, and (6) tighten gradually and maintain a sloped columellar base. One can also add columellar shaping sutures of 4–0 clears PDS. Widening nostrils in primary cases is both rare and difficult. ARS grafts are the best solution. I am not an advocate of nostril shaping excisions as the scarring is often significant.

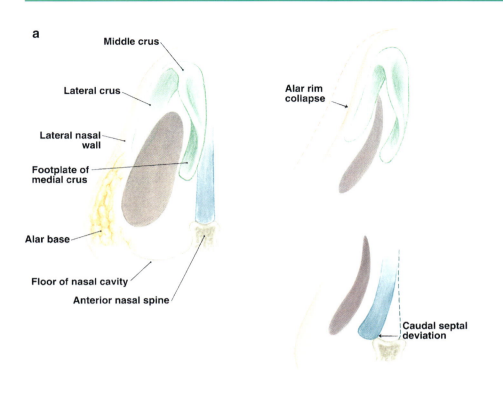

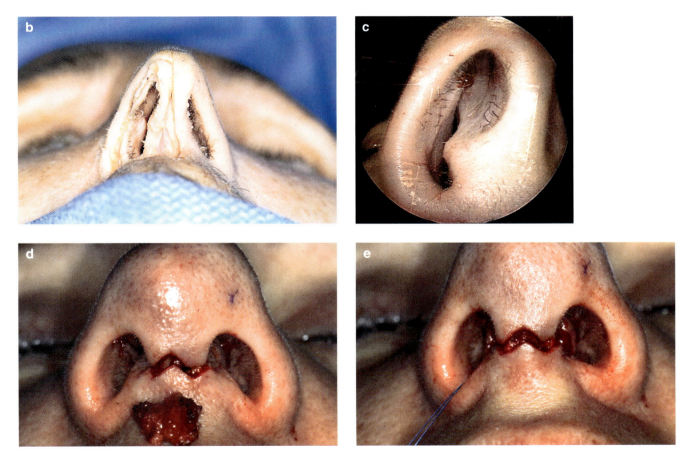

Fig. 6.10 (a–c) Nostril valve **DVD** (**e, f**) narrowing the columellar base

Vestibular Valve   The importance of the nasal vestibule and its role in respiration is well recognized. The classic paper of Cottle (1955) states clearly that the vestibule is an effective series of resistor baffles that slows down the air currents and directs them upward for warming and moistening. However, surgical correction of vestibular valve deformities is only now being extrapolated from secondary to primary cases. Anatomically, the vestibule sits between two narrow apertures – the nostril and os internum (Fig. 6.11). Although a variety of septal problems can impinge, most clinical cases consist of either lateral alar collapse or vestibular webbing with the latter in secondary cases.

Lateral Alar Collapse. There are essentially two types of lateral àlar collapse: the flaccid alar rim as seen in the parenthesis tip and the collapsed lateral crura–accessory cartilage junction. The lateral cartilage junction serves as the major baffle of the vestibule and it can be obstructive. It is important to distinguish the etiology, since a cartilage graft for support is the first choice with excision of the cartilage junction done only when indicated. For combined deformities, I use the following techniques: (1) the area of depression is marked on the skin and then its caudal border transferred internally, (2) the mucosa is injected and the incision made, (3) the mucosa is elevated off of the lateral crura–accessory cartilage junction, (4) a subcutaneous dissection is done, (5) the cartilage junction and any scar tissue is excised, (6) the recipient pocket is dissected down to the pyriform aperture, (7) a reciprocal split of the conchal bowl graft will provide sufficient material for both sides, (8) the wider portion overlaps the pyriform edge while the superior portion is tapered as it nears the alar cartilage, (9) the incision is closed with 5–0 plain catgut and the edge of the graft is incorporated into the suture, (10) a "sandwich splint" of silactic sheeting is placed on either side to decrease the dead space and to force the graft outward, and (11) the splints are removed after 3–5 days to avoid skin damage.

Vestibular Webbing. Traditionally, vestibular webbing was attributed to composite shortening of the upper lateral cartilages. Based on secondary cases, I feel the etiology is more complex and may well be related to contracture and scarring of undermined mucosa. Treatment of vestibular webs is difficult. I vary the operation depending upon the type and extent of the web. Minor webs tend to be thin and are corrected with three-dimensional Z-plasties similar to those used in lengthening a contracted thumb-index web space. Moderate webs tend to be thicker and the web is turned into a medially based flap and the mucosa is elevated from the lateral side wall toward the septum. The mucosal flap will allow restoration of the vestibular atrium and the lateral wall can be closed primarily or a thin mucosal graft applied. For major stenosis, a composite graft harvested from the anterior conchal bowl is inserted through an open approach.

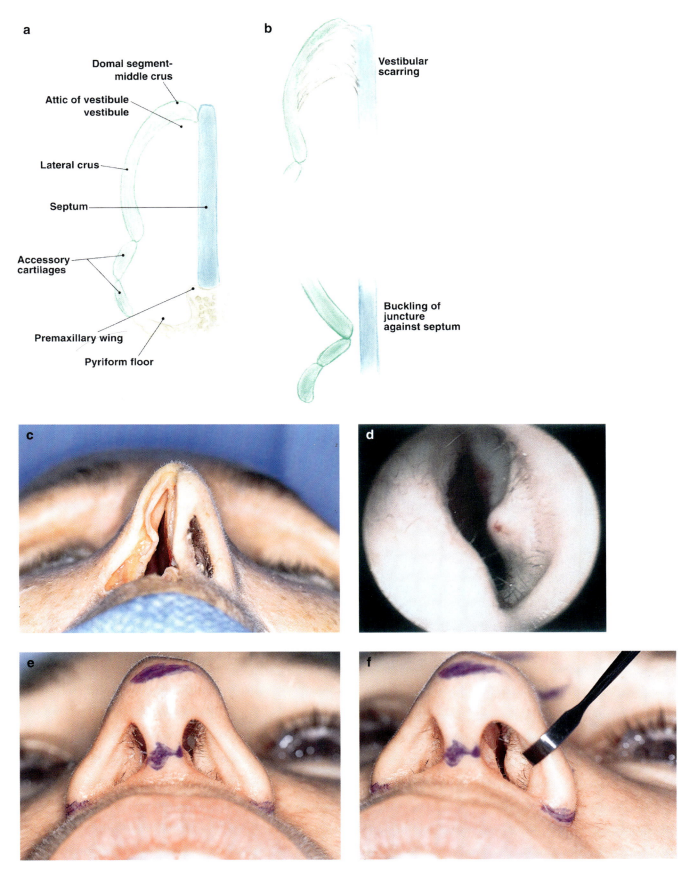

Fig. 6.11 (a–f) Vestibular valve anatomy

Internal Valve   In primary patients, the most common causes of internal valve problems are septal deviation, narrowing of the internal valve angle, turbinate hypertrophy, and lateral wall collapse (Fig. 6.12). Since septal and turbinate surgery are discussed separately, emphasis will be on the other two problems. Clinically, one can diagnose internal valve obstruction by retracting the cheek outward, which should open up the internal valve (positive Cottle test). Intranasal inspection before and after decongestant sprays is critical to determine the specific site of the obstruction.

Internal Valve Collapse (Primary). Arbitrarily, one may discuss "compromise" of the internal valve angle in which the angle is obstructed due to any of its three components: mucosal abnormalities, dorsal septal deviations, or upper lateral cartilage collapse. In most primary cosmetic cases, the etiology is collapse of the upper lateral cartilage against the septum over a vertical distance of several millimeters resulting in marked narrowing of the angle. Although initially asymptomatic, hump reduction followed by lateral osteotomies and shortening of the nose may well tip the balance from asymptomatic to symptomatic nasal obstruction. Preventive treatment with spreader grafts is the solution and should be an integral part of most cosmetic cases. Although discussed elsewhere, the important points in using spreader grafts are as follows: (1) septal cartilage or components of the excised hump are fashioned into "matchstick size" grafts whose width is determined by both functional and asymmetric aesthetic needs, (2) the caudal end does not extend into the angle, but rather forces the upper lateral cartilage outward, and (3) the grafts are sutured into place.

Internal Valve Narrowing (Secondary). In some secondary cases, marked narrowing of the valve is encountered and has the potential for multifactorial etiologies: surgically induced mucosal scarring deficiencies, untreated dorsal septal deviations, and upper lateral cartilage collapse. Obviously, one must correct the cause whether isolated or combined. Sheen evolved the spreader graft as an effective method of restoring the internal valve angle. Although many consider it to be a restoration of normal architecture, it is really a distraction outward of the upper lateral cartilage away from the septum and a lowering/blunting of the mucosal apex which results in a wider valve angle. In cases with an over-resected dorsum, placement of a large dorsal graft will distract the upper lateral cartilages and markedly improve the restoration.

a

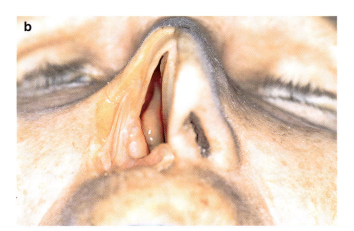

Nasal
valve
angle   10°-15°

Upper lateral
cartilage

Septum

Lateral wall
(fibro-areolar
tissue)

Inferior
turbinate

Floor of
nasal cavity

Anterior
nasal spine

Nasal valve area

ULC
collapse

Mucosa

Septal
bowing

Lateral wall
collapse

Inferior
turbinate
hypertrophy

Septal
deviation

b

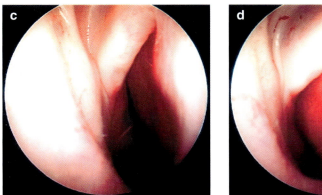

c 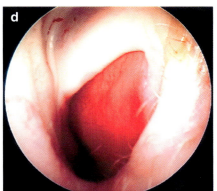   **d**

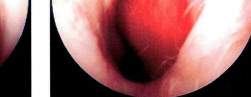

Fig. 6.12 (a–d) Internal valve **DVD**

Bony Valve   The concept of a bony valve evolved during examination of secondary rhinoplasty patients and was then confirmed in primary posttraumatic noses. In secondary rhinoplasty patients, excessive verticalization of the lateral bony wall can occur especially after medial osteotomies. In primary cases, the usual cause is trauma where the lateral wall is compressed against the septum. It is only by mobilizing the bone outward that one can open the airway.

Diagnosis. During the intranasal examination, one can see that the internal valve is blocked by a verticalization of the upper lateral cartilage. However, when the upper lateral cartilage is elevated, it is obvious that the airway is still blocked by the lateral bony wall. The etiology is primarily *medial movement and increased verticality* of the bony lateral wall; both of which compromise and narrow the nasal passageway. The importance of this diagnosis is that one cannot correct the problem with just spreader grafts.

Surgical Treatment. To correct the problem, one must mobilize the bony lateral wall outward to alleviate the narrowing. To achieve total mobilization of the bony wall, one often has to do medial oblique, transverse, and low-to-low osteotomies. Once the osteotomies are completed, a Boise elevator is then placed in the nose and the lateral wall moved outward and angulated. With concurrent external finger palpation, the surgeon can feel the bone being brought upward and outward. Stabilization in the desired position requires major spreader grafts extending high into the bony vault to force the wall outward. Doyle splints with the dorsal flange cut off permit the tube portion to be put high in the airway and provide outward distraction for 2–3 weeks.

In sever cases of instability, it may be necessary to place a pair of parallel drill holes in each nasal bone. The spreader grafts are then brought high into the bony vault and fixed with a #25 needle through the most cephalic holes. The distal portion of the spreader grafts are sutured to the ULCs or a strut. Then, a 4–0 PDS suture is placed through the caudal holes in the nasal bones and tied in an overlapping fashion. Then the upper needle is removed and a second suture is placed through the cephalic holes. These two sutures will stabilize the bony pyramid.

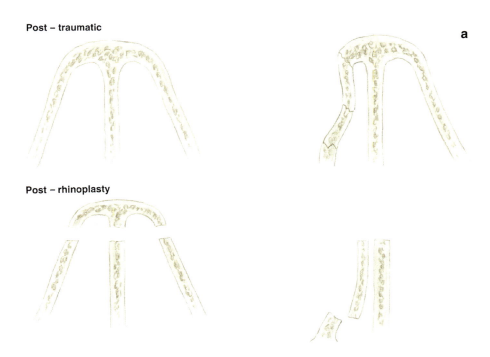

Post – traumatic

Post – rhinoplasty

a

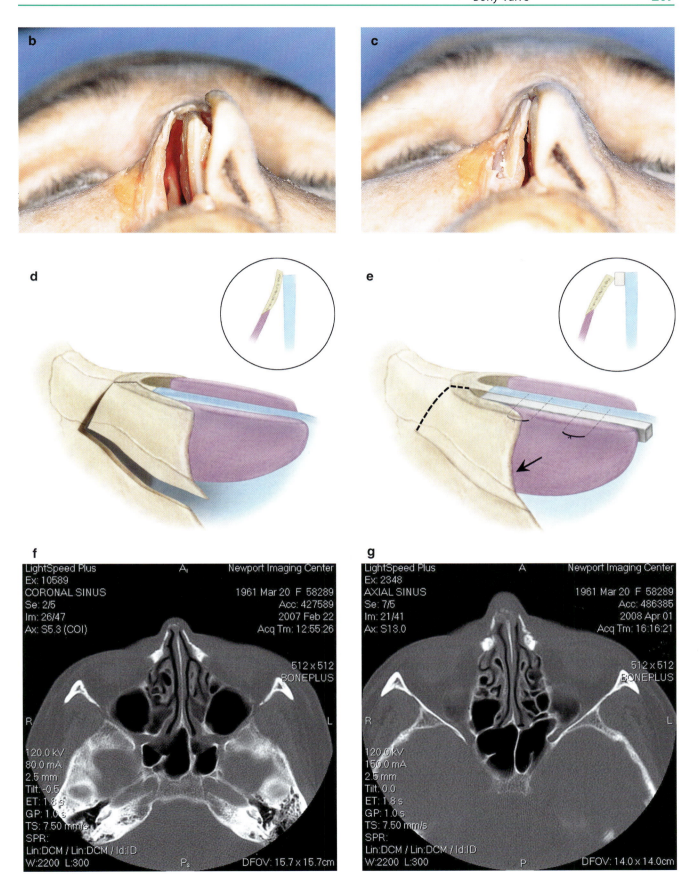

Fig. (**a**) Etiology of bony valve obstruction, (**b, c**) bony valve blockage (**d, e**) mobilizing bony wall with outward fixation using spreader grafts, (**f, g**) preop and postop CT-Scan with opening of the bony valve

Turbinates The inferior turbinate is a dynamic structure, which diverts nasal air flow and provides primary resistance (Fig. 6.13a). The head of the inferior turbinate is quite large (14 mm in height), extremely dynamic, and located in the critical internal valve *area*. The inferior turbinate is closest to the septum in its midportion before diverging away from the septum posteriorly. Examination of the nose with anterior rhinoscopy should focus on the size, shape, and color of the turbinates as well as the nasal mucosa and mucus. Next, the nose is vasoconstricted (Afrin) and anesthetized (tetracaine) with topical sprays. After several minutes, the patient is asked if the obstruction is improved. Complete relief indicates mucosal congestion, whereas partial improvement focuses attention on anatomical causes. On reexamination, failure of the turbinate to shrink most often indicates bony hypertrophy.

Indications. Ultimately, inferior turbinectomy is done in three groups of aesthetic patients: (1) unilateral compensatory hypertrophy associated with septal deviation, (2) chronic bilateral hypertrophy, and (3) preventative resection.

Technique. In most cases, I perform a partial anterior inferior turbinectomy (hereinafter: turbinectomy) near the end of the procedure as it minimizes any disruptive bleeding and allows immediate insertion of splints as required (Fig. 6.13b). The exceptions are cases of massive bony hypertrophy where access to the septum and airway mandates early excision. The disadvantage of performing turbinectomy after lateral osteotomies is the intraturbinate swelling that occurs after the lateral osteotomies. The preoperative plan is checked against the intraoperative finding and a final decision is made as to how the anterior middle and posterior portions will be treated. If the posterior obstruction is due to simple medial displacement of the inferior turbinate, then a lateral outfracture is done. The advantage of doing the outfracture at this point is that it allows confirmation of the diagnosis and permits subsequent alternative treatment if necessary.

Then the head of the turbinate is injected with 1–2 cc of local anesthesia. As modified from Mabry (1988), an incision is made in the head of the turbinate and the mucosa is elevated over a distance of 2 cm. Then using a modified Greunwald forceps, the hypertrophic glandular and bony tissue is excised submucosally. If the posterior portion is hypertrophied, then the prongs of the Elmed bipolar coagulator are inserted through the incision. Coagulation occurs between the two needle electrodes thereby reducing its size. Anteriorly, the redundant mucosa is excised from the lateral portion, which allows creation of a smaller "neoturbinate." The mucosa is then closed with one to two 5–0 plain catgut sutures. In all cases, an internal splint is used although three variations exist: (1) silastic sheet without side tubes for turbinectomy alone, (2) silastic sheet with side tubes for turbinectomy and concomitant septal correction, and (3) silastic sheet with gelfoam for extensive turbinectomy and in most males. The splints are removed after 7 days.

Problems

The three most common postoperative problems are bleeding, synechiae, and long-term failure. Bleeding after turbinectomy is a reality with ranges from 2% to 14% of patients but 5–6% is an accepted norm. It is tempting to speculate that the incidence of bleeding is related to the amount of excision especially in the highly vascular posterior region. Since I do not perform an extensive posterior resection, I was able to avoid a postoperative bleeding for almost 8 years. Subsequently, I had three in the last 6 months; two of which occurred when I did not use gelfoam in extensive resections and the other was patient medication induced. Immediate control was achieved in the office by removing the silastic splint and inserting an expansible splint (RhinoRocket) plus anxiety reduction with chlorpromazine. Reoperation or posterior packing was not necessary. The rate of synechiae formation ranges from 4% to 22% with reoperation occasionally required. This problem is easily avoided by the use of intranasal splints, which are left in for 7 days.

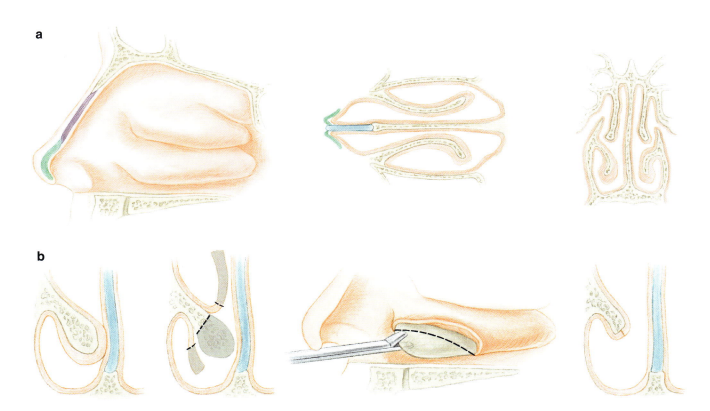

Fig. 6.13 (**a**) Turbinate anatomy, (**b**) submucosal resection

The functional result of a rhinoplasty is as important as the aesthetic result, a fact easily confirmed in dealing with secondary patients.

Nasal History. Nasal obstruction is a term, which is frequently used, but rarely defined. Nasal obstruction can be considered an alteration of normal function, which correlates with an increase in nasal resistance. The diagnosis is made by history and rhinoscopic examination. Question regarding onset, duration, frequency, exacerbating, and remitting factors, as well as the character and frequency of rhinorrhea are important in distinguishing allergic from anatomical nasal obstruction. Equally, one must pay careful attention to medications, environmental factors, as well as previous trauma or surgery. The most common symptoms are nasal stuffiness, postnasal drip, and recurrent bilateral sinusitis.

Nasal Exam. The patient is examined in the sitting position. I have the following instruments available: (1) a standardized examination sheet, (2) a fiber optic headlight, (3) Afrin and xylocaine sprays, (4) a nasal speculum and alar rim retractor, (5) cotton tip applicators, and (6) an endoscope. The external nose is examined in resting and deep inspiration for deviation, deformities, and dynamic collapse, as well as scars and skin conditions. A two-staged internal examination is done on both sides before and after vasoconstriction (Fig. 6.14). It is important to examine the nostril/vestibule and internal valve angle using an alar rim retractor rather than a speculum to avoid distortion of the structures. The valve angle is inspected during normal and deep inspiration. The turbinates are assessed for size, color, and surface changes. The septum is evaluated for deviations, displacements, and impactions. The mucosal lining is observed as well as the mucous. The findings are recorded and then the nose is sprayed with a decongestant. One is trying to eliminate the effect of mucosal congestion, which should reveal underlying fixed anatomical deformities. The internal exam is repeated and the operative plan for the internal nose is recorded.

Operative Planning. Most body deviations of the septum are corrected during the septal harvest. Caudal septal deviations are relocated away from the deviated side and routinely fixed to the ANS using a suture through a drill hole. Spreader grafts are the definitive treatment for internal valve collapse while preventing an inverted-V deformity. In general, I prefer out-fracturing of the inferior turbinates and reserve resection for cases of 3 + fixed hypertrophy or compensatory hypertrophy. In severe septal deviations, I have not been impressed with how quickly a compensatory hypertrophy resolves and feel that definitive turbinate reduction concomitant with septoplasty is warranted.

Septum CARTILAGINOUS GRADE I-V	
BODY	
CAUDAL	
DORSUM	
BONY DEFORMITY	

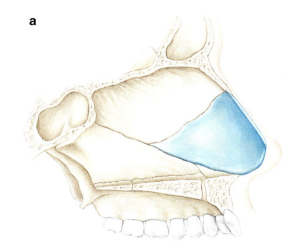

a

Turbinates GRADE I-IV	R	L
ANTERIOR MUCOSA BONE		
POSTERIOR MUCOSA BONE		

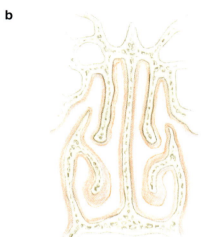

b

Valves	R	L
NOSTRIL		
VESTIBULAR		
INTERNAL ANGLE AREA		
BONY		

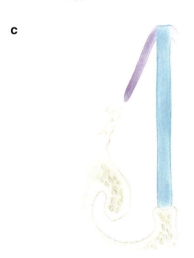

c

Fig. 6.14 (**a–c**) Intranasal exam

Case Study: Septal Deviation

Analysis

A 32-year-old woman presented with a history of marked nasal obstruction worse on the left than the right. There was no history of nasal trauma. Aesthetically, the patient wanted refinement of her existing nose rather than a significant change. Functionally, this case required all four of the basic techniques in Level 1 surgery. The caudal septum had to be relocated L to R and fixed to the ANS. The severe body deviation was resected and truly measured 14 mm across. The internal valves were opened with spreader grafts, which were asymmetric for aesthetic reasons. The markedly hypertrophic right inferior turbinate was partially resected including the bony hypertrophy. At 14 months post-op, her respiration is markedly improved (Fig. 6.15).

Operative Technique

1) Open approach
2) Incremental dorsal reduction (bone 0.5, cartilage 1.0)
3) A 5 mm caudal septal resection
4) Bidirectional septal exposure via transfixion incision and dorsum
5) Resection of quadrilateral cartilage and some vomerine bone
6) Caudal septal relocation L to R with suture fixation to ANS
7) Unilatreral L low-to-high osteotomy, no R osteotomy
8) Asymmetric spreader grafts (R 2.0, L 3.5)
9) Crural strut and tip sutures: CS, DC, DE, and TP
10) Partial resection of R inferior turbinate including bone

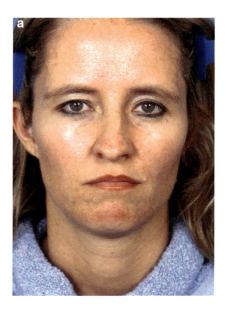
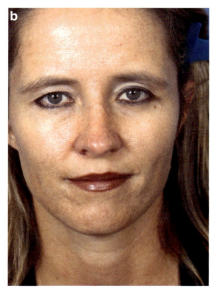
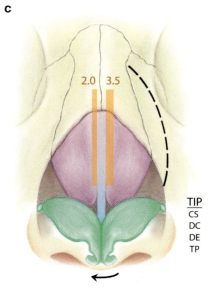

Fig. 6.15 (a–j)

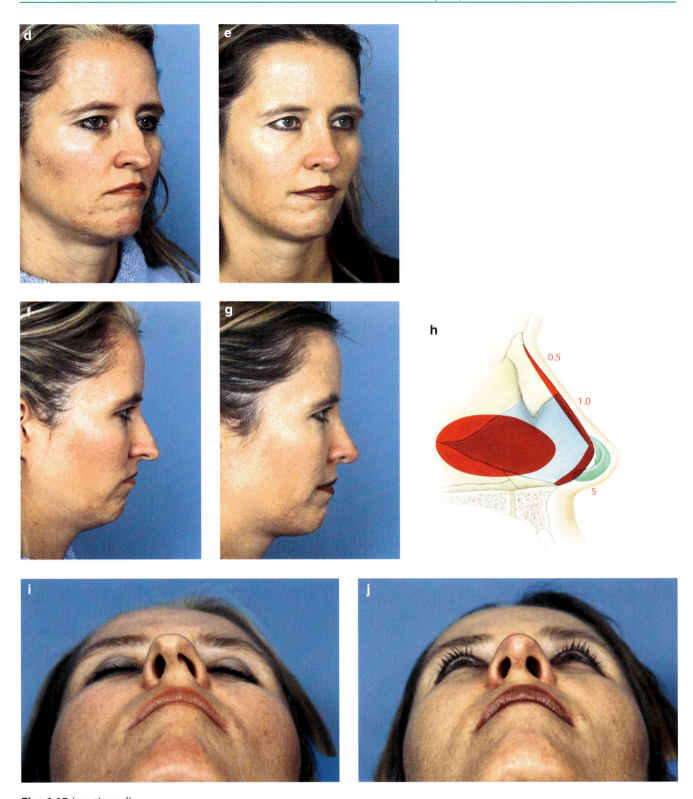

Fig. 6.15 (continued)

**Decision Making
Level 2**

These cases require a greater degree of sophistication, which is based on the building blocks from Level 1 surgery.

Advanced Septal Surgery. Straightening most dorsal deviations requires relocating the caudal septum first and then insertion of asymmetric spreader grafts. In more complex cases, a portion of the dorsal L-shaped strut will need to be resected (Fig. 6.16a). The three-step approach requires the following: (1)insertion of a single spreader graft on the concave side, (2) controlled excision of the deviated portion of dorsal septum, and (3) insertion of the second spreader graft with rigid five-layer fixation. The critical step is to get the septal strut stabilized before resecting any of the dorsal limb of the L-shaped strut. In the most severe posttraumatic and congenital ADDN cases, total septoplasty is warranted (Fig. 6.16b). The entire cartilaginous septum is removed, an L-shaped strut is created, followed by reinsertion with fixation to the ANS and dorsum. The caudal fixation is similar to a caudal septal relocation and the dorsal portion is a five-layer sandwich similar to that of repairing a dorsal disjunction.

Valvular Surgery. One must become comfortable with both alar rim grafts (ARG) and alar rim support grafts (ARS). These are essentially the same grafts, but the former is placed in a subcutaneous pocket following the alar rim, whereas the latter is sutured along the nostril rim via a separate rim incision. The choice of grafts is simple – an ARG is done unless the deformity is so severe that an ARS is required. Also, if the ARG does not work, then remove it, make a true rim incision and sew it in along the nostril border as an ARS. One of the more complex questions is the role of lateral crura strut grafts and the way in which they compare to alar batten grafts? I tend to think of the lateral crural strut grafts as a very precise graft designed to provide support to the lateral crura. As will be discussed in Chapter 8, there are three variations of alar extenders depending upon the orientation of the graft's distal end. One is restoring the tripod leg and providing support to the external valve. These thin grafts (4–5 mm wide) are sutured to the undersurface of the lateral crura medially. The lateral portion is inserted into one of three locations: pyriform, alar base, or nostril rim depending upon indication. In contrast, most alar batten grafts are quite large (15–20 × 8–12) and are used to support the entire lateral lobule.

Turbinates. The first choice for reducing turbinate obstruction is to out-fracture the turbinates. Turbinate resection is reserved for massively enlarged turbinates or those with compensatory hypertrophy.

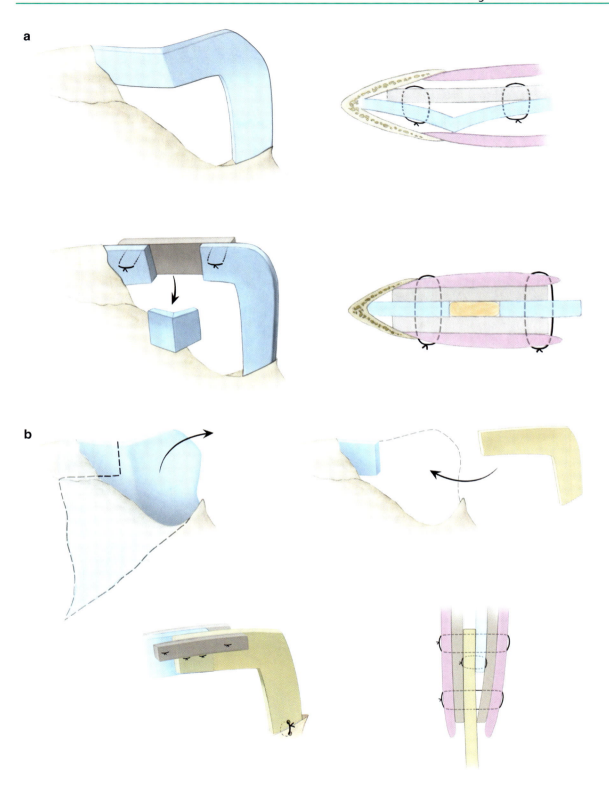

Fig. 6.16 (**a**) Dorsal straightening, (**b**) total septoplasty

Analysis

A 31-year-old woman presented with a history of nasal trauma at age 15 (Fig. 6.17). Intranasally, the caudal septum was deviated to the right while the body was deviated to the left. Since the external pyramid was also deviated, a total septoplasty with double shift reposition was planned. Based on my experience, any septal procedure short of a *total septoplasty* would not correct this degree of deviation. Removal of the septum eliminates the constricting septal and mucosal forces allowing a straight L-shaped strut to be configured and reinserted. Note: the septal replacement graft is a true *septal replacement* and not a septal extender graft. It is the addition of a columellar strut that gives the tip support and allows it to rise above the septum thereby avoiding a flat wide tip.

Operative Technique

1) Open approach with detachment of the upper lateral cartilages.
2) A right transfixion incision. Bidirectional septal exposure.
3) Incremental dorsal reduction (bone: smooth, cartilage 1.5 mm).
4) Caudal septum shortened 3 mm, but 7 mm at its most prominent.
5) Total septal excision leaving a 10 mm long dorsal component.
6) Immediate drawing of caudal septum, then 90° turn, and cut L-shaped replacement plus columellar and bilateral spreader grafts.
7) Transverse and low-to-low osteotomies, plus a double level on L.
8) Septal replacement graft inserted as a "double shift": caudal to left, dorsal to the right. Braced with spreader grafts.
9) Insertion of a columellar strut plus tip sutures (CS, DC, ID, TP).
10) Nostril sill excisions (R:2, L:3.5). Doyle splints for 12 days.

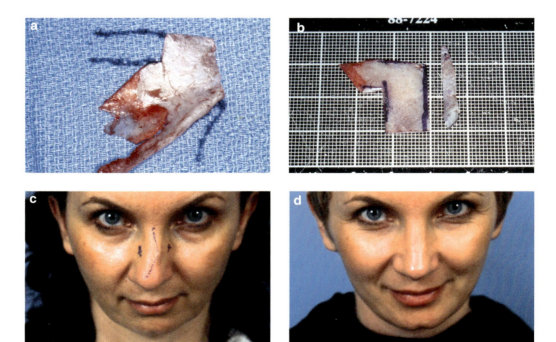

Fig. 6.17 (a–l)

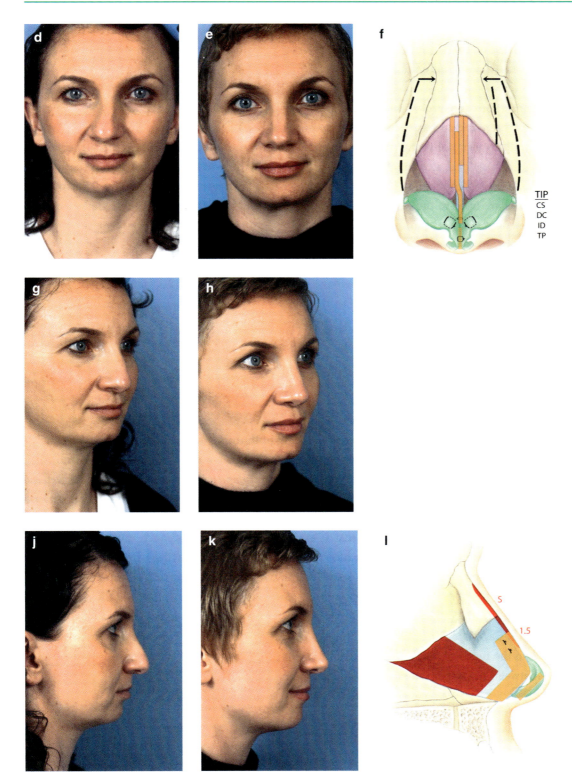

Fig. 6.17 (continued)

Case Study: Septal Support Surgery

Analysis

A 21-year-old student presented with a posttraumatic nasal deformity following an accidental blow to the nose (Fig. 6.20). She noted a significant flattening of the nose and rounding of the nasal tip and nostrils during the first 6 months. She had a positive septal collapse test. She was nasally obstructed due to septal deviation and intranasal polyps. Since the patient's septum was intact prior to the trauma, sufficient septum was expected, but the patient did give consent for a rib graft. Septal support and nasal appearance were restored using interlocked extended spreader grafts and a structural columellar strut. The angulation of the grafts restored the aesthetic dorsal profile line while the rigid fixation to the columellar strut provided septal support.

Operative Technique

1) Exposure and evaluation of the septum via a transfixion incision.
2) Open approach and reduction of alar cartilages to 6 mm strips.
3) Excision of septal body to correct obstruction and provide graft material.
4) Transverse and low-to-low osteotomies.
5) Separation of ULC for insertion of extended spreader grafts.
6) Insertion of a structural columellar graft.
7) Fixation of spreader grafts to columellar strut on an angled basis to restore dorsal profile line.
8) Fixation of alars to columellar strut, with CS .
9) Tip shaping with DC, DE.

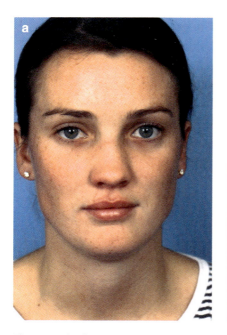
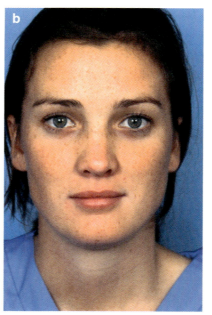
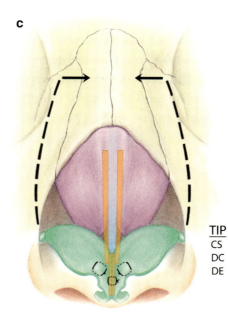

Fig. 6.20 (a–j)

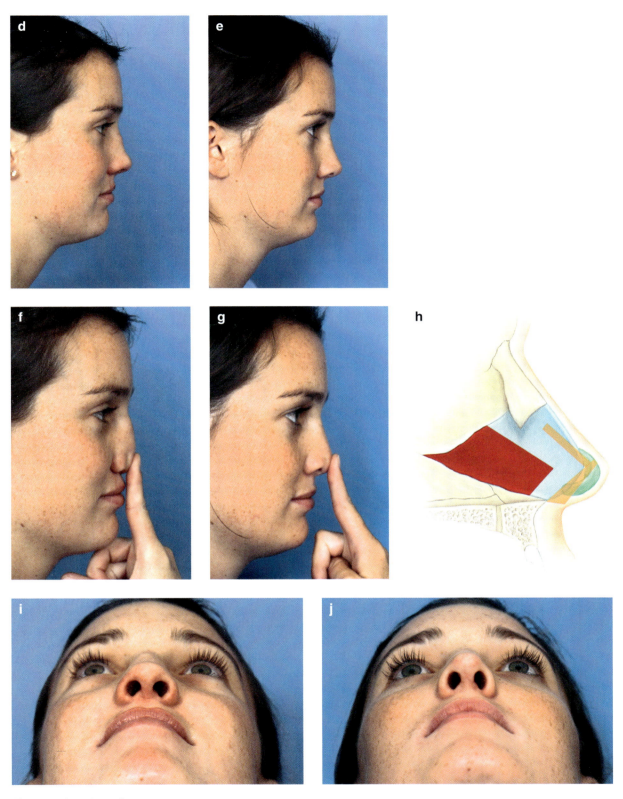

Fig. 6.20 (continued)

Technical Misadventures

Septal Disjunction. When the dorsal septum is divided or broken at the bony–cartilaginous junction the result is an unstable nose. One can encounter this problem for the first time in dealing with a twisted posttraumatic nose. The dorsum is reduced, the septum is exposed, and pressure is put on the cephalic bony septum to straighten it. Suddenly, the septum breaks at the bony–cartilaginous junction and one sees the cartilaginous septum slowly fall into the pyriform aperture – that is, a septal disjunction (Fig. 6.21). One should not panic. Rather, just assumes that a 10 mm L-shaped strut is present, but broken. If the body of the septum was previously harvested, then one fashions bilateral spreader grafts from the septum. Otherwise conchal cartilage is obtained. The goal will be to realign the strut components and brace them on either side with spreader grafts. Then two five-layer sutures are used to brace the septal division with the upper laterals in effect providing support for the strut. As seen in Fig. 6.21, I had harvested the septal body for spreader grafts in a very deviated nose and mobilized the caudal septum for relocation. Then I put pressure on the bony septum and heard a crack. As the L-shaped strut dropped into the pyriform aperture, I overcame my "photo phobia" and took a very rare picture – the patient's L-shaped strut on the backtable prior to reinsertion plus the previously resected septal body. As seen in the postoperative result, the nose was definitely straight and I was greatly relieved.

Mucosal Tears. Inevitably, one will make a significant mucosal tear, usually at the convex bony–cartilaginous vomerine junction or over a pointed septal spur. For small anterior tears, direct suture through the nostril is not difficult if one uses a small M-1 (#742) needle with 4–0 plain catgut. As the tears become larger and more posterior, I find the repair much simpler if I have used an open approach and can repair it from the top on the "septal side" rather than going through the nostril. However, when the tear is quite posterior and one must tie the suture deep in the dark, then I use Drumheller's "lasso technique"(Fig. 6.22). It consists of the following steps: (1) use the M-1 needle, (2) take the end of the suture and tie a surgeon's knot around the end of the suction tip (Fig. 6.22), (3) slip the suture off the suction tip leaving the circular "lasso," (4) using a bayonet needle holder, insert the needle across the cephalicend of the mucosal tear, (5) bring the needle out of the nostril and pass it thru the "lasso" (Fig. 6.21b), (6) place tension on the suture pulling the lasso into the nose snugging it down, and (7) continue sewing until the tear is closed and a knot can be tied anteriorly near the nostril aperture. The beauty of the lasso technique is its simplicity and avoidance of tearing the mucosa as one attempts to tie a knot deep in the nose.

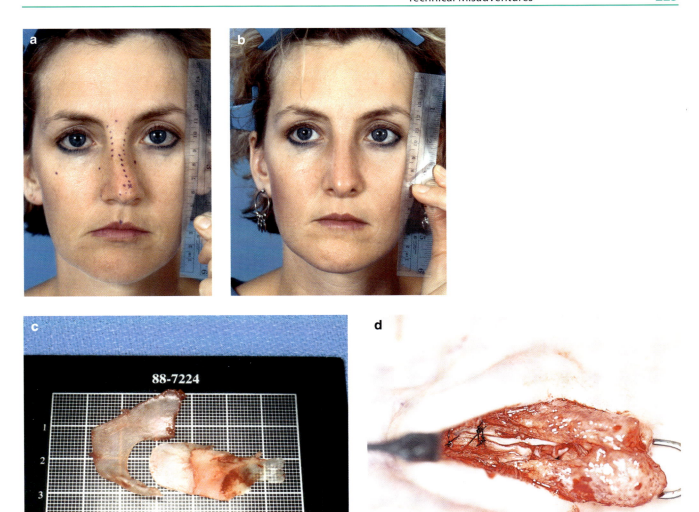

Fig. 6.21 (**a**) preop (**b**) 1 year postop, (**c**) septal disjunction (*left*) and septal harvest (*right*), (**d**) reinsertion

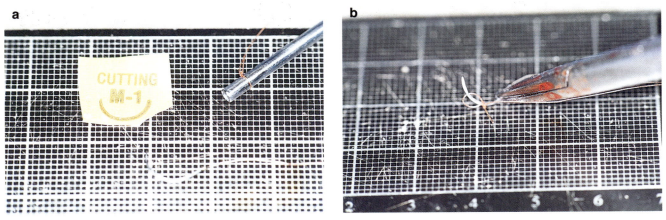

Fig. 6.22 (**a, b**) Repair of mucosal tears

Reading List

Adamson P, Smith O, Cole P. The effect of cosmetic rhinoplasty on nasal patency. Laryngoscope 100: 357, 1990

Bridger OP. Physiology of the nasal valve. Arch Otolaryngol 92: 54, 1970

Cole P. Nasal and oral airflow resistors. Site, function, and assessment. Arch Otolaryngol Head Neck Surg 118: 790, 1992

Constantian MB. The incompetent external nasal valve: pathophysiology and treatment in primary and secondary rhinoplasty. Plast Reconstr Surg 93: 919, 1994

Constantinides MS, Adamson PA, Cole P. The long-term effects of open cosmetic septorhinoplasty on nasal air flow. Arch Otolaryngol Head Neck Surg 122: 41, 1996

Cottle MH. The structure and function of the nasal vestibule. Arch Otolaryngol 62: 173, 1955

Cottle MH, Loring RM, Fischer GO, Gaynon IE. The "maxilla-premaxilla" approach to extensive nasal septum surgery. Arch Otolaryngol 68: 301, 1958

Daniel RK, Regnault P. Aesthetic Plastic Surgery: Rhinoplasty. Boston, MA: Little, Brown, 1993

Goldman JL. (ed). The Principles and Practice of Rhinology. New York: Wiley, 1987

Grymer LF, Hilberg O, Elbrond O, Pedersen OF. Acoustic rhinometry: evaluation of the nasal cavity with septal deviations, before and after septoplasty. Laryngoscope 99: 1 180, 1989

Gubisch, W. Twenty-five years experience with extracorporeal septoplasty. Facial Plast Surg 22: 230, 2006 (Note: entire Journal issue is devoted to septal surgery)

Gubisch W, Constantinescu HL. Refinements in extracoporeal septoplasty. Plast Reconstr Surg 104: 1131, 1999

Guyruron, B, Uzzo, CD, Scull H. A practical classification of septonasal deviation and effective guide to septal surgery. Plast Reconstr Surg 104: 2202, 1999

Haight JS, Cole P. The site and function of the nasal valve. Laryngoscope 93: 49, 1983

Haraldsson PO, Nordemar H, Anggard A. Long-term results after septal surgery submucous resection versus septoplasty. ORL J Otorhinolaryngol Relat Spec 49: 218, 1987

Jackson LE, Koch RJ. Controversies in the management of inferior turbinate hypertrophy: a comprehensive review. Plast Recosntr Surg 103: 300, 1999

Jost O. Post-traumatic nasal deformities. In: Regnault P, Daniel RK (eds) Aesthetic Plastic Surgery. Boston, MA: Little, Brown, 1984

Jugo SB. Total septal reconstruction through decortication (external) approach in children. Arch Otolaryngol Head Neck Surg 1113: 173–178, 1987

Jugo SB. Surgical Atlas of External Rhinoplasty. Edinburgh: Churchill, Livingstone, 1995

Kern EB, Wang TD. Nasal valve surgery. In: Daniel RK (ed) Aesthetic Plastic Surgery: Rhinoplasty. Boston, MA: Little, Brown, 1993

Lawson W, Reino AJ. Correcting functional problems. Facial Plast Surg 2: 501, 1994

Mabry RL. Inferior turbinoplasty: patient selection, technique, and long-term consequences. Otolaryngol Head Neck Surg 98: 60, 1988

McCaffrey TV, Kern EB. Clinical evaluation of nasal obstruction. A study of 1,000 patients. Arch Otolaryngol 105: 542, 1979

Mosher, JP. The premaxillary wings and deviations of the septum. Laryngoscope 17: 840, 1907

Pallanch JF, McCaffrey TV, Kern EB. Normal nasal resistance. Otolaryngol Head Neck Surg 93: 778, 1985

Pastornek NJ, Becker DG. Treating the caudal septal deflection, Arch Facial Plast Surg 2: 217, 2000

Pollock RA, Rohrich RJ. Inferior turbinate surgery: an adjunct to successful treatment of nasal obstruction in 408 patients. Plast Reconstr Surg 74: 227, 1984. Follow-up Pollock, RA, Rohrich, RJ. Inferior turbinectomy surgery; an adjunct to success Plast Reconstr Surg 108: 536, 2001

Sheen, JH. Spreader grafts: a method of reconstructing the roof of the middle vault following rhinoplasty. Plast Reconstr Surg 73: 230, 1984

Warwick-Brown NP, Marks NJ. Turbinate surgery: how effective is it? A long-term assessment. ORL J Otorhinolaryngol Relat Spec 49: 314, 1987

Grafts 7

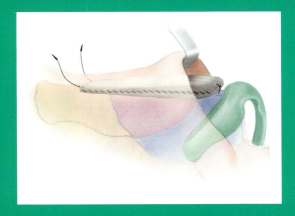

Introduction

After inserting several thousand grafts during rhinoplasty surgery, I have come to ten conclusions. First, grafts must be an integral part of analysis and operative planning, not an intraoperative necessity. For example, the decision to do a radix graft will influence the amount of dorsal reduction. Second, one must be adept at using all types of donor materials and not be dependent on just one. Although septum is usually sufficient in primary cases, it is often insufficient in complex secondaries thereby making rib grafts essential. Third, one should be able to harvest a graft quickly. If it is difficult to take a graft, then one will often rationalize why it is not needed. Four, graft shaping and recipient bed preparation are of equal importance. Five, the less done to a graft the better it is. I am dubious of the long-term survival of crushed and even bruised cartilage grafts. Six, fixation of the graft most often requires sutures during an open approach, as one does not have the tight pockets of the closed approach. Seven, antibiotic coverage is important including an intravenous dose during the operation and 5 days postoperatively. Eight, alloplasts may be a shortcut for the surgeon, but it increases the risk of failure for the patient. Nine, autogenous grafts rarely extrude, can withstand infection, and have definitely stood the test of time. One only needs to contrast the efficacy of autogenous cartilage versus the inevitable absorption of cadaver cartilage. Ten, grafts have dramatically improved the quality of our rhinoplasty results, allowing for a more natural functional primary result, and a heretofore unobtainable nonoperative look in secondary cases.

Allure of Alloplasts

The instant availability, absence of donor site morbidity requirements, adaptability, spectacular early results, as well as reduced cost and minimal surgical skills make alloplasts highly desirable. Yet their problems with infection, extrusion, displacement, mobility, and long-term failure are critical disadvantages. Three factors must be assessed: biocompatability of material, surgical application, and long-term result. Most alloplasts are quickly embraced only to be rejected once problems appear. Beekhuis (1974) championed Supramid mesh as a "miracle of modern chemistry" and an ideal material for nasal dorsal augmentation. Early problems were attributed to either technical error or poor patient selection. A decade later, surgeons reported disappearance of the material and biopsies showed its degradation. The second challenge is patient selection. In contrast to the favorable primary Asian nose, most surgeons need a dorsal graft for their secondary cases with a nonfavorable recipient bed. Thus, the implant is placed in a "subdermal" scarred nonvascular bed rather than a "subcutaneous" pocket. The third factor involves early versus long-term results. One of the more intriguing transformations in results is in the use of cadaver cartilage. Schuller et al. (1977) reported a complication rate of 5.5% early, 2% late, and partial absorption of 1.4% at 3-year follow-up. Subsequently, Welling et al. (1988) reviewed 42 of Shuller's original 107 patients and found that 100% of the grafts were absorbed when in place longer than 10 years. What is the rhinoplasty surgeon to do – alloplasts, yes or no? Based on 70 years of nasal surgery, alloplasts in the nose do not have a good track record, especially on the dorsum and in secondary cases. Therefore, I personally have decided to use only autogenous tissue in the nose. For this patient, the eyes convey the early happiness of an alloplastic dorsal implant and the misery that followed its failure 6 months later (Fig. 7.1).

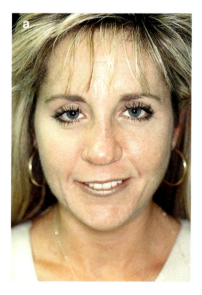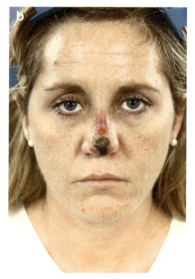

Fig. 7.1 (**a**) early result, (**b**) infected alloplast graft 6 months later

Fillers: Fantastic or Fantasy?

Most experienced rhinoplasty surgeons do not use allografts for one simple reason – they have seen too many disasters from Porex, silicone, Goretex, etc. Currently, we are faced with a new challenge – injectable fillers. As with previous promises of simple spectacular solutions to complex deformities, one should evaluate the consequences, both immediate and long term.

Advantages. The ability to correct localized depressions and blend in prominences is the most attractive aspect of fillers. If valid, it would mollify patients and possibly reduce revisions. The idea of major augmentation with fillers would help secondary patients with limited economic resources.

Disadvantages. I see the "filler influence" creating major problems for rhinoplasty patients and surgeons. For the patients, it will be a combination of false promises, competency, and results. Many patients want to believe that a "lunchtime rhinoplasty" is possible, but do they really understand that it is transitory? How can a *nonsurgeon* really understand what an "open roof" is in a secondary rhinoplasty patient? How exactly can the filler be placed below the dermis, but above the mucosa? For most injectors, it is a technical impossibility. I have personally seen the complications of skin slough and fungating infection following Radiesse injections in secondary cases. Just how long will the patient be happy, especially as the improvement fades? Will the injector then be under pressure to go up the ladder of permanency – Restalyne, Radiesse, Articol, or Silicone? For the rhinoplasty surgeon, there will be challenges throughout the perioperative period. Pre-op, many nonsurgeons and less-experienced surgeons will balloon out a deformed secondary nose in hopes of satisfying the patient. The result is a nose that is now a double disaster and may require a two-stage approach – Op #1 to remove the filler, Op #2 to reconstruct the nose. Intra-op, surgeons who are also injectors will see their commitment to operative perfection challenged and perhaps compromised. A little voice will be whispering: "Oh, I can smooth that area out later with a little filler, I don't really need to remove that graft or take a fascia graft." Short cuts are hard to resist. What do I suggest? I remain skeptical of fillers and do not use them. However, I remain seduced by their simplicity and hope that others will prove me wrong. For that reason, I have included a section on fillers written by experts in the section on revisions in Chapter 9. **Note: none of the patients in this text has had fillers put in their nose to enhance their result. This may be the last rhinoplasty text that will ever be "filler-free."**

Case Study: Why Do Grafts?

Analysis

A 33-year-old health care worker requested a major difference in her nose including a straight profile (Fig. 7.2). There were no respiratory complaints. However, the nostrils collapsed on deep nasal inspiration. The small tip suggested an occult alar malpositon that was confirmed at operation. It was emphasized that a "balanced approach" would be necessary to straighten her profile: radix augmentation, dorsal reduction, and tip augmentation. Major rim support would be necessary to prevent external valve collapse.

Operative Technique

1) Harvest of deep temporal fascia and septal exposure
2) Open approach then dorsal reduction (bone: 0.5 mm, cartilage: 3 mm)
3) Upper caudal septal excision (1.5 mm) followed by septal harvest
4) Transverse and low-to-low osteotomies. Insertion of spreader grafts
5) Reduction of alar cartilages to 6 mm, undermining of lateral crura, then transection and release of the lateral crura
6) Insertion of a columellar strut and tip sutures: CS, DC, and ID
7) Tip refinement grafts: folded infralobule and domal
8) Suture of lateral crural strut grafts to lateral crura
9) Insertion of a ball (radix) and apron (dorsum) fascia graft
10) Closure with suture of the lateral crural strut graft (LCSG) into the nostril rims

Number of grafts – five types with nine individual grafts.

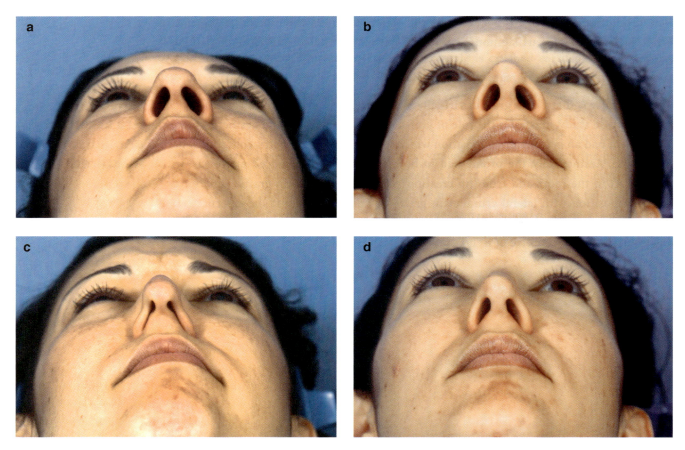

Fig. 7.2 (a–l)

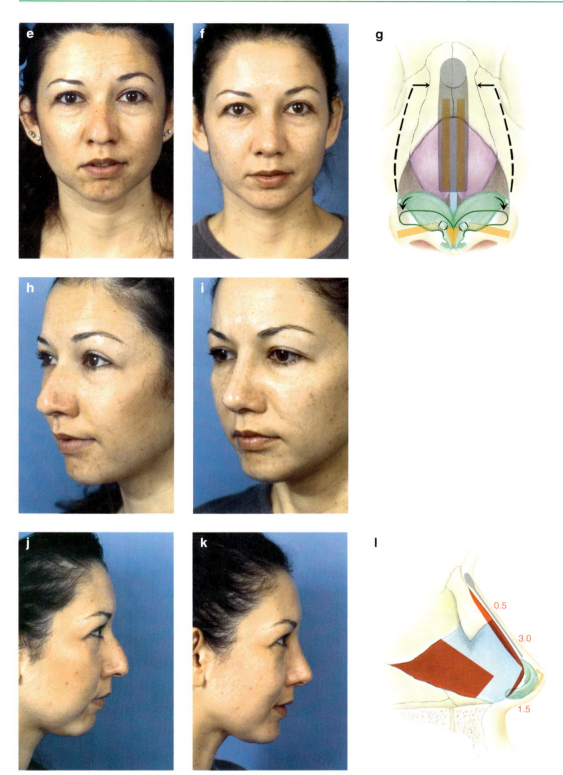

Fig. 7.2 (continued)

Septal Harvest   Septal cartilage is the graft material of choice because of its survival, strength, shaping, and availability. What are the disadvantages of septal cartilage? First, it must be harvested which risks a septal perforation. Second, it must be shaped, placed, and secured correctly. Third, it must survive long term. Technically, harvesting cartilage from a "normal" septum is far easier than doing a septoplasty on an "abnormal" deviated septum or reentering the septum during a secondary rhinoplasty (Fig. 7.3).

Technique. The septum is reinjected with local anesthesia (1% xylocaine with epinephrine 1:100,000) to produce hydrodissection. In general, the amount of cartilage to be resected is determined by the types of grafts required while preserving at least a 10 mm L-shape strut dorsally and caudally. Prior to the actual harvest, the following 3 things must be done: 1) the definitive dorsum and caudal septum established, 2) the mucosa elevated bilaterally back to the bony septum, and 3) the side with the septal spur identified which indicates the side with the septal extension. At this point, the following 5 step septal harvest is done:

1) Dorsal incision 10mm below and parallel to the dorsal septum,
2) Caudal incision 10mm back and parallel to the caudal septum,
3) Posterior dissection of the septum out of the vomerine groove,
4) A downward "push" disarticulation of the cartilaginous septum from the bony perpendicular plate of the ethmoid,
5 Careful mobilization of the cartilaginous tail of the septum which can be 10–15mm long.

At this point, the cartilaginous septum is completely disarticulated and easily removed. Although many surgeons close the mucosal leaflets with 4–0 chromic sutures, I prefer to use silastic nasal splints as they provide compression over a greater region and prevent synechiae between the septum and the turbinates. Access incisions are closed in the standard fashion. The goal is to remove septal cartilage only, not an osseocartilaginous piece of septum.

Problems. To date, there have been few problems with harvesting the septum. I am not aware of septal collapse. There have not been any functional problems due to a flaccid septum or chronic changes in mucosal integrity. I do warn all patients preoperatively that a 1–2% septal perforation rate is to be expected especially in difficult secondary cases – fortunately, it is an over estimation.

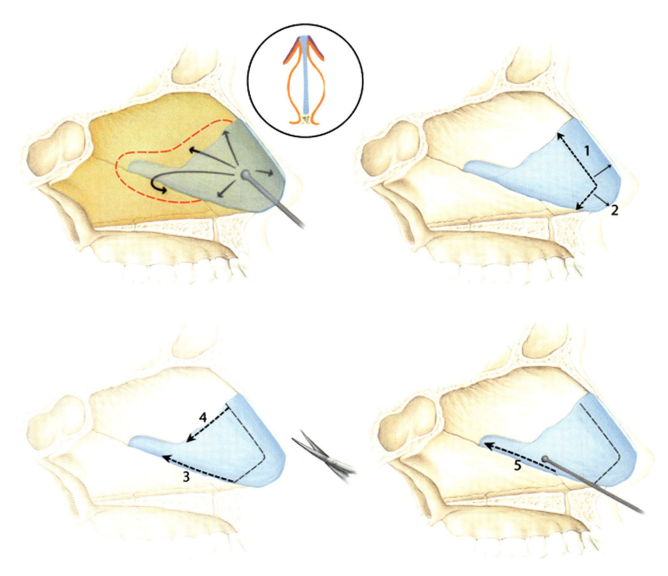

Fig. 7.3 Septal harvest **DVD**

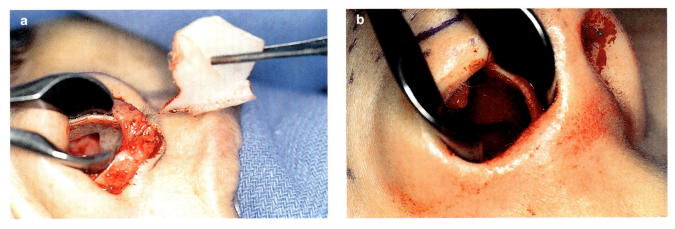

Fig. 7.4 (**a**) Bidirectional approach **DVD** (**b**) transfixion approach

Conchal Harvest   Ear grafts can be classified into two broad categories: cartilage grafts and composite grafts (skin and cartilage) (Fig. 7.5).

Technique. The ear is extensively prepped with Betadine to reduce bacterial count. I do not change instruments or gloves and have not had any infections in several hundred ear grafts during the past 15 years. A sheet of Xeroform gauze is cut into two pieces: a large three fourth piece is used to make a mold of the conchal bowl and serve as an anterior bolster, while the small one fourth piece is rolled up like a cigarette for a posterior bolster. The ear is infiltrated anterior and posterior with a total of 5 cc of 1% xylocaine with epinephrine 1:100,000. The skin of the anterior conchal bowl should turn white and balloon away from the cartilage under the force of the injection. With the ear retracted forward, a longitudinal incision is made above the planned incision site of the cartilage. The posterior concha is exposed. The cartilage is incised below the antihelical fold and the anterior skin is elevated. Once the skin is completely elevated, the entire conchal bowl can be removed. Hemostasis is repeated. Any sharp cartilage edges are rounded off. The incision is closed with a running locking 4–0 plain catgut suture. The tie-over bolster dressing is applied. Two 4–0 nylon sutures are inserted starting from the conchal surface of the crural strut, passing through the posterior surface of the ear below the suture line and then back through the ear above the suture line. The rolled-up gauze is inserted in the posterior loop and pulled snug both to cover the suture line and to serve as a bolster. The mold of gauze is then slipped into the anterior conchal bowl and the two sutures tied. The ear is not drained and no other dressing applied. The mold is removed at 1 week concurrent with nasal cast.

Problems. The patient must be informed of three expected occurrences: (1) pain, (2) scar, and (3) possible change in ear position. The ear donor site always hurts more than the nose and may be sensitive to cold for a year. The scar is generally insignificant when placed posteriorly in contrast to the anterior scar which has a wide variation–do not use an anterior incision. Asymmetry between the ears could occur, but it is rarely noticed. To date, there have been no donor site infections, persistent neuromas, nor hematomas. It is better to use up one ear before starting on the other. I have had retroauricular keloids in two Caucasian patients.

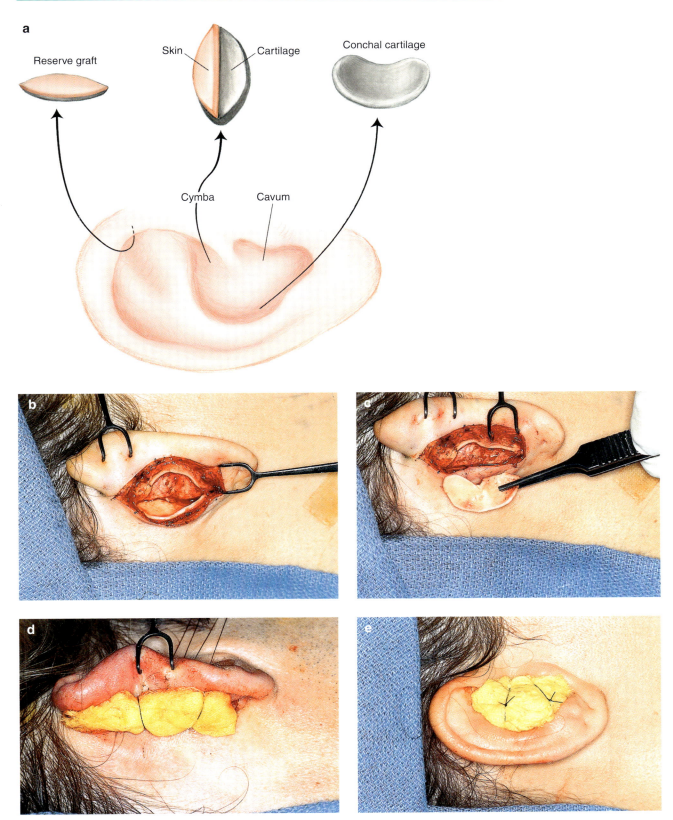

Fig. 7.5 (**a**) Types of conchal grafts, (**b–e**) conchal cartilage harvest

Composite Conchal Grafts

Three applications of composite grafts are seen which often represent a progression in size and difficulty: (1) alar rim lowering, (2) correction of vestibular stenosis, and (3) internal valve stenosis. The usual sequence is to define the defect, harvest the graft, close the donor site, and suture in the graft.

Technique. The most common donor site is the anterior surface of the ipsilateral cymba concha (Fig. 7.6). Traction on the helical root and the antihelix will expose the hidden medial extent of the cymba concha. The desired graft is then drawn most often with an elliptical shape. Several factors must be considered. If the cartilage needs to be straight as for alar rim then the upper border is placed lower towards the central strut, whereas if a curve is needed for the vestibule then the border is moved as high as possible. Skin to cartilage ratio will also influence location and method of closure. When large amounts of cartilage are required, the cephalic incision is the same for both skin and cartilage while the lower border requires a careful skin-only incision and then undermining of the skin downward toward the central strut. The cartilage is then incised inferiorly. The posterior dissection is done above the perichondrium. Hemostasis is meticulous and any sharp cartilage edges excised. Closure of the donor site defect consists of the following: (1) wide skin undermining, (2) horizontal mattress sutures of 4–0 plain catgut, which picks up centrally the underlying postauricular soft tissue thus recreating the natural depression, and (3) 5–0 plain catgut sutures at either end. No dressing is required. On occasion, the entire conchal bowl is harvested as a composite graft and the defect filled with a full-thickness skin graft.

Reserve Composite Graft. A small (12 × 5 mm) composite graft can be harvested from the anterior undersurface of the cephalic helical root when the concha bowl has been previously used (Fig. 7.7). However, the donor site often requires a full-thickness skin graft to close the defect.

Problems. Based on over 200 composite grafts in rhinoplasty patients, I have found composite grafts to be extremely effective at correcting alar rim notching and lowering the alar rim up to 4 mm. The disadvantages include its inherent greater thickness as compared to alar cartilage and "graft show" especially if the incision is made too close to the alar rim or the dissection is done downward toward the alar rim. Although the cartilage can be shaved, a better solution for the thin-skinned patient is to use the undersurface of the helical rim.

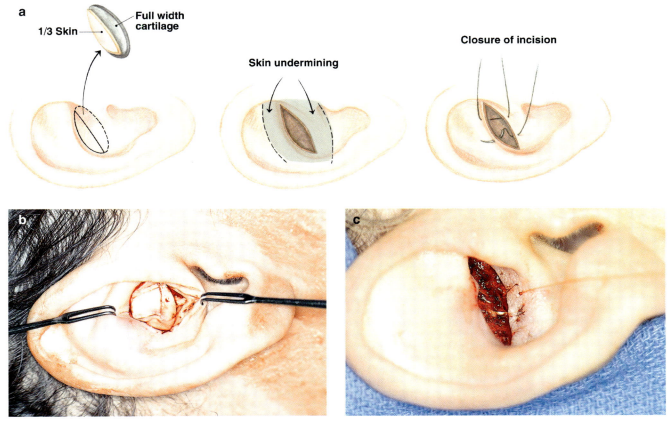

Fig. 7.6 (**a–c**) Standard composite graft **DVD**

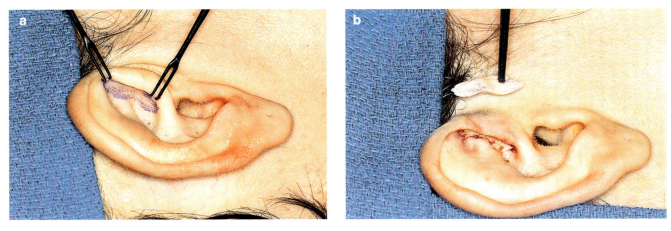

Fig. 7.7 (**a, b**) Reserve composite graft

Fascia Harvest   Autogenous fascia is an extremely valuable grafting material for nasal surgery when soft tissue padding is need as opposed to structural support. Deep temporal fascia is used exclusively due to its thickness and long term survival. Superficial temporal fascia is too thin and has little long term presence.

Technique. I routinely harvest a 5 × 5 cm piece of deep temporal fascia (DTF) through a 3.0 cm incision above the auricle (Fig. 7.8). Recently, I have converted from astraight line incision to a posterior angled V-incision. A straight line is drawn coming up from the tragus and the a posterior V with 1.5cm limbs is added. The hair is not shaved. The area is injected with local anesthesia containing epinephrine. The incision passes downward to the subcutaneous tissue which is spread transversely with the scissors. Haemostasis is checked at this point. The superficial temporal fascia is penetrated and the loose areolar layer is found with the gleaming white deep temporal fascia underneath. Then the scalp is retracted superiorly using two Ragnell retractors. The fascia will be incised as 4 arcs: 1) superiorly at the junction of DTF and perichondrium, 2) anteriorly at its split to accommodate the deep temporal fat pad, 3) inferiorly down to the top of the ear, and 4)posteriorly as far back as necessary. As the DTF is incised, one sees the underlying red temporalis muscle. The scalp is then retracted in each of the other three quadrants and the fascia incised. A large fascia graft is removed. Haemostasis is repeated. The incision is closed with staples. No drains or dressings are used. Antibiotic ointment is applied, and the patient is allowed to wash their hair on the second postoperative day. Fascia is used in a wide variety of configurations. Virtually all radix grafts are simple balls of fascia (Fig. 7-9). In thin skin patients, a full length dorsal graft of fascia in a single layer is employed for primary cases and a double layer for secondary patients. When both the radix and dorsum need extra padding, I use a "ball and apron" to fill the radix and pad the dorsum. In other secondary patients, the entire nose will be relined using a "fascia blanket" graft.

Problems. Donor site morbidity is more theoretical than real as the scar is extremely well-hidden by the unshaved hair. Any postoperative hematoma that occurs can be expressed after removing several staples and then a pressure dressing applied. There is no need to return to the operating room.

Perichondrium. Rib perichondrium is interesting for soft-tissue padding. It is significantly thicker than fascia and swells more. It is used concurrent with rib grafts to the nose and is not harvested separately. Rectus fascia is also tempting, but it contracts and thickens markedly which makes it of little value.

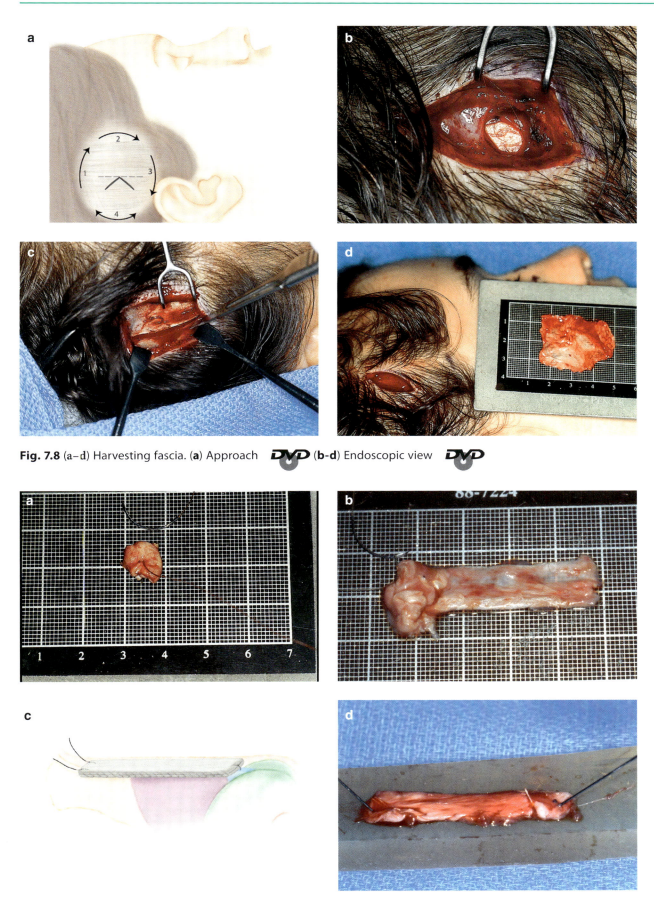

Fig. 7.8 (a–d) Harvesting fascia. (a) Approach *DVD* (b-d) Endoscopic view *DVD*

Fig. 7.9 (a, b) Radix and radix/dorsal graft *DVD* (c, d) dorsal graft *DVD*
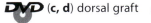

Rib Harvest   The term, "rib grafts," has a wide variety of meanings in rhinoplasty surgery. There are variations as regards donor site, composition, shaping and utilization [Daniel 1994]. Initially, rib cartilage was required to fashion a dorsal graft, but the indications have expanded dramatically. In complex secondaries, virtually every type of graft will be made from rib cartilage including tip, alar rim, spreaders, pyriform. Traditionally, rib cartilage grafts were harvested from the chondrosynschium of ribs 5-7 both for ear and nasal reconstruction (Fig. 7.10). In contrast, rhinoplasty surgeons want straight segments of rib cartilage. I use either the subcostal (9th & 8th ribs) or inframmary (5th & 6th ribs) incision depending upon the patient's preference for the location of the scar.

Harvesting Costal Cartilage: Subcostal Approach. The 9th rib is the first "floating rib" and thus a simple retrograde supraperichondrial dissection is possible (Fig. 7.11). The patient is placed in the supine position with a small sand bag under the hip. The 9th rib tip is palpated and a 2.5cm incision is marked between the 8th and 9th rib extending laterally from the 9th rib tip. The area is injected with 6cc of local anesthesia. The initial incision is carried down to the fascia. Palpation is repeated to confirm the rib location and dissection continues through the muscle and fascia til the distal 9th rib is fully exposed. Although it is possible to harvest the entire cartilaginous portion through a 2.5cm incision in thin patients, the incision is usually extended to 3.5cm especially when the 8th rib will also be harvested. Once the rib tip is revealed, it is grasped with forceps and then a retrograde supraperiosteal dissection is done back to the bony junction using the cautery. A Doyen elevator is placed beneath the palpable bony junction and a #15 blade is used to cut through the junction. Once the graft is removed, then the wound is filled with saline and the anesthesiologist maximally expands the chest to test for any pneumothorax. If additional cartilage is required, then a segment of the 8th rib is harvested subperichondrially similar to harvesting the 5th and 6th rib. The wound is partially closed in layers as extra cartilage can be banked for future use. The wound is not drained.

Harvesting Costal Cartilage: Inframmary Approach. It is important to mark the inframmary fold, especially its medial extent, preoperatively with the patient sitting. If the patient has breast implants, they must be warned that a rupture could occur. The standard incision is 3.5cm and is placed 1cm above the inframmmary fold which usually coincides with the 5th costal interspace (Fig. 7.12). With experience, a 1.5cm keyhole incision can be used, but it is very restrictive and is usually placed in the inframmary fold and obliqates excision of the adherent 6th rib. The wound is infiltrated with 6ccs of local anesthesia. The incision is made and then a cautery is used to dissect down to and through the rectus fascia. The muscles are "split," easily retracted and thereby left intact which minimizes postop pain. The 5th and 6th ribs are easily exposed. In general, one prefers to harvest a segment of the 5th rib as it rarely has a cartilage fusion to the 6th rib. In contrast, the 6th rib is fused on its caudal border to the 7th rib virtually 95% of the time which makes for a more tedious dissection. Next, one must decide whether to split or excise the anterior perichondrium as a possible graft for padding of the nasal skin envelope. The lateral perichondrium on either side is elevated using curved elevators. A complete circumferential dissection is done beneath the cartilage at either end. Once satisfied with the length of the graft, then the cartilage is divided at either end. A Doyen elevator is placed beneath the rib and the cartilage cut partially with a #15 blade and the cut completed with a Freer elevator. The graft is then dissected off the underlying perichondrium

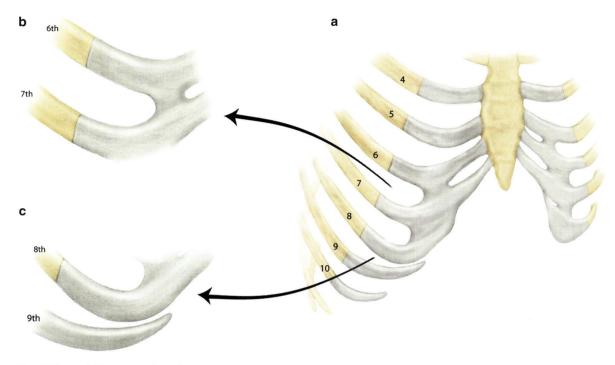

Fig. 7.10 (**a–c**) Costal cartilage harvest

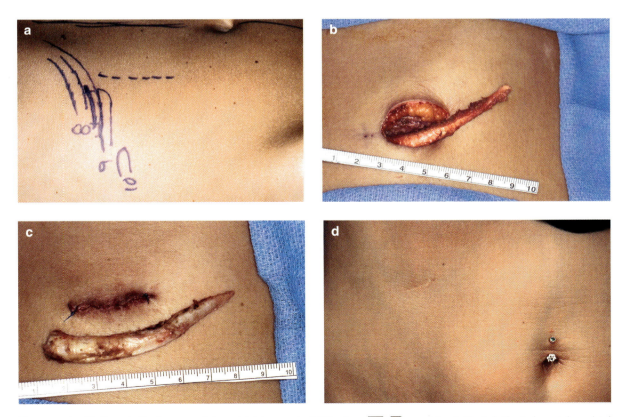

Fig. 7.11 (**a–b**) Costal rib: Supraperichondrial harvest of 9th rib **DVD**, and (**c-d**) Costal rib: Subperichondrial harvest of 8th rib **DVD**

from lateral to medial. Once the cartilage graft is removed, the wound is checked for a pneumothorax. Each of the intercostal nerves is blocked with 0.5cc of 1% Marcaine. The closure is multi layered, but no drain is required. How does the subcostal 8th harvest differ from an inframammary 5th & 6th harvest? The critical difference is the reality of " intermediary cartilage fusion" between 6 and 7. These bridges have to be carefully divided. One can not pass a Doyen rib stripper as it is a cartilage fusion not perichondrial attachments between the adjacent ribs, thus making the dissection more tedious.

Harvesting – Osseocartilaginous. When structural dorsal grafts are required (cocaine nose), I harvest an osseocartilaginous graft from the 9th rib (Fig. 7.12). The advantage is that there is no need for K-wires as warping is not a problem. Survival occurs because bone is placed over bone and cartilage over cartilage. The patient is turned into a right hemi-lateral position and held in that position with an inflatable bean bag mold. The incision is centered at the tip of the 10th rib and drawn in the intercostal space between the 9th and 10th ribs. The donor area is injected with 8 cc of 1% xylocaine with epinephrine 1:100,000. A 3cm incision is made and extended down through subcutaneous tissue to the muscle fascia using a blade tip cutting cautery. Then, the external oblique muscle is divided over the 9th rib. One enters an areolar space and the glistening rib is easily visualized. The osseocartilaginous junction is exposed and marked. The periosteum is divided over the bony portion of the 9th rib, elevated using a Cottle elevator, and then Doyen elevators. A minimum 4 cm of bone is taken and it is wise to confirm this distance using a ruler. With the bony rib supported away from the pleura, the rib is easily cut with two snips of a rongeuer. The cartilaginous portion is dissected free supraperichondrially using the cautery. A standard test for pneumothorax is done.

Problems. There are very few problems associated with harvesting the rib except for the expected scar. Pain is reduced with Marcaine intercostal blocks done prior to closure. Pneumothorax is rarely a factor, but is treated as follows: (1) insertion of a small Robinson catheter through the perforation, (2) closure of the surrounding muscle layer and then a purse string suture of 2-0 vicryl around the tube, (3) maximum chest expansion by the anesthesiologist, and (4) removal of the tube as the knot is tied. A postoperative chest x-ray is mandatory.

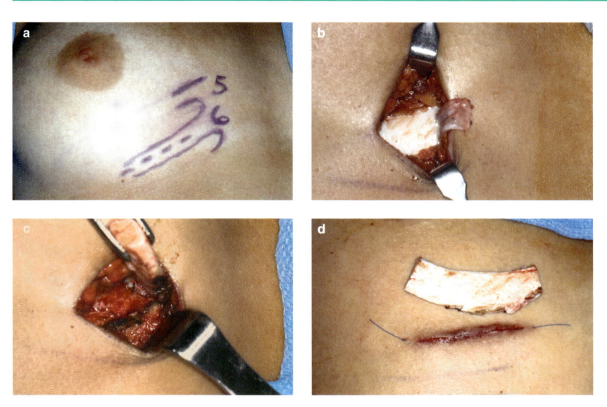

Fig. 7.12 (a–d) Inframammary rib harvest of full thickness segment and partial thickness piece **DVD**

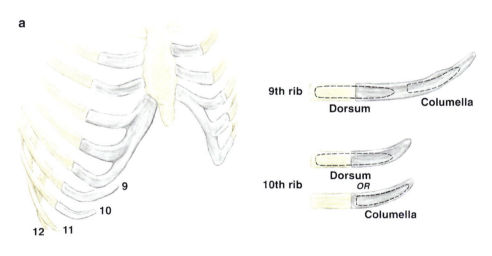

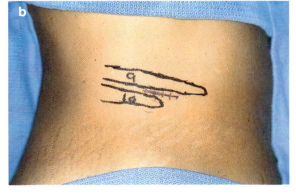

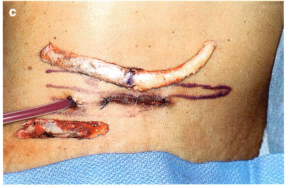

Fig. 7.13 (a–c) Osseocartilaginous rib harvest

Columellar Struts

Currently, I use a columellar strut in virtually all my open rhinoplasties to provide intrinsic columella shape, tip projection, and to counteract the contractual forces of the skin envelope. I classify three types of strut grafts: columellar strut, extended strut, and septocolumellar strut (Fig. 7.14).

Standard Columellar Strut. These struts measure approximately 20 mm in length and 2–3 mm in width with the thicker portion located inferiorly (Fig. 7.14a). I rarely use an angled strut. The strut is placed between the lateral crura with the inferior end short of the nasal spine. The crura are then advanced upward and rotated medially 90° before being fixed to the strut with a #25 needle just below the domes. A horizontal suture of 5-0 polydioxanone suture (PDS) fixes the crura to the strut and is placed in the middle crura above the columellar breakpoint. The superior portion of the strut can be cut to fit beneath the domes and the inferior portion cut off, if there is too much fullness in the columellar labial angle.

Extended Columellar Strut. These grafts tend to be longer (30 mm) and shaped to influence the columella labial angle. They measure 8–10 mm at their widest portion which is the junction between the upper two third and the lower one third of the strut (Fig. 7.14b). After its insertion between the crura, a distinct change should be seen at the columella labial angle. Again, the graft is kept short of the anterior nasal spine (ANS) to avoid clicking. These grafts are frequently used in ethnic noses and in the older patient with an acute columellar labial angle.

Septocolumellar Struts. Structural grafts are designed to provide support to the distal third of the nose and thus represent a replacement/reinforcement of both the caudal septum and the columella (Fig. 7.14c). In general, I insert large segments of osseocartilaginous septum (30 mm high × 20 mm long) via a combined dorsal/tip split. The structure graft is fixed to the septum at multiple points with 4-0 PDS. Then the crura are advanced upward on the strut, fixed with a #25 needle, and then sutured with 5-0 PDS. The strut is contoured cephalically to fit the supratip set off. The most common application is in Asian noses and lengthening of the upwardly rotated tip. I called these septocolumellar grafts in the Atlas (Daniel 2002) and Toriumi (1995) refers to them as septal extension grafts.

Problems. The most common problem is that the graft is too long and clicks across the ANS; a situation easily corrected by direct excision of its inferior portion. Structural grafts are very demanding and will be discussed in depth under upwardly and downwardly rotated tips.

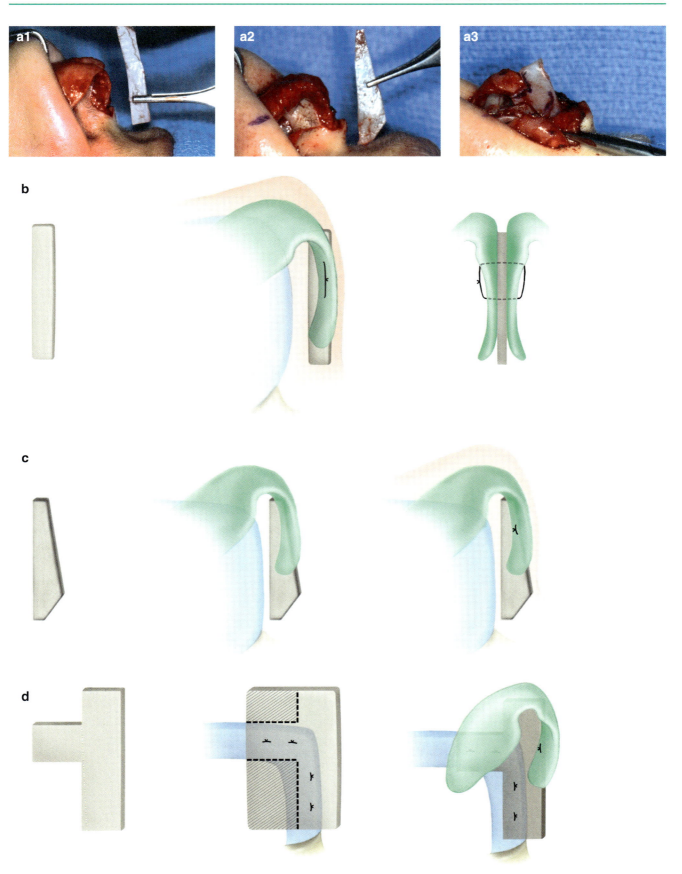

Fig. 7.14 (a) Types of columellar struts, **(b)** columellar strut 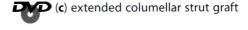 **(c)** extended columellar strut graft  **(d)** septo-columellar strut grafts **DVD**

Tip Grafts

In primary cases, tip grafts can be divided into two materials and two shapes. The material is either excised alar cartilage for add-on tip refinement grafts (TRG) or septal cartilage for structural grafts.

Tip Refinement Grafts (TRG)

Whenever possible, excised alar cartilage is used as it is quite pliable, easily shaped, and can be layered. These grafts have minimal risk of showing through the skin in contrast to rigid grafts of septal or conchal cartilages. There are 5 types:

1) *Domal TRG*. These grafts accentuate the dome defining points and are relatively small (8x4mm). They are sutured over the domes covering the domal creation sutures. Single or double layers are employed depending upon the desired definition.

2) *Shield TRG*. These are shield shape with a distinct dorsal edge to produce dome defining points. The shoulder of the graft is sutured to the domal notch. A second "booster" graft can be placed behind the shield to force the tip more caudal.

3) *Diamond TRG*. These grafts are diamond in shape and cover the entire tip diamond to set the tip off from the rest of the tip lobule. They are sutured at each domal notch, the columellar breakpoint, and the midline junction of the cephalic lateral crura.

4) *Folded TRG*. These grafts have the same shape as a long diamond, but are folded at their widest point with the shorter end folded behind. The graft is projected 1-2mm above the domes. Essentially, one is pushing the dome defining points caudally while achieving both increased definition and projection.

5) *Combination TRG*. Any combination of these 4 grafts can be used to achieve a specific goal. One variation is to insert multiple shields and diamonds to increase volume. Another grouping is to add a domal graft first, then bend a diamond over it which accentuates the tip diamond under thicker skin.

Structured Tip Graft. In contrast, septal cartilage is used for major tip changes. A tapered golf-tee-shape graft is used with dimensions measuring 12–16 mm long, 8–10 mm wide at the top tapering to 4 mm inferiorly, and 1–3 mm thick with greatest thickness superiorly. The goal is to have the superior edge of the graft create the tip definition while the columellar portion blends in with the crura. Prior to suturing the graft in place, two critical steps have been completed: the crural strut has been inserted and the domes have been modified. Before suturing the graft to the stable columella platform, a major decision must be made: integrate the graft into the existing tip configuration or project the graft above the domes to create definition through the skin (Fig. 7.16). The thinner the skin the more the graft must integrate into the alar architecture and be highly beveled. The thicker the skin the more the graft projects above the domes and the sharper the edges (Fig. 7.17). The graft is sutured in place using 4–6 sutures of 5–0 PDS.

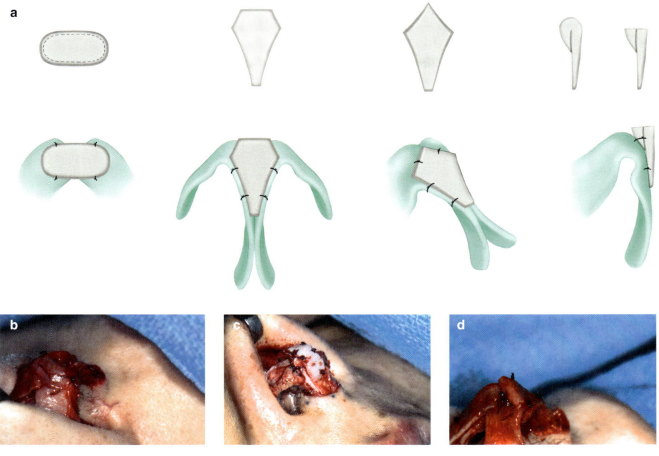

Fig. 7.15 Add-on tip refinement grafts (TRG) **DVD**

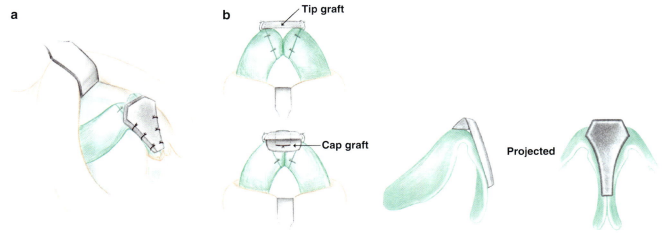

Fig. 7.16 (**a, b**) Integrated tip graft   **Fig. 7.17** Projected tip graft

Spreader Grafts

Put simply, spreader grafts are a functional and aesthetic necessity (Fig. 7.18). Following resection of the dorsal hump, the superior portion of the septum is converted from a broad "T," which distracts the upper lateral cartilages, to a narrow "I," which allows the upper lateral cartilages to collapse inward. Spreader grafts reestablish the broad "T" of the septum thereby achieving two critical factors: (1) functionally, the internal nasal valve angle is opened and (2) aesthetically, the dorsal lines are supported thereby avoiding a collapsed inverted-V deformity.

Technique. The grafts are cut from the donor material using a #11 blade. Thickness varies from the usual 1.5 mm up to 4 mm depending upon narrowness and asymmetry. The height is 2–3 mm to facilitate suturing and the length is 15–25 mm depending on availability. A true "pocket" as Sheen originally envisioned is not possible caudally in most cases but is very desirable cephalically, especially under the bony vault. The grafts are inserted one at a time making sure to have a smooth dorsum. They are held in place with two #25 needles placed percutaneously through the skin. The needles pierce all five layers: the upper lateral cartilage, then the spreader graft, the septum, spreader graft, and opposite upper lateral cartilage. The caudal end is sutured first with 5–0 PDS often incorporating just the spreader grafts and the septum (three layers), whereas the cephalic suture incorporates the upper lateral cartilages as well (five layers). Suturing avoids accidental disruption or dorsal displacement.

Application. I tend to think of spreader grafts having different widths to correct dorsal asymmetries. Different lengths are used for various purposes. The standard length is primarily filling the cartilaginous open roof. After a high bony reduction, longer grafts are needed to extend high into the bony open roof to maintain ideal dorsal width. For the upwardly rotated tip, longer grafts can be placed more caudally in an "extended" position to brace a structured columellar strut which allows the tip to be derotated.

Problems. To date, the benefits of spreader grafts have been extraordinary while the problems have been few. The most worrisome is the 1% incidence of dorsal displacement, which creates a small bump in the keystone area that requires a revisional shaving down. Sometimes, one can do this in the exam room with local anesthesia using a 16 needle. Without question, the major problem with spreader grafts is surgical reluctance. Ultimately, this is one graft where the answer is "just do it." I have never regretted inserting spreader grafts, but I have regretted not doing them.

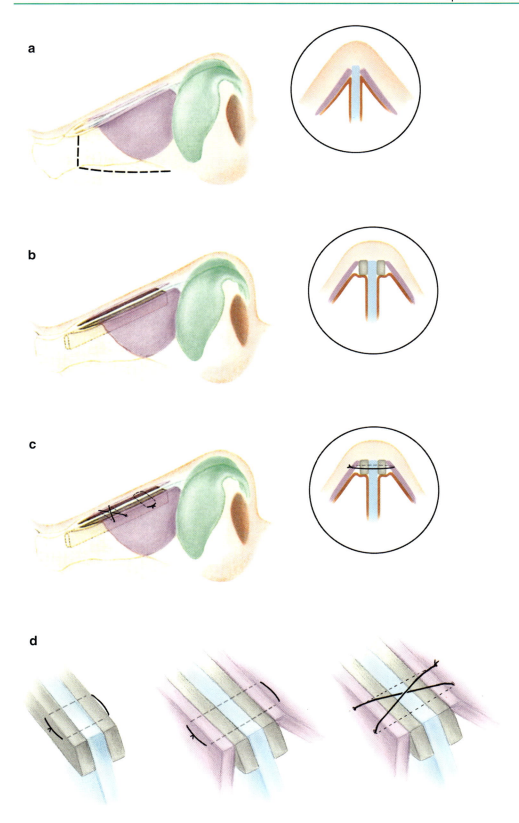

Fig. 7.18 (a–d) Spreader grafts

Radix Grafts

Early in my practice I went through the usual progression of radix grafts – crushed septum then excised alar and finally fascia with a dramatic decline in revision rate from 20% to 5% to virtually 0%. Currently, I use fascia in all my radix grafts, but do it in three configurations.

Radix Graft: Fascia (F). A sheet of deep temporal fascia is harvested, bunched into a ball, and sutured together with a 4–0 plain catgut suture (Fig. 7.19a, d, g). The recipient pocket is elevated, the attached needle is brought out at the nasion, and the fascial ball pulled into the pocket. A steristrip tape is placed across the bridge keeping the fascia in the radix pocket.

Radix Area Graft: Diced Cartilage and Fascia (DC+F). When the entire radix area must be augmented, I use a two-step method: (1) a small fascia graft is slipped into the pocket with a percutaneous suture, (2) a small amount of diced cartilage (0.1–0.3 cc) is placed against the bone (Fig. 7.19b, e, h). The cartilage will fuse to the bone while the fascia will provide a soft contour and avoid any visibility of the graft.

Radix/Upper Dorsum: Diced Cartilage in Fascia (DC-F). As the length of the defect extends below the nasion and down to the rhinion, a diced cartilage in fascia (DC-F) graft is created. The fascia is penned to a silastic block, filled with diced cartilage (0.3–0.5 cc), and then the fascial edges are sutured together with 4–0 plain catgut. This cartilage filled "bean bag" is slipped into the recipient pocket using a percutaneous suture on the cephalic end (Fig. 7.19c, f, i). The caudal end is sutured to the cartilaginous dorsum.

Problems. There have been virtually no problems with fascia grafts in the radix. In contrast to solid septal grafts which are designed to extend the dorsal lines cephalically, fascial grafts are only filling the radix area and moving the nasion outward from the corneal plane. As the "area deficiency" increases, greater fill is required and hence the diced cartilage grafts. Unless the diced cartilage is covered with fascia, it will be palpable and may become visible long term. Historically, a half-length dorsal graft was the greatest nightmare of all grafts as they always showed under the thin skin of the rhinion. However, diced cartilage in fascia grafts has solved the challenge. It is always wise to be conservative in how much diced cartilage to put in under the tight skin of the radix. If revision is necessary, bevel it in situ with a #15 blade.

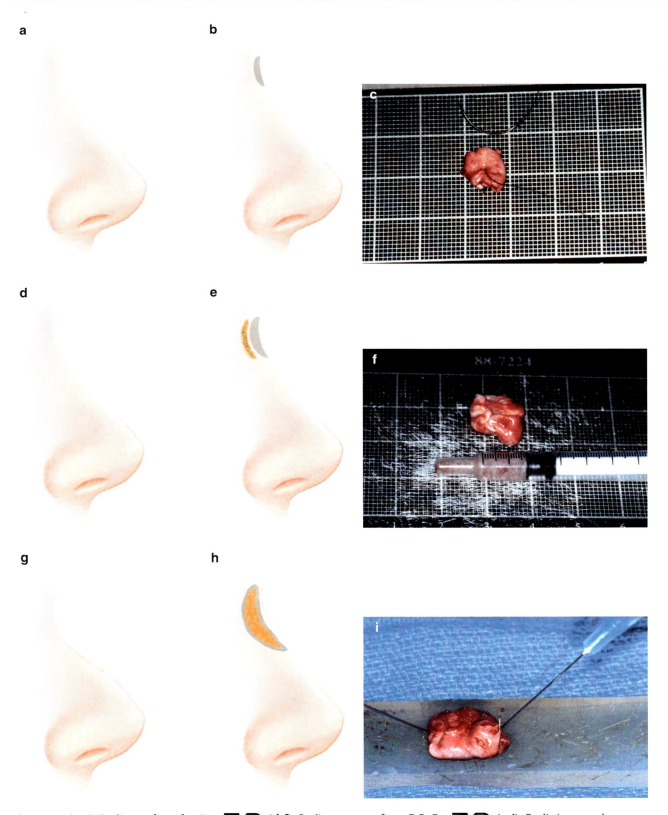

Fig. 7.19 (**a-c**) Radix graft – fascia *DVD* (**d-f**) Radix area graft – DC+F *DVD* (**g-i**) Radix/upper dorsum – DC-F *DVD*

Dorsal Grafts: The Designer Dorsum

During the last 8 years, the greatest advance in nasal grafting is dorsal augmentation. Solid dorsal grafts are rarely used due to their inherent risks of visibility, sharp edges, or warping. Three types of grafts are used to correct dorsal deficiencies. Fascia is used to pad the dorsal skin envelope and augment minimally the dorsum (0.5–1.5 mm). Diced cartilage in fascia (DC-F) is used for virtually all dorsal augmentations in the 1–8 mm range. It is inserted either by itself or as the aesthetic layer of a composite reconstruction. Osseocartilaginous rib grafts (OC) are reserved for contracted cocaine noses where structural support is critical. A brief description of the latter technique will be given next with additional discussion in the section on The Cocaine Nose.

Osseocartilaginous Grafts (OC). Once the OC graft is harvested, it is shaped using #11 blade for the cartilage portion and a power drill burr for the bony portion (Fig. 7.20). The graft is repeatedly placed into the recipient bed and the skin redraped until the ideal shape is achieved. In most cases, the graft is a 60:40 composition of bone to cartilage. The graft is then inserted and tightly held on the sides while two percutaneous K-wires are drilled through the graft down to the nasal bones with the wires removed at 7–10 days. The basilar part of the columellar strut is fixed to the ANS. Then a tongue-in-groove technique is used to join the strut to the cartilaginous portion of the dorsal graft. Follow-up MRI scans indicate that both bony fusion and survival occurs. Warping is rarely a problem in osseocartilaginous grafts. Malalignment is the major concern.

Fascia (F). I use fascia as a dorsal graft whenever the dorsal skin is thin or minor augmentation of less than 1.5 mm is needed (Fig. 7.21). The fascia is pinned on a silastic block, trimmed to an 8 mm width, and then fixed with 4–0 plain catgut on straight needles (SC-1) at the cephalic end. The needles are passed through the skin at the nasion level and guided into the pocket and then the caudal end is sutured to the cartilaginous vault. When a double layer is required, the fascia is folded, fixed at either end, and closed with a running suture along its open edge. Insertion and fixation is similar to a single layer graft. Note: the double layer fascia graft is essentially the same technique that is used for the "container" of a DC-F graft.

Diced Cartilage in Fascia (DC-F). Diced cartilage has revolutionized dorsal grafting. The basic concept is to dice cartilage into small bits (<0.5 mm) which can be put into a fascial sleeve that is slipped into the dorsal defect. The technique will be described in detail followed by an in-depth analysis of experienced gained from over 300 DC-F grafts done in the past 7 years. Once again, the DVDs are of inestimable value in showing the actual technique.

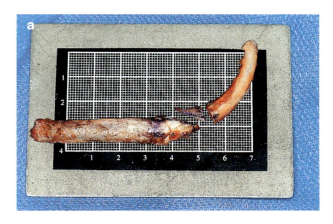
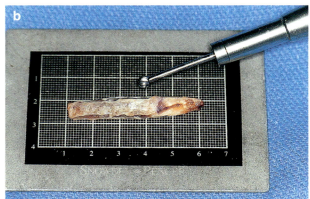
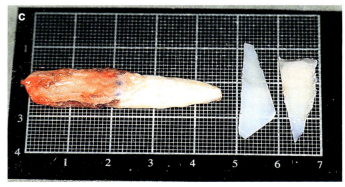
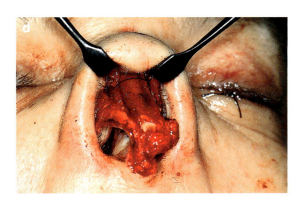

Fig. 7.20 (**a–d**) Osseocartilaginous dorsal graft

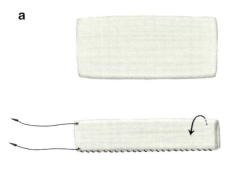
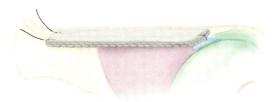
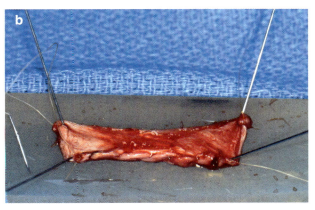
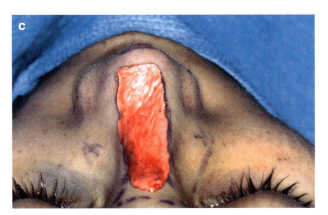

Fig. 7.21 (**a–c**) Fascial dorsal graft

Step #1: Fascial Harvest. The largest possible sheet of deep temporal fascia is harvested. The resection extends superiorly to the periosteal junction, anteriorly to the deep temporal fascial split, then inferiorly toward the concha, and posteriorly as far back as possible.

Step #2: Dicing the Cartilage. Cartilage is diced into <0.5 mm bits using excised cartilage (dorsum, alar), septum, concha, or rib. In general, the *circulating nurse* puts on sterile gloves and dices the cartilage into <0.5 mm squares while the surgeon continues to operate. It is important to cut the cartilage with two #11 blades without traumatizing the cartilage – do not morselize or crush it. A 1.0 cc tuberculin syringe is filled with diced cartilage. The plunger is inserted and the cartilage is compressed maximally. The cartilage should be diced so fine that it can pass through the hub – the *spurt test*. Since the cartilage is so finely diced, the hub does not have to be cut off the syringe with a #10 blade.

Step #3: Constructing the Fascial Sleeve. Measurements of the dorsal defect allow an exact DC-F *construct* to be made on the back table and inserted into the defect. The fascia is pinned on a silastic block and folded into an 8–10 mm wide × 20–35 mm long sleeve. The cephalic end is sutured at its corners using two sutures of 4–0 plain on SC-1 needles. Then the free edge is trimmed and the free edge sutured partially closed with a locking suture of 4–0 plain. Note: this is similar to a double layer dorsal fascia graft.

Step #4: Filling the Construct. The syringe is slipped into the open side of the sleeve and filled to the desired thickness. The critical step is to achieve very specific dimensions: thickness (1–8 mm), length (10–40 mm) and shape (tapered or uniform). It is done by using the nondominant hand to mold the DC as it is slowly injected into the sleeve with the dominant hand. Alternatively, one can use an elevator to "stuff" the sleeve, but one wants a solid shape. The length of the dorsal graft is trimmed to the exact length required. It is important to mold the graft to the exact dimensions on the back table and not over-graft the nose.

Step #5: Inserting the Graft. The percutaneous sutures are inserted at the nasion level and the shaped graft slipped into the recipient bed. In most cases, the graft has been made quite accurate and thus minimal molding in-situ is done. If I am concerned about the shape, I do not hesitate to remove the graft and modify it on the back table. If necessary, diced cartilage can be expressed out of the fascial sleeve. The graft is then closed and fixed to the cartilage vault with a 4–0 plain suture (Fig. 7.22).

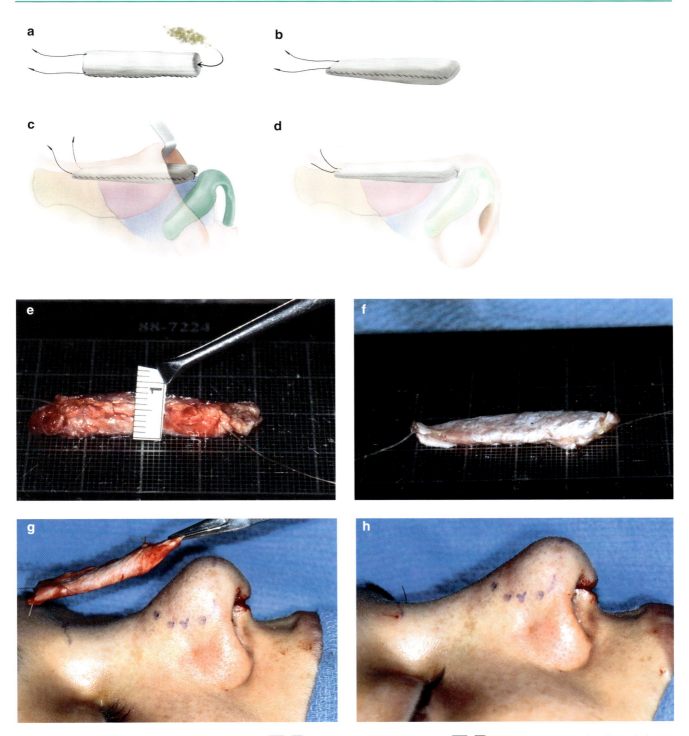

Fig. 7.22 (**a**) Diced cartilage in fascia (DC-F) 📀, (**b**) dicing the cartilage 📀 (**c**) constructing the fascial sleeve 📀 (**d**) filling the sleeve to measure 📀, and (**e-h**) inserting the graft 📀

Post-op Course. Once the nose is closed, the dorsum is gently taped with steristrips. When the cast is removed at 6 days, the nose is inspected and gentle molding can be done to insure a smooth dorsum. If required, the patient is seen every 2 days and the graft molded up to 14 days. The patient should not wear glasses for 6 weeks. If there is any asymmetry at 1 year, it can be easily shaped by beveling with a #15 blade. When complex revisions are done, the now solid graft is removed, shaped, and reinserted.

Diced Cartilage and Fascia (DC+F)

When highly tapered or localized grafts are required, then a DC+F graft is done. Essentially, a standard fascial dorsal graft is inserted first, either single or double layer. Then diced cartilage is placed beneath the fascia to achieve a very specific shape. Obviously, this step is done immediately prior to closure to avoid any dispersal.

Why Diced Cartilage Grafts?

There are numerous advantages and very few disadvantages for DC-F grafts. The top ten advantages are as follows: (1) These are autogenous grafts using viable cartilage with no risk of rejection. (2) One can use any combination of excised, septal, conchal, or rib cartilage. In contrast to solid grafts, one does not have to harvest the perfect, and rarely found, 35 × 8 mm piece of septal cartilage nor fuse together two pieces of curvy conchal cartilage. (3) There is neither a risk of warping nor a need for foreign material (K-wire). (4) The graft is easily and quickly prepared with the circulating nurse or a junior assistant dicing the cartilage and loading the syringe. (5) The shape is easily "customized" as regards thickness (1–8 mm), shape (tapered or uniform), and length (Fig. 7.23). The ability to mold a graft with a specific shape for a specific defect is extraordinary. (6) Molding of the graft is possible both intraop and early post-op. (7) The graft can be easily revised using a percutaneous #16 needle to remove a sharp edge, or a #15 blade to shave off any prominence. (8) Infection has not been a problem. (9) Absorption has not been seen in over 300 cases with a maximum follow-up of 7 years. (10) Over a period of months, the diced cartilage "solidifies." The interspace between the diced cartilage bits is filled with fibrous tissue within the fascial sleeve (Fig. 7.24a, b). When removed the graft is quite solid and semirigid. Any pieces shaved off for shaping purposes are sufficiently solid that they can be used even for tip grafts. Histological studies confirm that the individual pieces of cartilage have survived and suggest that the fascia has become a neoperichondrium (Fig. 7.24c, d).

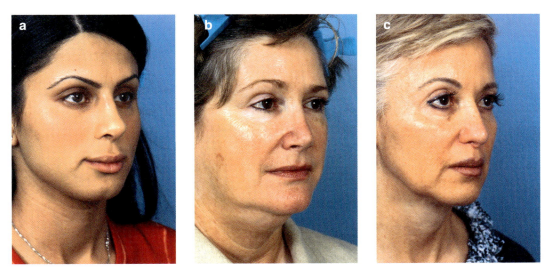

Fig. 7.23 Range of augmentation and duration with DC-F grafts, (**a**) 2 mm, 2 years, (**b**) 4 mm, 6 years, (**c**) 6 mm, 3 years

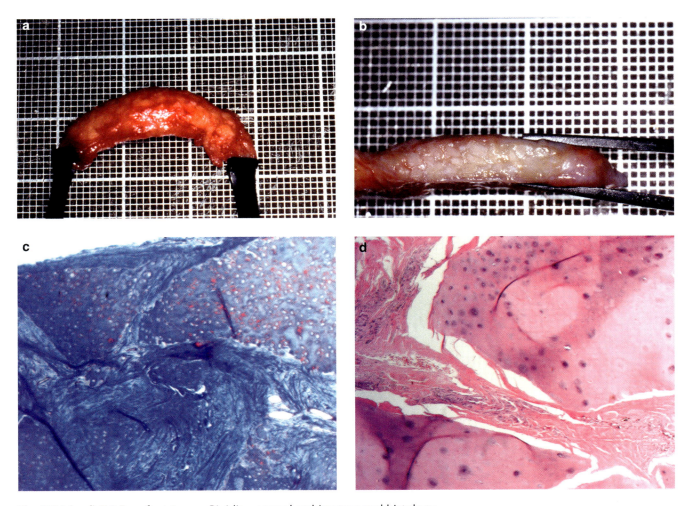

Fig. 7.24 (**a–d**) DC-F graft at 1 year: Rigidity, normal architecture and histology

Alar Rim Graft and Alar Rim Support Graft

For patients with a retracted alar rim or a high potential for developing it, alar rim grafts of septal cartilage are dramatically effective and technically simple. What is the difference between *alar rim grafts* (ARG) and *alar rim structure grafts* (ARS)? Basically, it is the same graft, but placed along the alar rim in two different ways. The ARG is inserted into a subcutaneous pocket while the ARS is sutured into a marginal rim incision along the full-length of the nostril. In general, ARG grafts are used for minor weaknesses and slight retractions of the alar rim. In contrast, ARS grafts are used for major retractions and to fundamentally change the shape of the nostrils (Daniel 2002, 2004).

Technique (ARG). The grafts measure approximately 10–14 mm in length by 2–4 mm in width with the thinnest end tapered significantly (Fig. 7.25). The contour of the alar rim is marked, especially the high point of the alar rim notch which often corresponds to the alar base/lobular junction. Then, a short intra nostril 4 mm incision is made at the level of the alar base posterior and transverse to the alar rim. A subcutaneous pocket is dissected that is parallel and 2–3 mm posterior to the alar rim. The graft is pushed into the pocket tapered end first and then the incision is closed. There should be an immediate improvement in the alar rim border. However, it is important to check the nostril shape from the basilar view and to palpate for the graft near the domes. If there is any distortion, the graft is backed out, shortened, and reinserted. One must balance lowering the alar rims, while avoiding distortion of nostril shape.

Technique (ARS). The exact same graft can be sutured along the alar rim rather than placed in a subcutaneous pocket (Fig. 7.26). In the majority of cases, a true rim incision is made 2 mm back from the alar rim beginning laterally and ending medially at the infracartilaginous incision. A pocket is dissected posterior to the incision – one never unfurls the alar rim. The graft is placed into the pocket. The incision is closed with 4–0 chromic but picking up the graft in each bite. It is essential to check the cephalic end of the graft and make absolutely sure that it is not overriding the domes. Postoperative nostril splinting is done for 2–3 weeks at night.

Problems. Most of the problems with alar rim grafts have been minor. If thick cartilage is used, there is a tendency for it to show in the area of the soft-tissue facets. The primary failure is expecting it to do too much. This type of graft is excellent for alar rim support or lowering the rim 2 mm at the very most. Any more than 2 mm of lowering requires a composite graft.

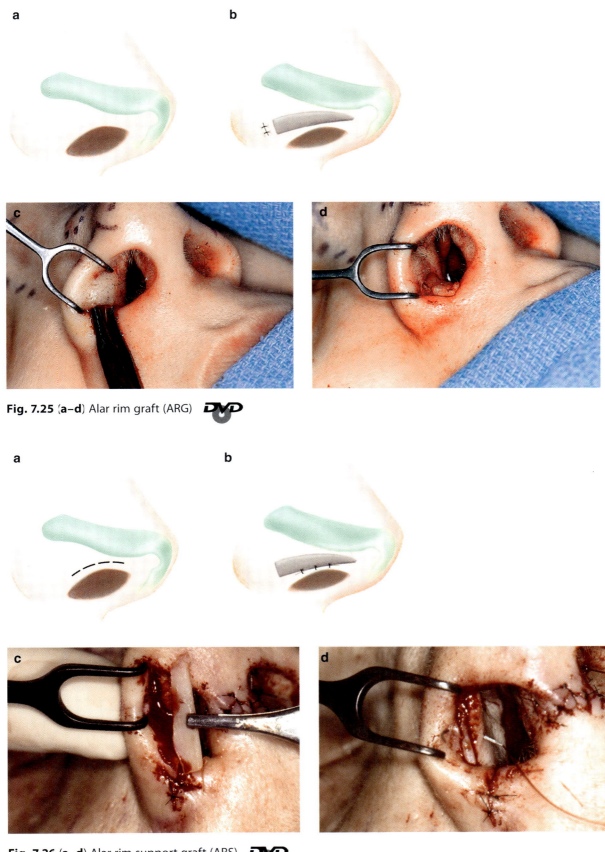

Fig. 7.25 (**a–d**) Alar rim graft (ARG)

Fig. 7.26 (**a–d**) Alar rim support graft (ARS)

Lateral Crural Strut Grafts

These grafts were developed by Gunter (1997) to reshape, reposition, or reconstruct the lateral crura while providing support for the external valve. Essentially these are straight strong pieces of cartilage measuring 3–4 mm in width by 14–20 mm in length. Although used in different ways, the medial portion of the graft is sutured to the *undersurface* of the alar cartilage while the distal end is placed in a lateral pocket. I insert the lateral portion into one of three locations: pyriform, alar base, or nostril rim depending upon indication (Fig. 7.27). Whenever possible, septal cartilage is used.

Technique: Shaping or Salvaging the Alar Cartilage. Deformed or mangled alar cartilages can be straightened and shaped by placing a short lateral crural strut graft beneath them and fixing the graft to the alar with several sutures of 5–0 PDS. This maneuver is particularly helpful in severely concave lateral crura. These grafts tend to be uniform in thickness.

Extended Lateral Crural Strut. In primary cases, the lateral crural strut is added once the tip suture surgery is completed. Essentially, the desired pocket is undermined in one of the three positions: Type (1) underneath the accessory cartilages, Type (2) in the alar base, or Type (3) along the nostril rim. These grafts are highly tapered and thin at the cephalic end to avoid distorting the domal area while thick laterally. The graft is inserted into the pocket, shortened laterally if necessary, and then sutured to the lateral crura at two points. One should avoid placing the lateral strut graft underneath or cephalic to the alar groove as it will be visible.

Lateral Crural Strut and Alar Transposition. These are very complex cases where one wants to make a fundamental change in tip shape and provide support to the external valve (Fig. 7.28). Alar transposition implies dividing the lateral crura at its junction with the A-1 accessory cartilage, undermining the entire lateral cartilage up to the domal segment, and then transposing it from a cephalic position to a more caudal position paralleling the nostril rim. In these cases, I have found it important to transpose the alars *prior* to insertion of the columellar strut. Once the alars are transposed the surgical sequence is as follows: (1) columellar strut, (2) tip suturing with optional TRG grafts, (3) suturing the lateral crural strut graft to the lateral crura, and (4) placing the lateral crural strut graft along the nostril rim or into an alar base pocket. In certain secondary cases, additional composite grafts may be required.

Problems. During the learning curve, the most common problems are distortion of the nostril rim, graft visibility in the alar grove, and palpability. These grafts must "flow" with the alar contour while providing support. Tapering of the medial end is critical. Mark the alar groove prior to surgery and place the pyriform extension caudal to it whenever possible. Warn patients in advance that they will be able to palpate the grafts.

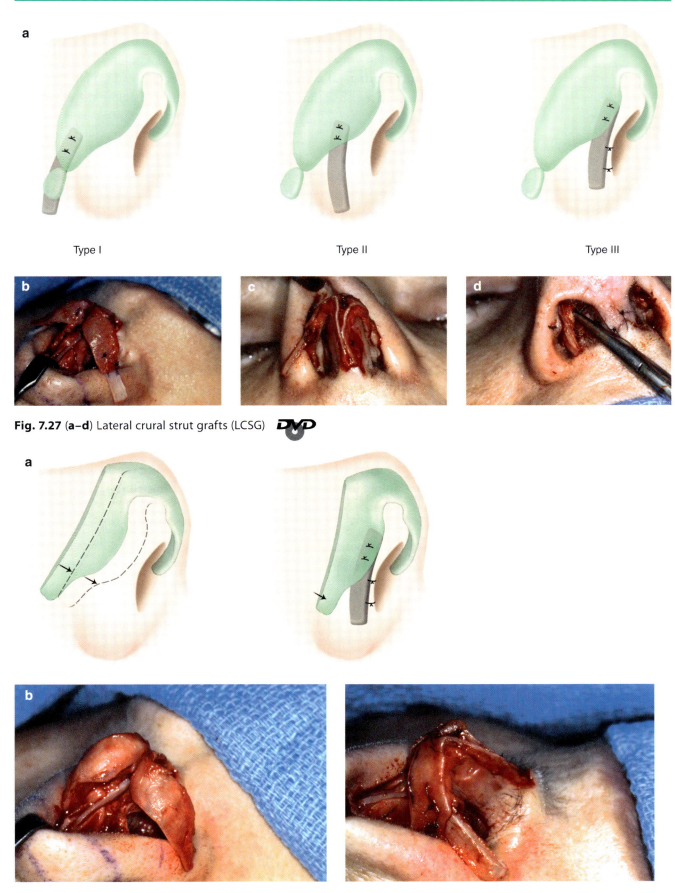

Type I   Type II   Type III

Fig. 7.27 (**a–d**) Lateral crural strut grafts (LCSG) **DVD**

Fig. 7.28 (**a, b**) Alar transposition and LCSG **DVD**

Specialized Grafts

Certain grafts are utilized rarely or almost exclusively in secondary cases.

Lateral Wall Grafts. Grafts to the lateral wall are associated with asymmetric noses or large dorsal grafts (Fig. 7.31a, b). To avoid visibility, the graft should be anatomically precise to correct a specific problem and placed in a pocket with suture fixation. A lateral wall graft is shaped like the upper lateral cartilage and then placed in a pocket directly over the upper lateral cartilage (ULC). The dorsal edge is precisely aligned with the dorsum. Full-length lateral wall grafts are not used as they tend to be visible.

Alar Spreader Grafts. This graft, which I refer to as an alar bar graft, was devised by Gunter (1992) to provide support for the pinched tip as seen on basilar view (Fig. 7.31c, d). Although conceptually simple, it is technically demanding. If lateral crura are 2 mm in width or more, then the cartilage is undermined from the vestibular lining. A #25 needle is placed across at the point of greatest collapse. The alar cartilages are slid along the needle until the desired correction is achieved. Then a piece of septal cartilage, often measuring 14 × 4 mm, is shortened to fit the desired length. The graft is sutured underneath the alar cartilages with 5–0 PDS. The graft must not be excessively long or nostril flare will occur. I have not found triangular alar spreader grafts effective as they create excessive supratip fullness.

Dermal Grafts. I have found dermal grafts to be extremely valuable in restoring defects resulting from loss of the dermis (Fig. 7.31e, f). The donor site is retroauricular for small defects and suprapubic for large defects. It is important to excise subcutaneous fat and hair bulbs from the under surface of the graft. For a heavily scarred tip, the entire lobule is undermined and then packed with the dermis graft which can measure 9 × 2.5 cm. The donor site scar will resemble a C-section scar in the supra pubic region. Smaller defects can have a two-layer stacked graft cut slightly bigger than the defect and guided into position with percutaneous sutures using SC-1 needles.

Banking and Harvesting. Any significant pieces of left over cartilage are banked beneath the scalp (Fig. 7.31g, h). The location is the temporal region, if fascia was harvested or in the lower retroauricular mastoid area. Any extra rib cartilage is placed in the sub costal rib donor site, but not in the inframammary site. In the latter cases, small pieces of costal contilage can be placed in the temporal region. I have harvested grafts up to 6 years post-insertion and all grafts have retained their rigidity, shape, and volume. Histologically, the cells are viable and stain for chondrocyte activity.

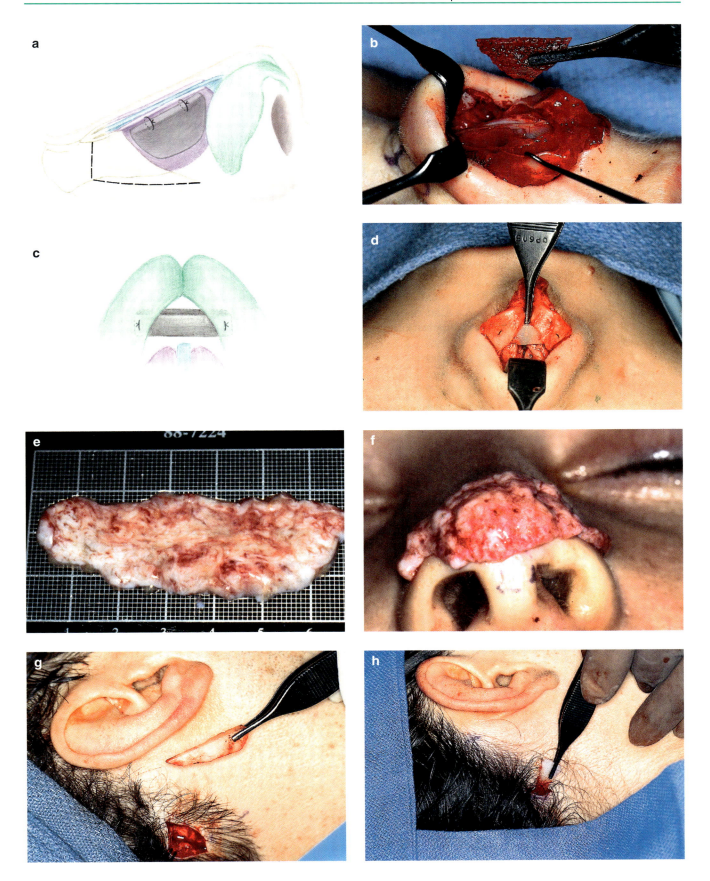

Fig. 7.31 (**a**, **b**) Lateral wall graft, (**c**–**d**) alar spreader graft, (**e**, **f**) dermal grafts **DVD** (**g**, **h**) banking/harvesting

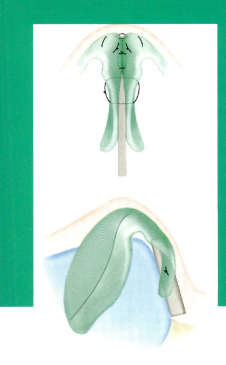

Primary Rhinoplasty: Decision Making

8

At this point in the text, the surgeon should understand and feel comfortable with each step in the basic rhinoplasty operation. The challenge now is how to progress from Level 1 cases to more complicated deformities, which require a broader array of surgical techniques. What is a logical progression? Surprisingly, many Level 2 nasal deformities are simply Level 1 cases, but with one component being markedly more difficult. For example, many patients with underprojecting tips require a standard approach to the rest of the nose, but sophisticated use of columellar struts and add-on grafts for the tip. Fortunately, the surgeon can progress to Level 2 cases using the basic skills mastered in Level 1 cases. This chapter will emphasize tip surgery because the reality of private practice is that "as the tip goes so goes the rhinoplasty" for both patient and surgeon. In addition, the surgeon will learn how to recognize Level 3 cases. Ultimately, each surgeon will develop their own grading system for Level 1–3 cases, which will facilitate selection of cases and techniques resulting in an expansion of their comfort zone.

Introduction

Case Study: Tip Definition

Analysis

A 30-year-old student requested a significant change in her nose, especially the tip (Fig. 8.2). She emphasized that she wanted a small refined tip while the surgeon emphasized tissue limitations. The size and thickness of the skin envelope were discussed as was the width of the nasal base. The goal was to achieve a maximum change in the tip and nasal base while taking a balanced approach to the dorsum. Excision of a cephalically tapered segment of the caudal septum improved tip rotation. The use of a columellar strut prevented tip droop postoperatively. Placement of the shield-shape add-on graft insured tip definition and a longer infralobule.

(Level: 2.0)

Operative Technique

1) Small intraoral chin implant and fascial harvest
2) Open approach and reduction of alar cartilages to 6 mm rim strips
3) Incremental dorsal reduction (bone: 0.5 mm, cartilage: 1.5 mm)
4) Upper caudal septal resection of 2.5 mm, followed by septal harvest
5) Low to high osteotomies; insertion of fascial radix graft
6) Crural strut and tip sutures: CS, DC, ID, DE
7) Shield-shape add-on graft using excised cephalic lateral crura
8) Bilateral spreader graft and out-fx of turbinates
9) Combined nostil sill/alar base excision (R:1.5/2.0, L 3/3)
10) Alar rim support grafts sutured into marginal incisions

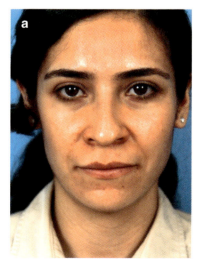
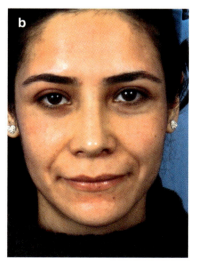
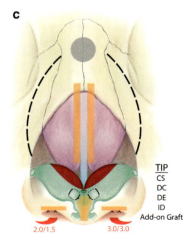

Fig. 8.2 (a–j)

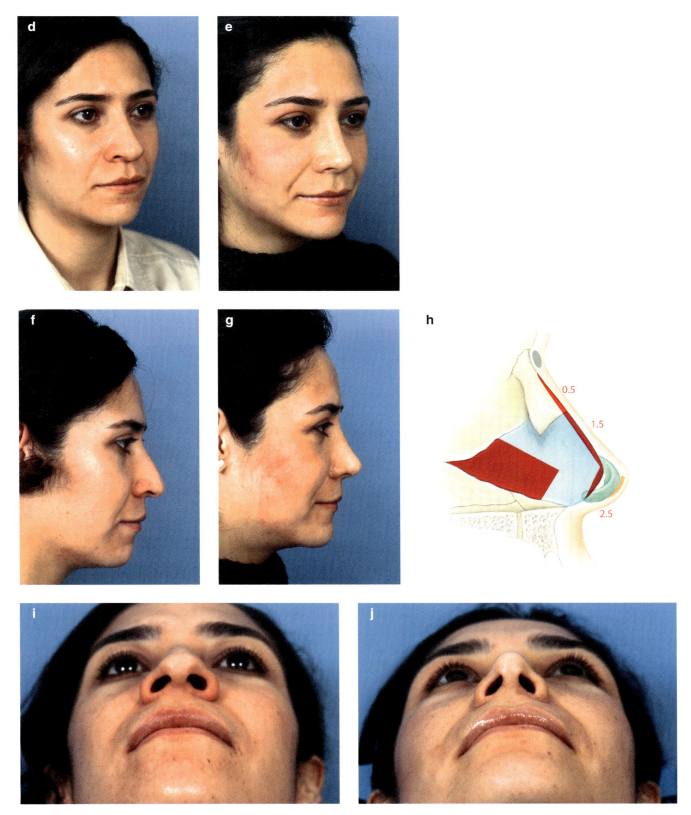

Fig. 8.2 (continued)

Tip Width   Tip width is generally accepted to be the distance between the dome defining points (Fig. 8.3). For most primary noses, excessive narrowness is rarely an issue. I can only conceive of it being present in association with a major concavity of the adjacent lateral crura or an abnormal tip shape. Treatment would consist of correcting the entire structure of the lateral crura and possibly adding a columellar strut to separate the domes. In contrast, excessive tip width is a common complaint among primary rhinoplasty patients. Often, it is associated with poor tip definition.

Decision Making. One must first analyze tip width as well as the related characteristics of definition and projection. Anatomically, tip width is the distance between highly defined tip points, which is accentuated by concave rather than convex lateral crura. I will often mark tip width and show it to the patient pre-op. It is the combination of excessive tip width and lack of definition that leads most patients to request tip surgery. Palpation is important in determining the rigidity of the alar cartilages and how well it will respond to tip suturing.

Level 1. Aesthetically, the tip-defining points are too wide (6-10m) and yet definition is reasonable. The usual method of reducing tip width is the interdomal suture with optional addition of a domal equalization suture. At the cartilage level, it is important to leave the domes 3–4 mm apart. This is one reason to be careful in using a single unifying transdomal suture, which can create a "monopoint" tip. On rare occasions, the anatomical cause is the width of the abutting middle crura. This rare problem is corrected by excising cephalic crura medially behind the domes and onto the middle crura.

Level 2. Aesthetically, these deformities are a combination of excessive width and lack of definition. Visually, one tends to see a tip width approaching (14-18 m) with poor definition. Anatomically, it is associated with a smooth domal segment and a convex lateral crura. These cases are easily treated with tip sutures beginning with the strut, domal creation, and interdomal sutures. Next, any lateral crural convexities are corrected using the lateral crural convexity suture. The tip position suture insures a supratip break. Add-on grafts can be added to further refine the tip (Daniel, 2009).

Level 3. Major tip deformities represent a shift in how we perceive tip width aesthetically. Often, the true tip is present, but our eye concentrates on a more lateral "pseudotip" produced by the retrograde curvature of the lateral border of a convex lateral crura (20-24m). Often these problems are further complicated by rigid cartilages or over projection. Tip suturing runs the risk of creating a smaller version of the original and therefore the solution may be domal excision plus a structured tip graft.

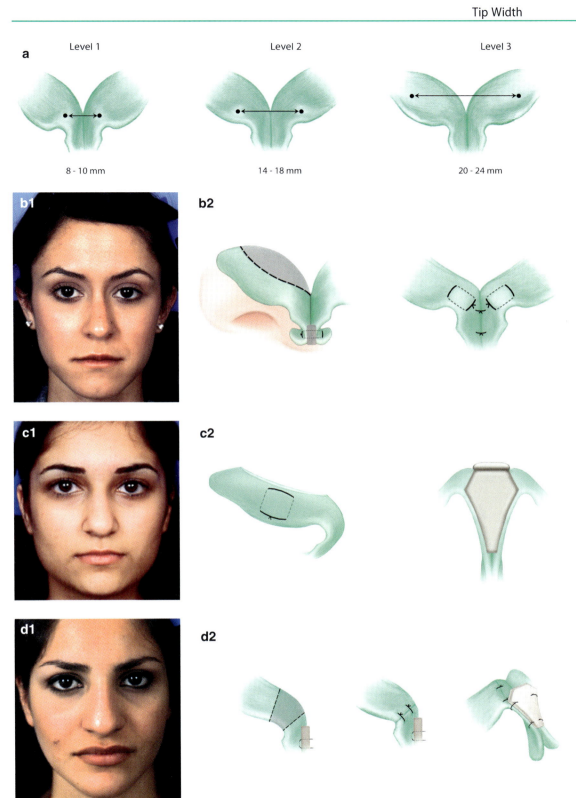

a

Level 1   Level 2   Level 3

8 - 10 mm   14 - 18 mm   20 - 24 mm

b1   b2

c1   c2

d1   d2

Fig. 8.3 (**a**) The wide tip, (**b**) Level 1, (**c**) Level 2, (**d**) Level 3

Case Study: Wide Tip

Analysis

A 35-year-old woman felt that her nose was too wide and deviated (Fig. 8.4). It was emphasized to her that she had a significant asymmetric developmental deviation as opposed to a deviated septum. Surface measurements were the following: intercanthal width (29.5), alar flare (32), and tip width (25). Her tip width was within 4.5 mm of her intercanthal width – a truly wide tip especially on oblique view. The profile indicated the third major problem – a very low radix and bony dorsum. The critical step was to achieve an absolute reduction in tip width toward the ideal and then to augment the dorsum until the nose was balanced. Extensive tip suturing was done and then an add-on shield graft was added to produce a refined tip. The patient was warned – better not perfect, very limited improvements possible.

(**Level 3.0**) Everything about this nose was difficult and every area required surgery.

Operative Technique

1) After the open approach, the alars were reduced to 6-mm wide rim strips.
2) Fascia and septal cartilage was harvested. Caudal septum relocated R to L.
3) Bilateral low-to-high osteotomies.
4) A 2.5-mm spreader graft was inserted on the L side only.
5) A crural strut was inserted followed by tip sutures: CSx2, DC, DE, ID, TP.
6) LCCSx2 were used on each side to reduce tip width followed by add-on graft.
7) Glabellar graft of DC + F inserted and then a DC – F graft (0.8 cc) for the dorsum.
8) Bilateral combined nostril sill/alar wedge resection.
9) Alar rim support grafts.

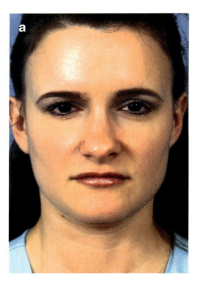
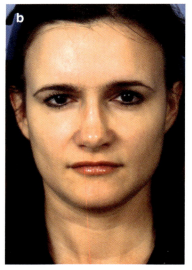
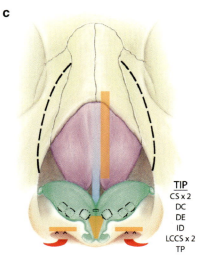

Fig. 8.4 (a–j)

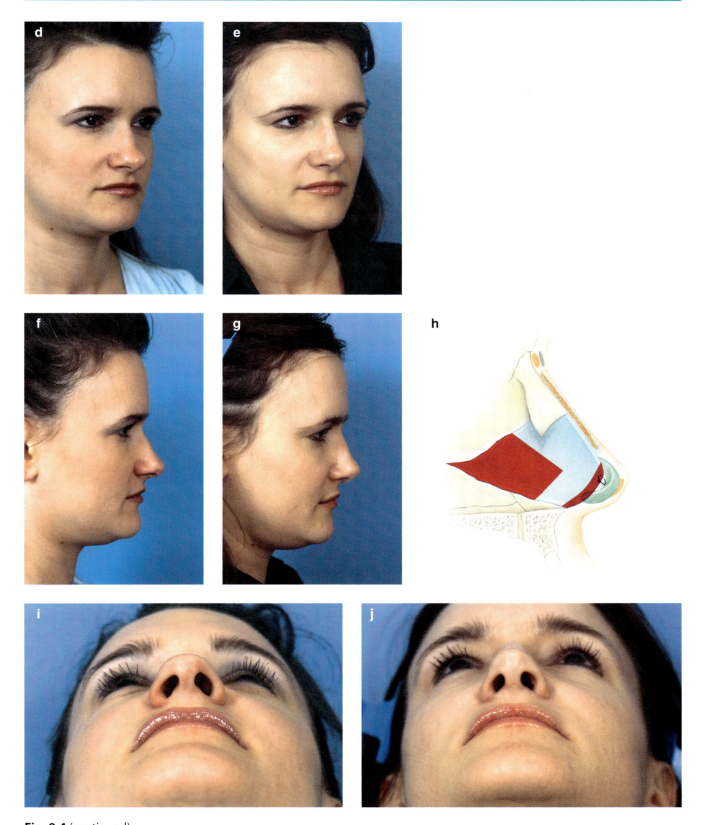

Fig. 8.4 (continued)

The Wide Nose

Interestingly, patients perceive of the "wide nose" at multiple points besides the tip – bony width, dorsal width, and alar base width (Fig. 8.5). Width is two of the three reasons why most patients seek a rhinoplasty: (1) a wide poorly defined tip, (2) a wide osseocartilaginous vault, and (3) a prominent profile.

Decision-Making. Essentially, one must decide on the best type of lateral osteotomy to narrow base bony width and whether any dorsal modification other than reduction is necessary. The most common problems include the following: x-point width beyond the intercanthal line, intrinsic convexity of the lateral walls, an excessively wide bony vault, or the combination of a wide nose and normal profile height. Frequently, the wide base will require combined nostril sill and alar base excision with the appropriate alar rim support grafts.

Level 1. As base bony width increases (x-points), transverse and low-to-low osteotomies become the right solution. The ability to rotate a straight osteotome against the lateral nasal wall while forcing the osteotome against the maxilla will insure definitive narrowing. As dorsal reductions exceed 6 mm, the resulting open roof often extends above the intercanthal level. In these cases, spreader grafts must extend high into the bony vault to avoid an inverted-V deformity.

Level 2. One will encounter noses with a wide bridge at the osseocartilaginous junction, which can become even more visible following dorsal reduction. The most effective way of insuring parallel dorsal lines is the medial oblique osteotomy. A curved osteotome is placed in the open roof and driven at 45° outward and downward. It is usually combined with a low-to-low osteotomy to insure narrowing of the entire complex. Another common deformity is the nose whose width is accentuated by convex lateral walls. A straightforward solution is the "double level" osteotomy. Essentially, one is breaking the lateral nasal wall at its mid portion and converting it from convex to straight or even slightly concave. It consists of the following sequence: (1) a perforated type osteotomy using a 2 mm osteotome along the fusion line of the nasal bone and the frontal process of maxilla, (2) a standard transverse osteotomy, and (3) a low-to-low osteotomy.

Level 3. The most interesting deformity is the wide nose with normal height on profile. Essentially, one must narrow the dorsum without changing the profile. This challenge is easily solved by doing a *paramedian narrowing of the dorsum*. The technique is as follows: (1) the dorsum is exposed through an open approach and extramucosal tunnels are made, (2) the midline is marked, (3) the ideal dorsal width is marked on the osseocartilaginous vault (5–8 mm), (4) paramedian cuts are made on the dotted lines along the cartilaginous vault up to the keystone area), (5) these cuts are extended through the bone using a straight guarded osteotome, (6) lateral osteotomies are done usually consisting of transverse and low-to-low osteotomies, (7) after the infractures, the excessive height of the upper lateral cartilages are trimmed (often 3–6 mm), and (8) the upper lateral cartilages can be sutured adjacent to or underneath the T-shaped septum.

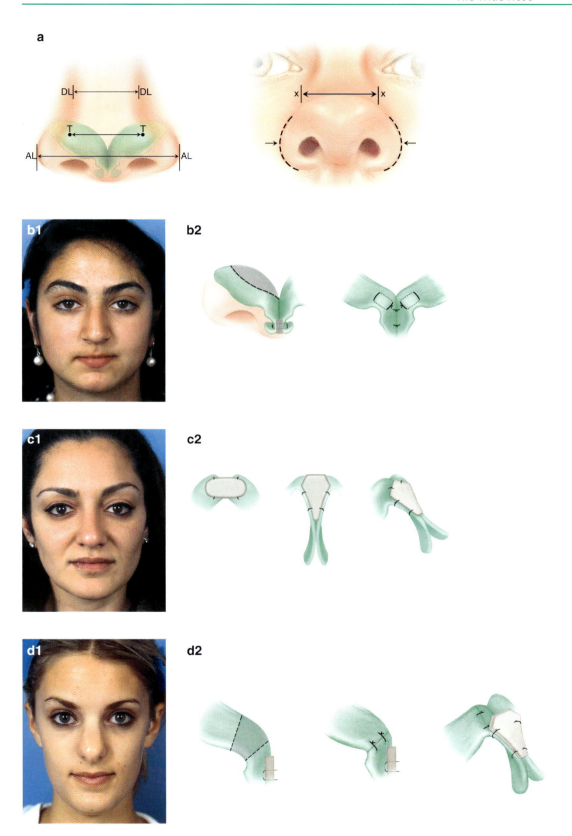

Fig. 8.5 (**a**) The wide nose, (**b**) Level 1, (**c**) Level 2, (**d**) Level 3

Case Study: Wide Nose/Wide Tip

Analysis

A 20-year-old student requested a rhinoplasty because of her wide tip and unattractive nose (Fig. 8.6). Of course, she wanted a thin narrow nose with a delicate tip. Further complicating the analysis was that her profile was essentially ideal and thus the nose needed to be narrowed without changing the profile. Controlled narrowing of the dorsum was done using paramedian osetotomies, which were marked 2.5 mm from the midline and represented a reduction from 19 to 5 mm at the keystone. Once all six osteotomies were completed, the ULC rose 3 mm above the dorsum and had to be excised. Tip sutures plus a two-layer infralobular add-on graft was effective at narrowing and triangulating the tip. ARS grafts were used to change the nostril shape from round to tapered.

(**Level: 3.0**) Every anatomical component of this nose was wide and amorphous. The analysis was complex and the surgical techniques were demanding.

Operative Technique

1) Harvest of fascia and septum.
2) Open approach with excision of the "scroll junction" only.
3) Minimal smoothing of the keystone area with a rasp.
4) Paramedian dorsal ostotomies 2.5 mm from the midline. Transverse and low-to-low osteotomies.
5) Three millimeter excision of overlapping ULC and suture fixation ULC to septum.
6) Cural strut and tip sutures: CS, DC, ID, DE. Two-layer shield-shape add-on graft.
7) Insertion of fascial radix graft and alar rim support grafts.

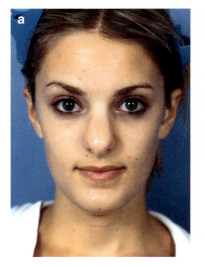
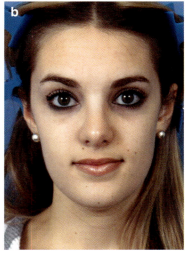
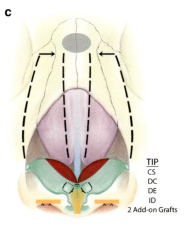

Fig. 8.6 (a–j)

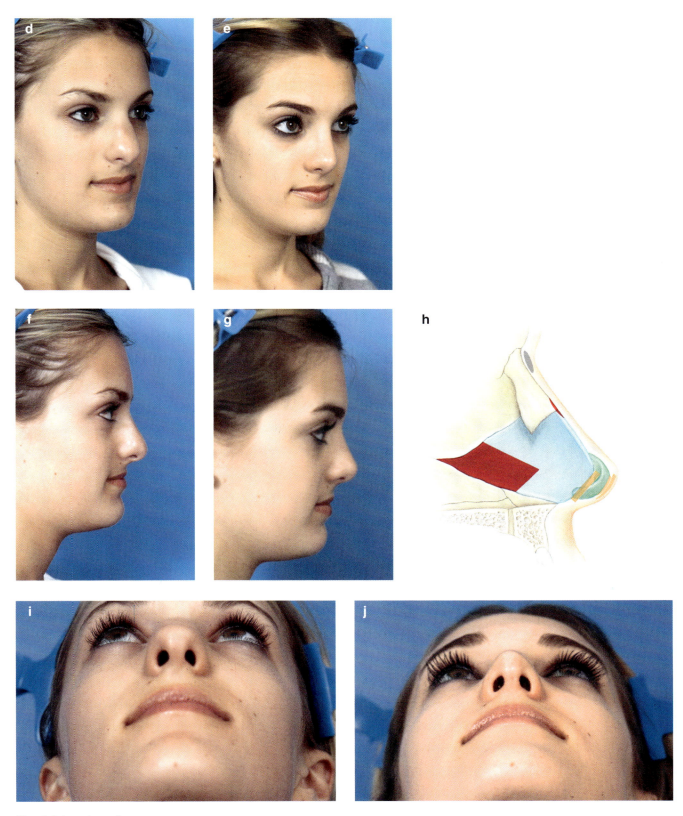

Fig. 8.6 (continued)

The Over Projecting Nose

Decision Making. Assessing projection often comes down to two factors: tip projection and the ideal dorsal profile line. Tip projection is defined as the distance from alar crease to tip (Fig. 8.7). It is composed of both intrinsic alar components and extrinsic influences from the osseocartilaginous vault. For those who enjoy photographic analysis, it is very easy to use Byrd's (1993) ratios of measuring midfacial height (MFH) and then using two thirds of its value for ideal dorsal length (N-Ti) and two thirds of N-Ti for ideal tip projection (AC-Ti). Two angles are drawn: the tip angle from the alar crease and the nasofacial angle from the ideal nasion. Where the two lines intersect determines tip projection, dorsal length, and ideal dorsal profile. In most cases, I place the greatest weight on tip projection and tip angle.

Level 1. These cases are often a "strong nose" where one wants to drop overall projection by 2–3 mm and the etiology is primarily extrinsic. Essentially, the tip is stretched outward on the dorsum and caudal septum. Thus, incremental dorsal reduction achieves the ideal profile line and drops both nasal and total tip projection. Additional subtle reductions in tip projection can be achieved by bilateral transfixion incisions (a loss of an additional 1–1.5 mm).

Level 2. These cases represent a challenge as the amount of deprojection is greater (3–6 mm), and the etiology is often combined. My goal is to eliminate the extrinsic forces (dorsum) first, which defines the remaining intrinsic (tip) component. The dorsum/radix is lowered appropriately until the ideal profile line is obtained. Then, the caudal septum/ANS is usually resected. At this point, all of the external forces, which influence the tip have been eliminated and one must reassess the operative plan. Can I drop tip projection using segmental excisions of lateral crura or do I need to excise the domes? In Level 2 cases, I create the ideal tip configuration with sutures and then reduce tip projection with segmental excision of the lateral crura. Isolated excisions of middle crura are not done as they are extremely destabilizing and fraught with complications.

Level 3. In these cases, the overprojection is quite great (>6 mm) and the intrinsic factors are significant including deformities of the alar cartilages. In these cases, suture modification is virtually impossible, and I prefer an open structure tip graft. The excess cephalic lateral crura is excised and then a cural strut is inserted. Next, a point 6–7 mm above the columellar breakpoint is marked. A transverse cut is made through the middle crura and the lateral component is undermined submucosally. An appropriate domal segment is excised (4–8 mm), which drops projection dramatically. The domal excision is closed with 5-0PDS. A tip graft is fashioned and then sutured into place. This is a very flexible operative technique and has worked well in cases requiring up to 12 mm of tip deprojection.

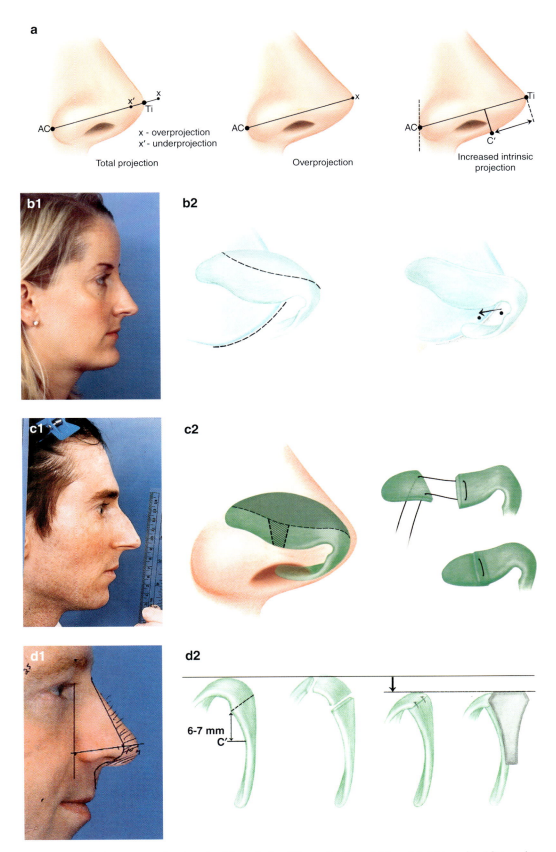

Fig. 8.7 (**a–d**) The over projecting tip. (**a**) analysis of tip projection, (**b**) Level 1, (**c**) Level 2, (**d**) Level 3

Case Study: Overprojecting Tip

Analysis

This 5' 7" patient wanted a significantly smaller nose. Lateral photographic analysis indicated that a 10-mm tip deprojection would be necessary (Fig. 8.7d). Surgically, the choice is – Can the tip be set back using lateral crural excision or do the domes need to be excised? This case was done in sequential fashion. First, the extrinsic forces were eliminated by reducing the dorsum and shortening the caudal septum (Fig 8.8 a, b). Second, careful alar analysis indicated that lateral segment excision would not be adequate and thus a domal excision would be required (Fig 8.8 c). Therefore, a direct 6 mm excision of the middle crura was done to drop projection. (Fig 8.8 d) Third, tip creation was necessary using a shield-shape graft plus a cap graft. The overall tip reduction approached 10 mm (Fig. 8.8).

(**Level: 3.0**) This was truly a functional reduction – eliminating the extrinsic forces first then the intrinsic. The difficulty was the magnitude of the reductions.

Operative Technique

1) A closed-open approach. Dorsal reduction (bone 1.5, cartilage 7).
2) Caudal septal excision of 5 mm.
3) Open approach and reduction of alar cartilages to 6 mm.
4) Harvest of septal body. Low to high osteotomies.
5) Insertion of spreader grafts.
6) Insertion of columellar strut. A 6-mm middle crura excision 6 mm above the columellar breakpoint.
7) Insertion of a shield-shape tip graft and cap graft.
8) Closure of all incisions and nostril sill excision.
9) A unilateral left ARG.

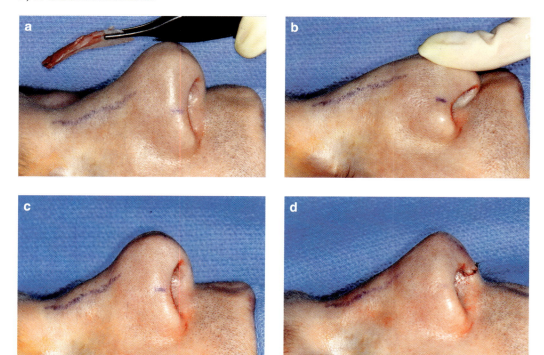

Fig. 8.8 (**a–l**) Extrinsic factors (**a**, **b**), intrinsic factors (**c**, **d**)

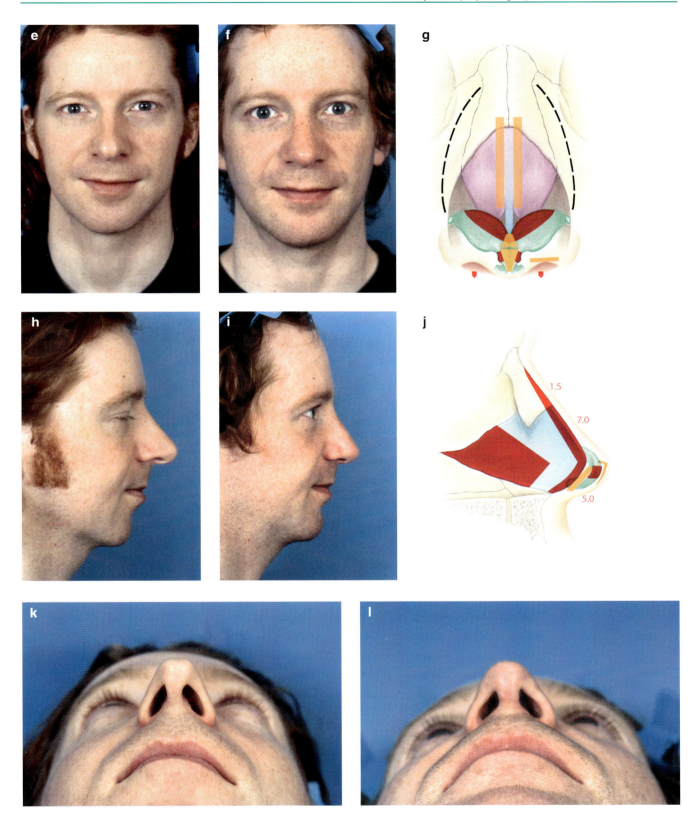

Fig. 8.8 (continued)

**Case Study:
Under
Projecting Tip**

Analysis

A 17-year-old student presented with a succinct complaint –"I hate my tip." Since the dorsum would be lowered minimally, it would be necessary to add volume and projection to the tip (Fig. 8.10). The tip was wide, downwardly rotated, hypoplastic, and intrinsically underprojecting. The columellar strut provided projection and prevented drooping postoperatively. The dorsal reduction was minimal and no spreader grafts were required. The interdomal suture narrowed the tip. The double-layer add-on graft provided intrinsic projection, tip volume, and domal definition. The triangulation of the tip is evident on basilar view. The power of TRG grafts should not be under estimate (Daniel, 2009).

(**Level: 2.0**) A classic example of "how the tip goes, so goes the rhinoplasty."

Operating Technique

1) Open approach with alar cartilage analysis.
2) Dorsal reduction (bony 0.2 mm, cartilage < 1.0 mm).
3) Harvest of septum and temporal fascia.
4) Low to high osteotomies. Insertion of radix fascial graft.
5) Insertion of crural strut and tip sutures: CS, DC, ID, DE.
6) Double layer domal add-on graft (6 × 3 mm).
7) ARS grafts to lower alar rims.

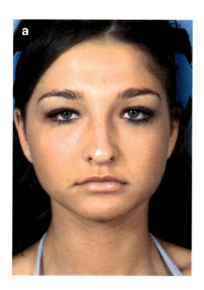 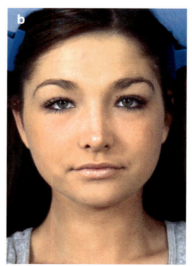

TIP
CS
DC
DE
ID
Add-on x 2

Fig. 8.10 (a–j)

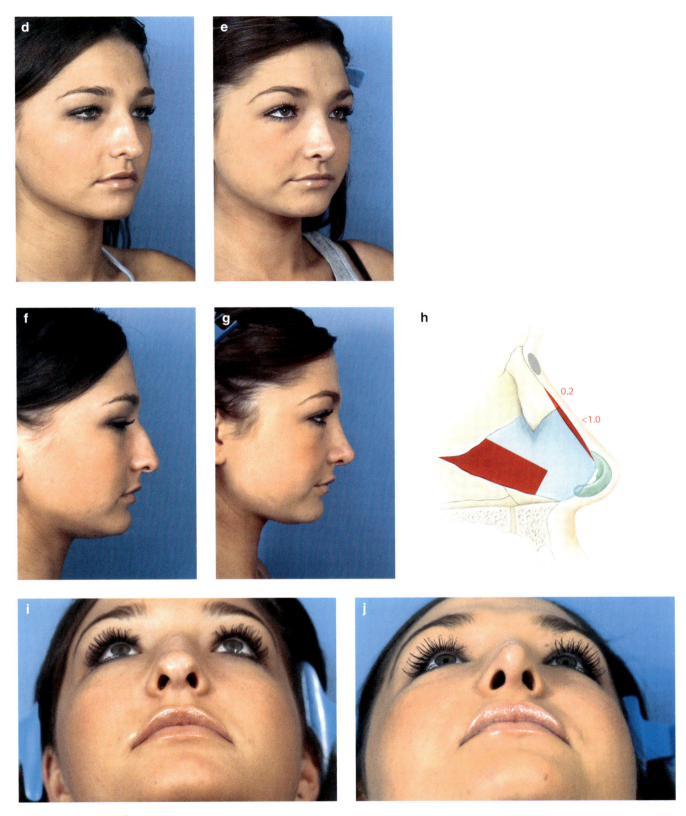

Fig. 8.10 (continued)

Downward Rotating Long Nose

Decision Making. Tips can be in downward rotation due to either extrinsic factors (extended caudal septum/ANS) and/or intrinsic factors (a long lateral crura or a long middle crura) (Fig. 8.11). Although everyone recognizes a long nose, it can be extremely difficult to classify. The first step in analyzing the long nose is to mark both the current nasion (N) and ideal nasion (Ni). The three distal points are marked (T, C′, SN) and measured. Obviously, N-T is dorsal length and the ideal N-Ti = .67xMFH. In general, N-SN is longer (5–6 mm) than N-T, whereas N-C′ is about 2 mm shorter than N-SN. Whenever N-C′ is longer than N-SN, then a hanging columella is present. The key factor is how "crowded" is the upper lip by the nose and will shortening of the caudal septum result in a long upper lip?. Also, assessment in static and smiling positions is required as well as palpation. Clinically, I classify downwardly rotated tips based on their severity into dependent, plunging, and plunging "plus."

Level 1. Most relatively long noses with downwardly rotated tips can be corrected by the following sequence: (1) excision of excess cephalic lateral crura, (2) conservative resection of caudal septum (3–4 mm) and occasionally the ANS, (3) tip suture including tip position suture for rotation and projection. Judicious excision (2–3 mm) of caudal border of the upper lateral cartilages can be considered.

Level 2. When suturing is not enough, then segmental excision of the lateral crura is added. For upward rotation, a cephalically based triangle is excised approximately 10 mm from the dome. The cephalic base is about 5 mm and tapered to the caudal rim either as a true triangle or 1–4 mm to also drop projection. The edges are then brought together with 5-0 PDS. I think that sutures from lateral crura to upper lateral or septal cartilage are very risky and not recommended.

Level 3. In certain cases, an open structure tip is the only solution including a domal segment excision, which includes the intrinsic deformity of the alar cartilage. The excised edges are repaired with 5-0 PDS and then an open structure tip graft is added.

Note: A relatively rare cause of the downwardly rotated tip in primary cases is caused by retrusion of the lower caudal septum/ANS (see Fig. 8.12). It is indicated clinically by an acute columella labial angle and a downward inclination of the columellar, especially in the older patient. Careful examination including palpation is critical. Correction requires insertion of a major columella strut to push down the columella as well as the SN point. The result is conversion of the columellar labial angle from acute to smoothly tapered. One can also add plumping grafts to the SN area.

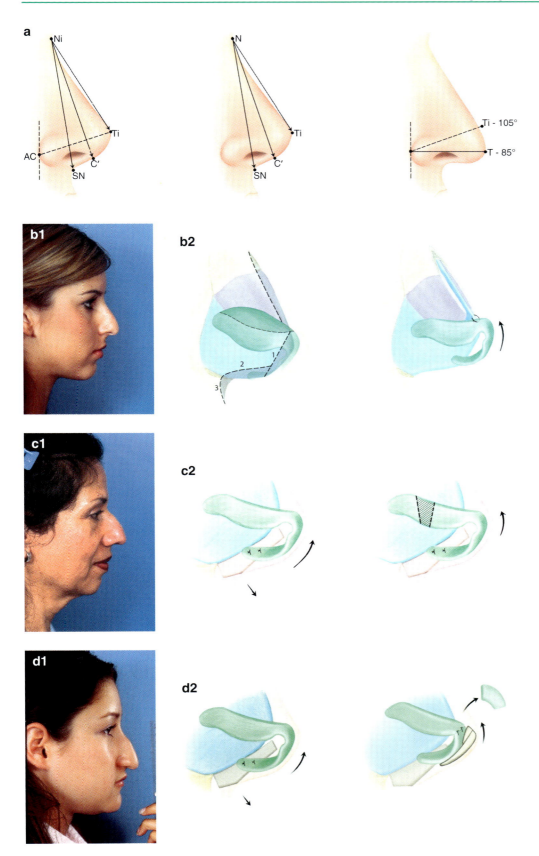

Fig. 8.11 (**a**) Long downwardly rotated nose, (**b**) Level 1, (**c**) Level 2, (**d**) Level 3

Case Study: Downward Rotation

Analysis

A 55-year-old woman sought improvement in her appearance, especially her nose. Obviously, the nose would need to be made smaller, but the real challenge would be the plunging tip on profile (Fig. 8.12). This deformity is emphasized by the retracted columellar. One must understand different concepts of the "long nose." The surgical procedure effectively shortened the nose as measured at N-T, but lengthened it at N-SN. The tip angle was raised from 90° to 100° and the columellar labial angle was raised from an acute 80°. A "teeter totter" approach was used – a major columellar strut pushing down the columellar labial segment and a tip position suture rotating the tip upward. To further reduce the signs of aging, a lower lid blepharoplasty and chin implant were done.

(**Level 2.0**) The analysis and operative planning were critical, while the actual surgery was straight forward except for the essential 7 mm wide columellar strut.

Operative Technique

1) A medium chin implant and lower lid bleph were done. Fascia was harvested.
2) Open approach with reduction of alars to 6 mm rim strips.
3) Incremental dorsal reduction (bone: 1.5 mm, cartilage 7.5 mm).
4) A 1 mm upper caudal septal resection followed by septal harvest.
5) Low to high ostotomies followed by spreader graft insertion.
6) Insertion of a structured columellar strut measuring 7 mm at CLA.
7) Tip suturing: CS, DC, DE, DP.
8) Insertion of combined "ball & apron" radix/dorsum fascia graft (F).
9) Alar wedge excision of 3.5 mm and ARG grafts to nostril rims.

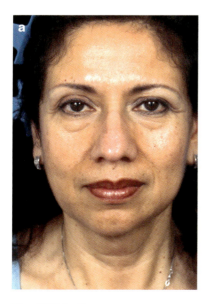 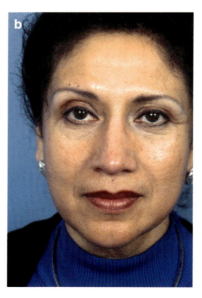 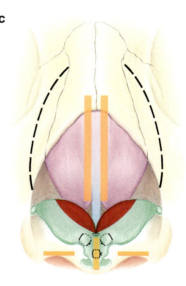

Fig. 8.12 (a–j)

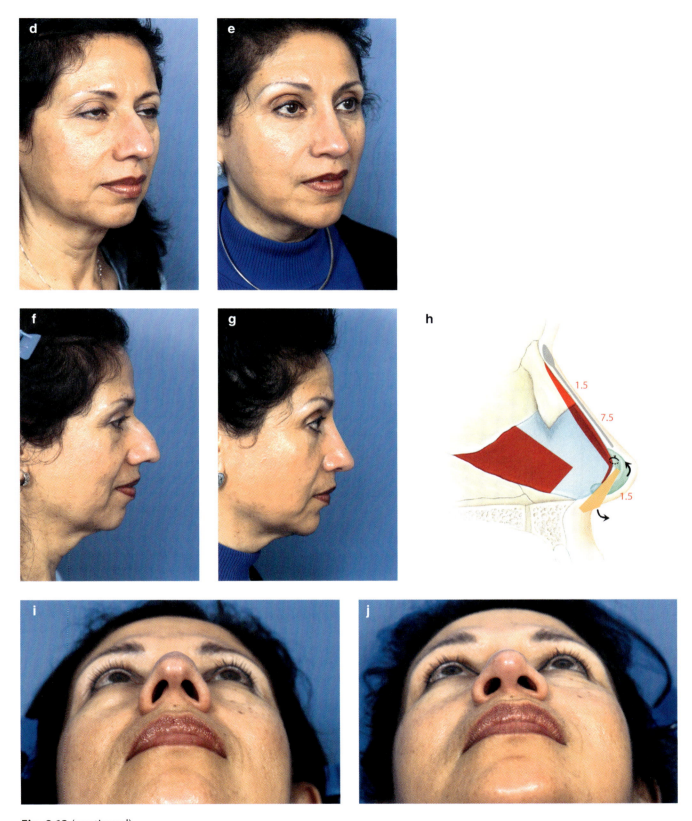

Fig. 8.12 (continued)

Upward Rotating Short Nose

Decision Making. Essentially, any tip angle greater than 105° with confirmation from the columella inclination signals an upwardly rotated nose (Fig. 8.13). In most short noses with an upwardly rotated tip, a triad is present: (1) tip angle > 110°, (2) a prominent dorsum with a nasofacial angle > 40°, and (3) an obtuse columella labial segment due to a prominent caudal septum. Of greater difficulty are cases where the nasofacial angle is essentially normal, but the tip is upwardly rotated and the dorsal length is short.

Level 1. Put simply, there is no such thing as a Level 1 short upwardly rotated primary nose. All of these cases are demanding and require sophisticated insertion of complex grafts. When first starting out, avoidance is the best option.

Level 2. These tips are upwardly rotated due to a deficiency in septal length or a deformity in the alar cartilages. Dorsal lengthening of the septum is necessary to derotate the tip. The septal cartilage is harvested via an open approach using a "top-down" dorsal split leaving the membranous septum intact. For most surgeons, the easiest method of lengthening a nose is a combination of extended spreader grafts and a triangular "pennant" shape columellar graft. The concept is to lengthen the cartilaginous dorsum 6–10 mm at the anterior septal angle. The spreader grafts are 20–25 mm long and extend caudally beyond the anterior septal angle by 6–10 mm. The strut is placed in between the extended spreaders and sutured into place, which will force the columellar downward. Then, the routine tip suturing onto the pennant columellar strut is done.

Level 3. These cases are extremely difficult as the challenge is severe in both the caudal septum and the alar cartilages. In Caucasians, this deformity is rare, but it is often the norm in Asian patients. In these cases, a massive (20 × 20 mm) septocolumellar graft is inserted between the alar cartilages and overlaps the caudal septum. The goal is to both lengthen the dorsal septum while providing a rigid strut for supporting the alar cartilages. It is fixed to the caudal septum using #25 needles. It is important to decide whether the goal is a pure derotation (no extension of the columellar below the SN/ANS) or derotation and lengthening are required (extension of the strut beyond the SN/ANS). Following insertion, the graft is sutured to the septum at three points using 4-0 PDS – dorsal, septal angle, and caudal septum. Then the dorsal component is shaped allowing for a 6–8 mm projection of the domes above the dorsal line. The excised septal cartilage is often used for a tip graft in the infralobule, which further derotates the tip.

Level 4. These cases are nasal reconstruction requiring rib grafts for lengthening. Whenever the soft tissues are pliable then a composite reconstruction is done. However, when the entire nasal lining is rigidly contracted then lengthening with a tongue-in-groove rib fixation is necessary.

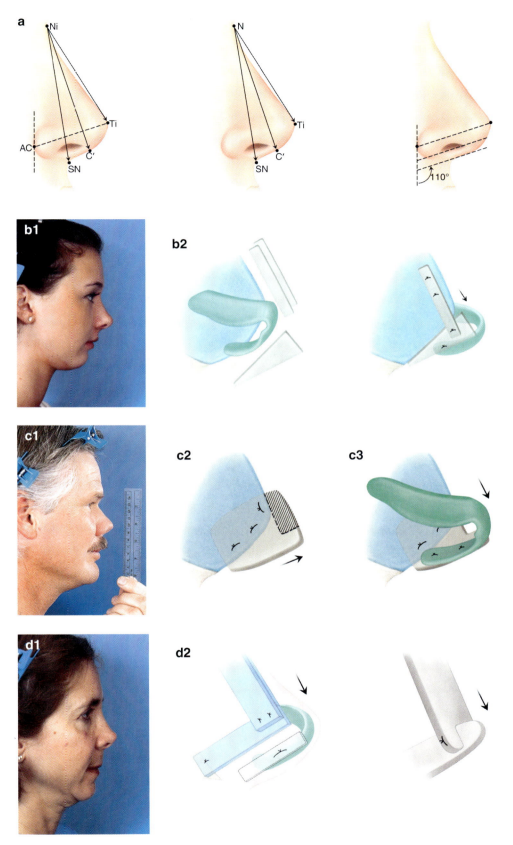

Fig. 8.13 Short upwardly rotated nose. (**a**) Analysis, (**b**) Level 2, (**c**) Level 3, (**d**) Level 4

Case Study: Short Upwardly Rotated Nose

Analysis and Commentary

A 6' 4" contractor complained that his nose was too turned up and everyone looked up his nostrils (Fig. 8.14). This was his natural nose, no prior trauma. Based on photo analysis, the tip angle needed to be derogated from 115° to 95° and the dorsum lengthened from 37 to 45 mm. A septocolumellar graft was used to lengthen the nose and provide a strong support for the heavy soft tissue envelope. A major radix/dorsal graft with DC beneath it elevated the root of the nose. This balanced approach resulted in correction of this very difficult problem.

(**Level 3.0**) Everything was difficult and reminded me of a cleft lip nose where major septo-columellar grafts are essential.

Operative Technique

1) Tip analysis showed a severe inward folding of a concave domal segment. Only a 3-mm scroll was excised.
2) Keystone area smoothed (<0.5 mm) and minimal cartilaginous excision (1.5 mm).
3) Insertion of a 22 × 15 mm septocolumellar graft.
4) Addition of a 25 × 8 mm pennant graft for a dorsal lengthening of 15 mm along the dorsal plane.
5) Advancement and suture fixation of the alar cartilages to pennant columellar strut.
6) Major radix/dorsal half-length graft with DC boost.
7) Combined nostril sill/alar wedge excisions.

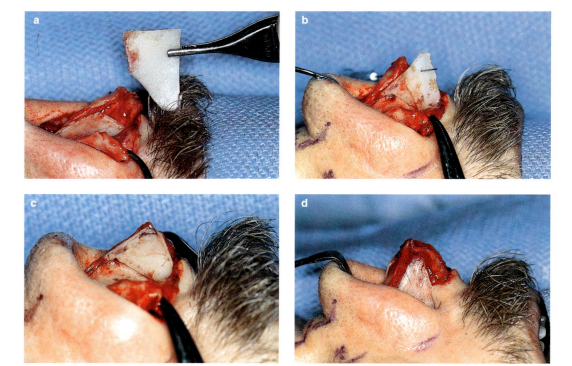

Fig. 8.14 (a–l)

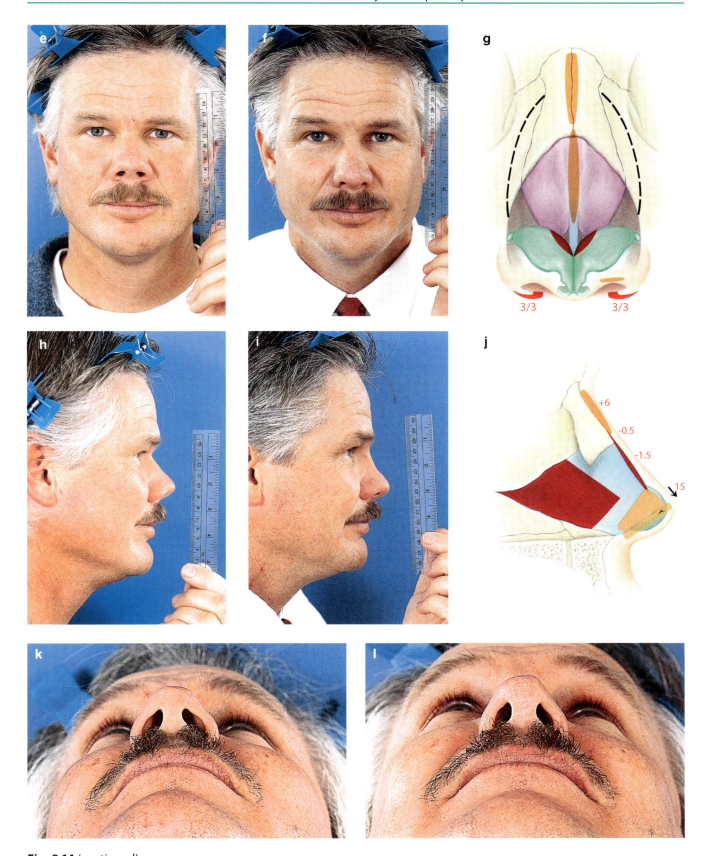

Fig. 8.14 (continued)

Broad, Ball, and Bulbous Tips

Abnormal tip shapes present a major challenge for the rhinoplasty surgeon, both technically and analytically (Fig. 8.15). Accurate definitions are impossible as the identical tip is considered by one surgeon to be bulbous, while another considers it boxy. These two sections will attempt to distinguish these tips based upon their intrinsic anatomy, external valve support, and surgical treatment.

Broad Tip. This is most easily distinguished on oblique view where the sheer volume of the tip of the alar cartilages is apparent. Anatomically, the domal segment is flat and continues into a broad convex lateral crura. Aesthetically, one is seeing the tip-defining points not at the domes, but rather at lateral crura convexities. The critical surgical steps within the tip suture technique are as follows: (1) decrease volume by cephalic lateral crura excision, (2) increase domal definition with domal creation sutures, and (3) decrease crural convexities with lateral crural mattress sutures. This approach is highly effective and represents a normal extension of Level 1 tip surgery to Level 2 cases.

Ball Tip. This is most easily diagnosed on anterior view as the lateral border of the alar cartilages gives the tip a circular or ball appearance.. Anatomically, the tip-defining points are on the lateral crura near the scroll formation, and not at the domes. Many ball tips can be sutured with LCCS being effective provided the lateal crus is malleable. If the alars are quite rigid or overprojected, then an open structure tip graft with *domal segment excision* is necessary. Once the columellar strut is sutured into place, the line of excision is marked 6–7 mm above the columellar breakpoint. There are three possible locations for the segmental excision: vertical to reduce projection, central to reduce projection and width, and lateral to primarily reduce width. Excising the domal segment eliminates the broadness of the lateral crura, while the open structure tip graft creates new tip-defining points.

Bulbous Tip. This is evident on any view as the tip looks like a "blob" due in large part to a very large thick skin envelope. There is no evidence of any underlying anatomy or any aesthetic tip characteristics. The first step is to make sure that the patients understand their anatomical limitations and accept a limited improvement. Surgically, the first step is to thin the soft tissue envelope. Infracartilaginous incisions are made and the lobular skin is elevated in the subdermal plane. Then, the skin envelope is elevated from the transcolumellar incision. The entire intermediate fibrofatty layer is elevated off the underlying alar cartilages. Second, a major structural columellar strut is inserted between the alars, which are advanced upward under tension and fixed with #25 needles. Usually, two crural strut sutures are used – one below and one above the columellar break point. The domes and lateral crura are modified as necessary. Third, a full-length structure tip graft is inserted, usually in the projected position with a supporting cap graft. One is doing everything to create "tip show" through thick skin. Often, a 7Fr drain will be inserted to shrink wrap the skin around the new tip.

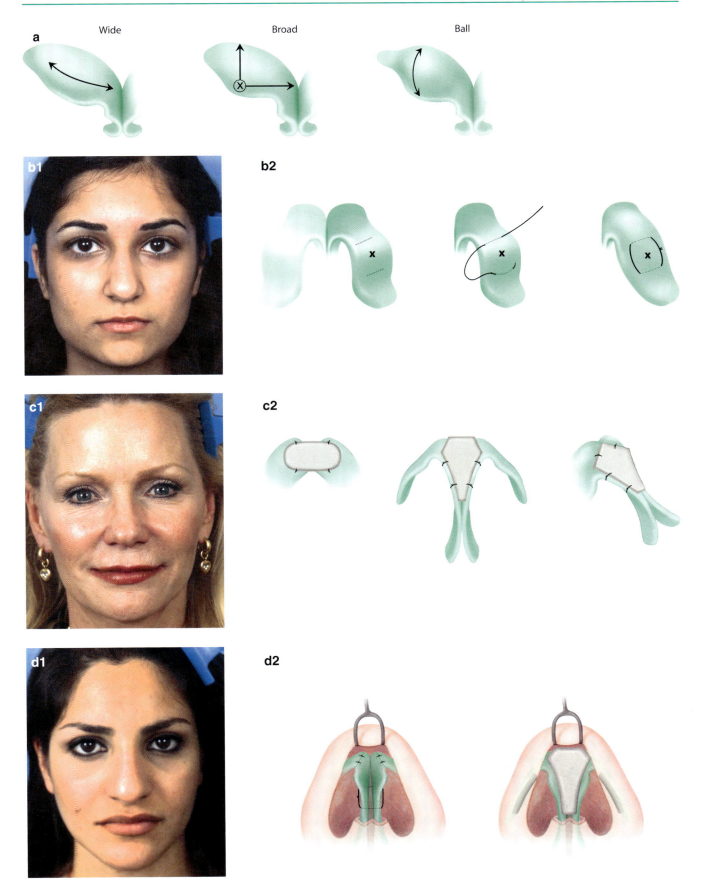

Fig. 8.15 (**a**) Broad, ball, bulbous tips, (**b**) broad, (**c**) ball, (**d**) bulbous

**Case Study:
Ball Tip**

Analysis

An executive requested an aesthetic rhinoplasty, which would reduce her ball tip (Fig. 8.16). She had no respiratory complaints. Her alar cartilages were quite rigid while her alar side walls were quite weak. When asked to take a deep nasal inspiration, her external valves collapsed. The alar cartilages were massive and no matter how much suturing could be done, the tip would still look like a "ball." Direct excisions removed the deformed domes and narrowed the tip significantly. The concealer tip graft covered the suture repair and prevented the show of any edges. The lateral crural strut grafts were sutured to the caudal border of the lateral crura and then along true rim incisions to prevent external valve collapse. At one year postop, the patient breaths well without nostrill collapse, but the vascular blush on her columellar remains unchanged from pre operative status.

(**Level 3.0**) Domal excision and concurrent lateral crural strut grafts are demanding technical maneuvers. A true form and function case.

Operative Technique

1) Open approach and septal exposure.
2) Dorsal reduction (bone: smooth, cartilage 2 mm), caudal septum 2.5 mm.
3) Septal body harvest.
4) Low to high osteotomies and spreader grafts.
5) Columellar strut Creation 6 mm rim strips.
6) Domal segment excisions 6 mm above columellar breakpoint (R 4.5 mm, L 6 mm). Repair of excisions with 5-0 PDS (see Fig. 8.17c for intraop).
7) Diamond shape concealer tip graft of excised alar cartilage.
8) Lateral crura strut grafts (T 3) sutured into a marginal rim incisions.

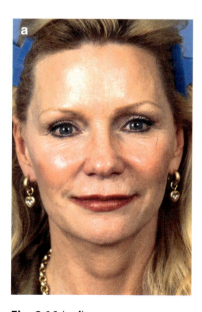 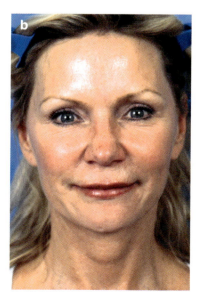 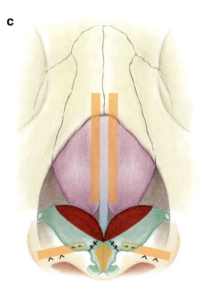

Fig. 8.16 (a–j)

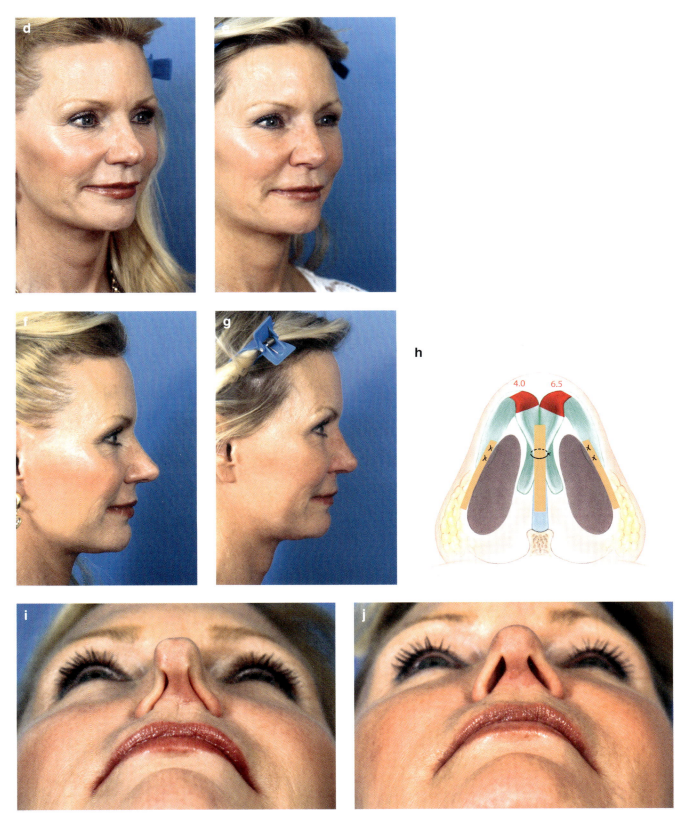

Fig. 8.16 (continued)

Boxy Tip and Alar Malposition

These tips are characterized by a lack of support for the external valve due in large part to a cephalic displacement of the lateral crura away from the nostril rim (Fig. 8.17). Cartilage grafts are essential to provide nostril rim support.

Boxy Tip. This is most easily diagnosed on basilar view, where the basilar perimeter is square and the nostril rim is concave rather than straight or convex. The alar cartilages can be highly variable, ranging from splayed small alars to wide rigid ones requiring excision. Once the tip surgery is completed, cartilage grafts are used to support the nostril rim. Although, alar rim grafts (ARG) are simpler these cases most often require alar rim support grafts (ARS). These grafts are ideally made of septal cartilage and measure 14 × 3 mm with a tapered cephalic end. Due to severe weakness of the external valve, I will frequently make a true rim incision 2 mm behind the nostril rim. The cephalic skin is undermined, but the nostril rim is never unfurled. The dissection continues laterally into the alar base. The thick end of the graft is inserted into the alar base pocket and then the graft is sutured at two points along the alar rim. A final check is made of the cephalic end of the ARS to insure that it is not overlapping the alar cartilages. Nostril splints will be used at night for 1–2 weeks to maintain the desired shape.

Alar Malposition (AMP). These cases represent a triad of anatomical and aesthetic problems: a parenthesis tip deformity, large abnormally shaped nostrils, and collapsible external valves. Defining alar malposition is difficult and many surgeons simply say that they "recognize it when they see it." The problem is that in thick skin patients, AMP can be present without any visible stigmata. Sheen defined AMP as "any displacement of the lateral cura from the usual parallel alignment with the nostril rims … most often the caudal edge of the lateral curs is parallel to the alar rim for half the length of the nostril." In a series of 50 primary rhinoplasties, I measured the distance of the lateral crura away from the midpoint of the nostril and found that 7 mm appeared to be the critical distance. Often, this simple measurement is all that is needed to suggest a diagnosis of AMP.

In severe cases, surgical treatment requires alar transposition plus lateral cural strut grafts. On several occasions, I have sutured an AMP in situ and found no change in the aesthetic deformity once the skin was redraped. Elevating the alar off the underlying mucosa is critical in making a permanent change in the tip deformity. The following surgical tip sequence is recommended: (1) reduce the lateral crua to 6-mm wide rim strips, (2) elevate the lateral crura off the underlying mucosa, (3) insert and suture the columellar strut, (4) tip refinement with either tip sutures or a structured tip graft depending upon the degree of overprojection, (5) attachment of lateral crural strut grafts, (6) temporary skin closure, (7) alar base excisions as indicated, (8) definitive placement of the lateral cura strut grafts usually along the rim (Type 3), and (9) closure and insertion of short temporary nostril sill splints. The patient will use nostril sill splints for 2–3 weeks while taping at night. Tip overprojection is quite real and domal excision plus a structured tip graft may be necessary. In thin skin patients, a "fascial blanket" will be used to cover the entire tip. One should never underestimate the difficulty of these cases.

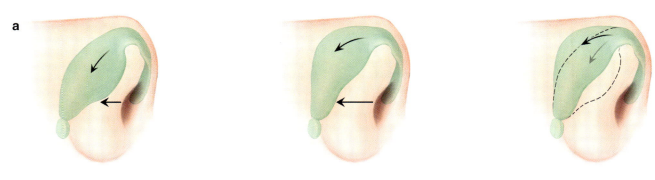

Fig. 8.17 (**a**) Normal anatomy, Alar malposition, and over lap.

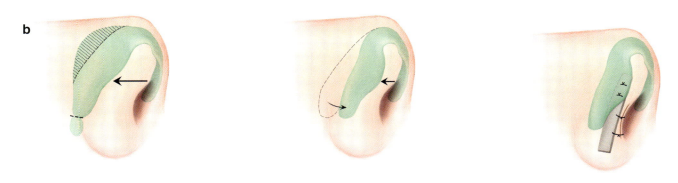

Fig. 8.17 (**b**) Treatment of Alar malposition using Alar transposition plus LCSG T3

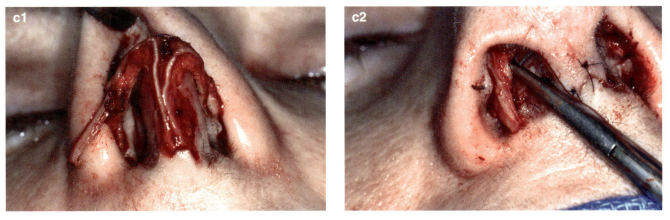

Fig. 8.17 (**c**) Intraop photos of Alar transposition plus LCSG T3   **DVD**

Case Study: Alar Malposition

Analysis

A 31-year old woman presented with a most unusual and severe triad of nasal tip deformities (Fig. 8.18). The tip was overprojected with a boxy configuration and alar malposition. Further complicating the challenge was her significant long face syndrome. Obviously, she should have had a LeForte II and mandibular advancement, but she was not interested. She did agree to a large chin implant. The basilar view of this patient confirmed the severity of the boxy deformity and nostril rim weakness. Since alar transposition and lateral crural strut grafts were planned, the normal open approach was altered. True rim incisions were made rather than the conventional infracartilaginous incisions. Undermining of the lateral crura allowed the tip to be fundamentally changed. This was a very aggressive tip operation for a very severe tip deformity, which produced a profound change in the nostril shape.

(**Level 3.0**) Perhaps the most difficult primary tip imaginable – consisting of an aesthetic deformity, overprojection, alar malposition, and external valve collapse.

Operative Techniques

1) Confirmation of pre-op alar malposition (10/19).
2) Open exposure using true rim incisions rather than infracartilaginous incisions.
3) Dorsal reduction (bone: 1 mm, cartilage: 5 mm). No caudal septal or ANS excision.
4) Septal harvest. Low to high osteotomies.
5) Creation of rim strips 6 mm in width. Release and transposition of the lateral crura.
6) Insertion of crural strut. Domal excision to drop projection 5 mm. Repair of excision.
7) Open structure tip graft of septal cartilage.
8) Suturing of lateral crural strut graft to lateral crura.
9) Out fracture of turbinates.

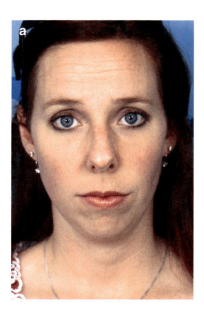
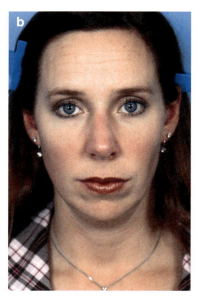
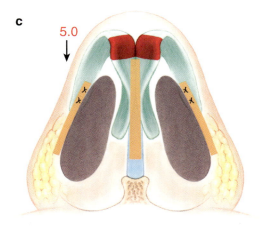

Fig. 8.18 (a–j)

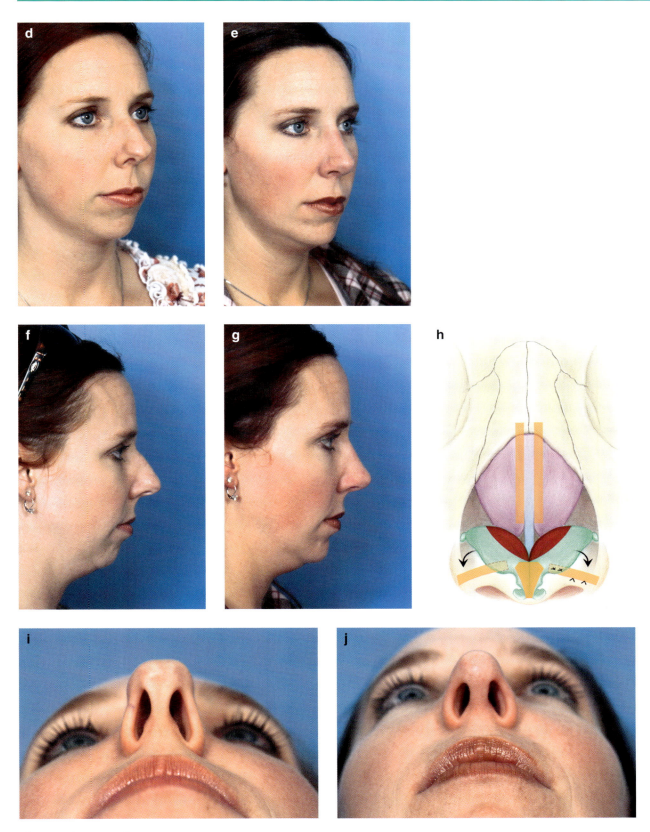

Fig. 8.18 (continued)

Reading List   Byrd HS, Hobar PC. Rhinoplasty: a practical guide for surgical planning. Plast Reconstr Surg 91: 642, 1993

Byrd HS, Andochick S, Copit S, Walton KG. Septal extension grafts: a method of controlling tip projection shape. Plast Reconstr Surg 100: 999, 1997

Cole P. Nasal and oral airflow resistors. Arch Otolaryngol Head Neck Surg 1: 18, 1992

Constantian M. The boxy nasal tip, the ball tip, and alar cartilage malposition: variations on a theme – a study in 200 consecutive primary and secondary rhinoplasty patients. Plast Reconstr Surg 116: 268, 2005

Constantian MB. Functional effects of alar cartilage malposition. Ann Plast Surg 30: 487, 1993a

Constantian MB. Experience with a three-point method for rhinoplasty. Ann Plast Surg 30: 1, 1993b

Constantinides M, Adamson PA, Cole P. The long-term effects of open cosmetic septorhinoplasty on nasal air flow. Arch Otolaryngol Head Neck 122: 41, 1996

Daniel RK. Rhinoplasty: Creating an aesthetic tip. Plast Reconstr Surg 80: 775, 1987

Daniel RK. Anatomy and aesthetics of the nasal tip. Plast Reconstr Surg 89: 216, 1992

Daniel RK. Analysis and the nasal tip. In: Daniel RK (ed) Aesthetic Plastic Surgery: Rhinoplasty. Boston, MA: Little, Brown, 1993

Daniel RK. Rhinoplasty: nostril/tip disproportion. Plast Reconstr Surg 107: 1874, 2001

Foda HM. Management of the droop tip: a comparison of three alar cartilage – modifying techniques. Plast Reconstr Surg. 112: 1408, 2003

Gorney M. Patient selection rhinoplasty: practical guidelines. In: Daniel RK (ed) Aesthetic Plastic Surgery: Rhinoplasty. Boston, MA: Little, Brown, 1993

Gunter JP, Rohrich RJ. Lengthening the aesthetically short nose. Plast Reconstr Surg 83: 794, 1989

Gruber RP, Friedman GD. Suture algorithm for the broad or bulbous nose. Plast Reconstr Surg 110: 1752, 2002

Guyuron B. Precision rhinoplasty. Part 1: The role of life-size photographs and soft tissue cephalometric analysis. Plast Reconstr Surg 81: 489, 1988

Johnson CM, Toriumi DM. Open Structure Rhinoplasty. Philadelphia, PA: W.B. Saunders, 1990

Peck GC. Techniques in Aesthetic Rhinoplasty, 2nd ed. Philadelphia, PA: JB Lippincott, 1990

Rees TD, La Trenta OS. Aesthetic Plastic Surgery, 2nd ed. Philadelphia, PA: W.B. Saunders, 1994

Rorhrich RJ, Adams WP Jr. The boxy nasal tip: classification and management based on alar cartilage suturing techniques. Plast Reconstr Surg 107: 1849, 2001

Sheen JH. Spreader graft revisited. Perspect Plast Surg 3: 155, 1989

Sheen JH, Sheen AP. Aesthetic Rhinoplasty, 2nd ed. St. Louis, MO: Mosby, 1987

Tardy ME. Rhinoplasty: The Art and the Science. Philadelphia, PA: W.B. Saunders, 1997

Tebbetts JB. Shaping and positioning the nasal tip without structural disruption: a new systematic approach. Plast Reconstr Surg 94: 61, 1994

Toriumi DM. Structural approach to primary rhinoplasty. Aesthetic Surg J 22: 72, 2002

Advanced Primary Rhinoplasty 9

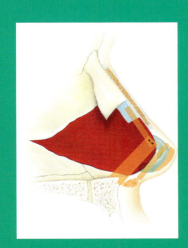

Introduction

What constitutes a difficult rhinoplasty? Traditionally, the answer is whatever rhinoplasty you are doing at that moment, or any operation that pushes you beyond your comfort zone. Objectively, I think the major differences between Level 2 and 3 cases are the following: (1) severity of deformity, (2) complexity of operative technique, and (3) requirement for intraoperative flexibility. Essentially, these cases mandate that something be done to all parts of the nose. One must modify and integrate the entire nose rather than simply lower the profile or refine the tip. The operative plan is often complex consisting of a myriad number of grafts, infrequently performed techniques, and asymmetric design. Intraoperative findings may require one to make major changes in the original plan. How does one progress from Level 2 to Level 3 cases? For many surgeons, it is the challenge of ethnic rhinoplasties which can have a spectrum of deformities that range from Level 2 to Level 3. Also, one will on occasion realize intraoperatively that the problems are greater than anticipated thereby increasing the grade from Level 2 to Level 3. When first entering practice, 33% of your rhinoplasty consults may appear to be Level 3 cases. As your gain experience and your comfort zone expands, the percentage of Level 3 cases will decrease. Ultimately, you will enjoy the challenge and the technical demands of these cases.

Asymmetric Nose and Tip

In contrast to posttraumatic cases, the asymmetric nose is often developmental in origin and thus the component parts are anatomically dissimilar (Fig. 9.1). These observations must be pointed out to the patient preoperatively using a mirror and emphasizing that only a "limited improvement" is realistic. Equally, a careful internal exam must be done as septal deviation and internal valve collapse are common.

Localized. Although slight discrepancies may be present in the bony and alar bases, the most obvious asymmetry is usually in the dorsal lines and tip. The dissimilarity may begin at the junctional "bumps" of the osseocartilaginous vault, be accentuated along the dorsum, compounded by a concavity/convexity contrast of the two upper lateral cartilages, and further highlighted by juxtaposition of a concave upper lateral cartilage and a convex lateral crura. For minor and moderate deformities, asymmetric spreader grafts are often a judicious solution coupled with the usual dorsal reduction and cephalic lateral crura resection.

Generalized. Approximately 25% of my cosmetic rhinoplasty patients have some degree of Asymmetric Developmental Deviated Nose (ADDN). I coined this term to distinguish developmental from posttraumatic deviations. In these cases, there is no history of significant nasal trauma. Virtually the entire face and nose have significant differences: usually a vertical and angular side of the nose while the face has a stronger/wider side versus a weaker/longer side. The most common combination is an angular wider nasal half on the short wide facial side and a vertical narrow nasal half on the long narrow facial side. If these discrepancies are pointed out preoperatively with the patient holding a mirror, there will be far fewer complaints postoperatively.

As regards the asymmetric nose, any underlying septal deviation is corrected first. Individual operative steps are modified to adjust for the asymmetries: (1) quantitative differences in resection, (2) unilateral steps, and (3) opposite procedures. For example, quantitative differences would be a combined alar base resection in which a 2.5 mm resection was done on one side and 3.5 mm on the other. A unilateral maneuver would be an onlay graft over the upper lateral cartilage on the concave side with nothing done contralaterally. An opposite procedure is rarely performed, but an example would be an out-fracture on the concave side and an in-fracture on the convex side.

Major tip asymmetries are very difficult and one begins from the crural strut insertion upward. Again, sutures followed by concealer tip grafts are the first choice. Frequently, lateral crural strut grafts will be placed beneath concave or distorted lateral crura. In worst case scenarios, it is necessary to excise the domes and insert an open structure tip graft.

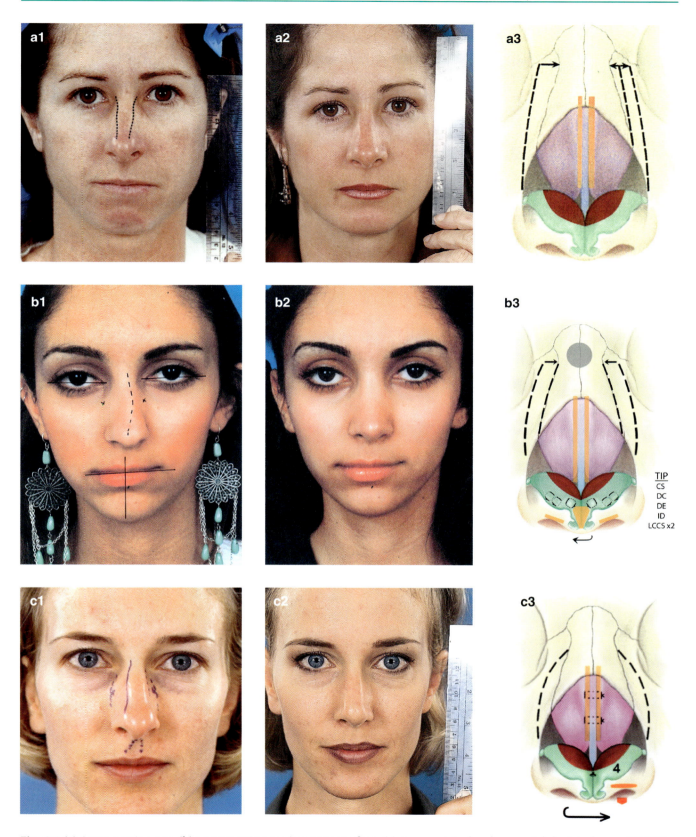

Fig. 9.1 (**a**) Asymmetric nose, (**b**) asymmetric nose/asymmetric face, (**c**) asymmetric developmental deviated nose (ADDN)

**Case Study:
Asymmetric
Deviated Nose**

Analysis

A 28-year old requested correction of her deviated nose and nasal obstruction. There was no previous trauma (Fig. 9.2). A diagnosis of severe asymmetric developmental deviated nose (ADDN) was made with its severity noted by the deviated philtral columns. The anatomical obstruction included septal deviation to the left with blockage of the internal valve plus turbinate hypertrophy. Aesthetically, she simply wanted the nose straighter, her dorsum lower, and a slight reduction in tip volume. A closed approach was planned. The unplanned conversion from closed to open was an intraoperative necessity to deal with a septal disjunction. Sandwiching the septum between spreader grafts and upper lateral cartilages provided rigid support and prevented postoperative saddling. At 1 and 7 years post-op, the patient has retained both nasal support and normal respiration.

Operative Techniques

1) Closed approach with volume tip reduction
2) Septal exposure with creation of extramucosal tunnels
3) Incremental dorsal reduction (bone: 2 mm, cartilage: 4 mm)
4) Caudal septal shortening (5 mm). Septal harvest. Caudal septal relocation L to R
5) Attempt to straighten bony septal deviation results in disjunction between the bony and cartilaginous septum
6) Conversion to an open approach
7) Stabilization of septum with spreader grafts and five-layer suture fixation
8) Low-to-high osteotomies
9) L 2.5 mm nostril sill excision. Alar rim graft (ARG) on left
10) Bilateral partial inferior turbinectomy including bone on L

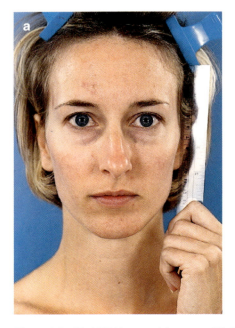 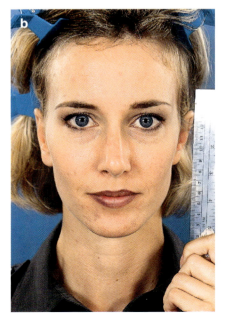 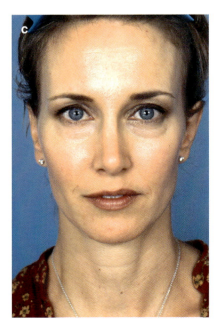

Fig. 9.2 (a–k) ADDN nose, (**a**) preop, (**b**) 1 year postop, (**c**) 7 years postop

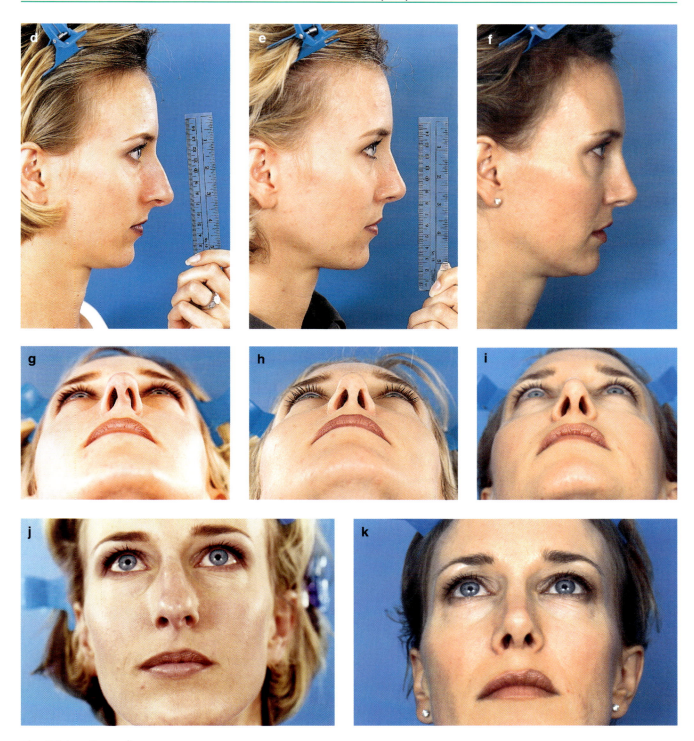

Fig. 9.2 (continuned)

Posttraumatic Nose

The posttraumatic deviated nose is exceedingly complex. One must be skilled with both complex septal surgery and multiple techniques for modifying the osseocartilaginous vault. A detailed history is obtained of the accident, age at injury, initial surgical treatment, and any follow-up procedures, as well as current problems. In general, I classify them externally into three types: straight line, C-shape, and S-shape. I do not hesitate to get CT-scan of the nose to help sort out the residual deformity of the nose.

Straight Line. These deviations are often related to underlying septal deviation culminating in caudal septum/anterior nasal spine (ANS) displacements to one side (Fig. 9.3a–d). They are the epitome of Cottle's dictum that "as the septum goes, so goes the nose." Essentially, standard techniques with emphasis on caudal septum relocation should yield a good result. These cases are very similar to ADDN.

C-Shape. The C-shape nose requires separate analysis of both the bony and cartilaginous vaults as well as the septum. Essentially, one must decide on the types of osteotomies and how severe the cartilaginous deformity is. If any reduction is planned, it is done prior to the septal work. It is important to detach the upper lateral cartilages and then individually adjust each upper lateral. Once the profile line is set, then the definitive septal work is performed. Lateral osteotomies are done as indicated. Osteotomies may facilitate outward repositioning of the inwardly displaced side. Often, the laterally deviated side will rise above the profile line and require additional lowering. The cartilaginous vault is then corrected beginning with straightening and reinforcement of the L-shape septal strut with asymmetric spreader grafts.

S-Shape. The S-shape nose is a step up in complexity with the bony vault on one side, the cartilaginous vault pushed to the opposite side, and then caudal septum crossing back to the opposite side; hence a double cross of the midline (Fig. 9.3e–h). Certain variations from the C-shape nose must be considered. First, the septal problems can be extraordinarily challenging and a total septoplasty is often warranted. The bony vault may well require asymmetrical rasping; more on the long angulated side, less on the short vertical side. Asymmetrical osteotomies are often necessary with two low-to-low osteotomies to shorten the long angulated side and a double-level out-fracture to correct the fixed concave lateral wall in the cartilaginous vault. Following removal of the total septum, an L-shape septal replacement graft is inserted. The reinserted L-shape graft is stabilized by the appropriate application of spreader grafts for the dorsal component and fixation to the ANS for correct alignment of the caudal component. A columellar strut will support the alars above the dorsal line and provide the desired tip projection. I do no advocate supporting the alars on the L-shape replacement graft.

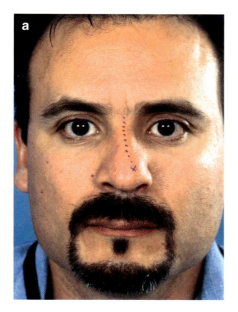
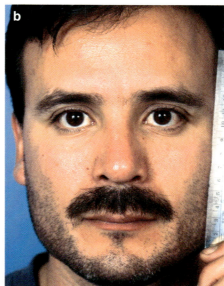
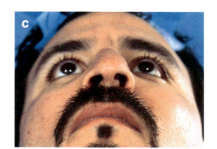
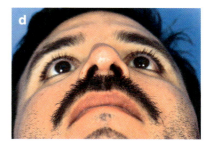

Fig. 9.3 (**a-d**) Deviated nose, straight line deviation

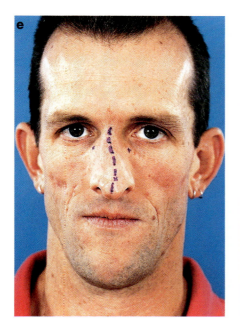
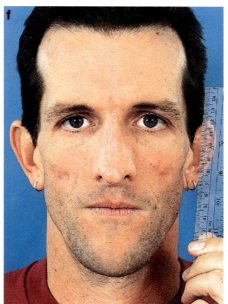
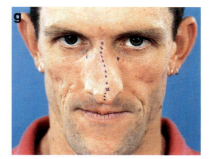
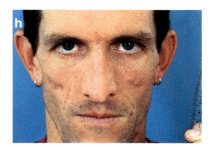

Fig. 9.3 (**e-h**) Deviated nose, S-shape deviation

Case Study: Posttraumatic Nose

Analysis

This patient had a severe nasal deformity following trauma in early childhood with possible extension onto the left maxilla (Fig. 9.4). The nasal obstruction was quite sever. The septum was collapsed longitudinally wiping out all support from the caudal septum. The destruction of the septum precluded doing a total septoplasty and left a rib graft as the only method of obtaining structural graft material. The extended spreaders and septal strut restored support to the nose. The columellar strut and multiple tip grafts allowed the tip to project above the dorsum which was reconstructed with DC-F. The double-level osteotomies narrowed the nose effectively.

Operative Techniques

1) Septal exposure with confirmation of extensive destruction.
2) Harvest of cartilaginous portions of the eighth and ninth ribs.
3) Open approach with *bidirectional approach* to the septum. The entire cartilaginous septum was excised leaving a 15 mm long by 10 mm high dorsal portion.
4) Transverse and double-level osteotomies.
5) ANS exposed via a gingival incision and a drill hole placed.
6) Foundation layer inserted: septal strut fixed to ANS, extended spreader grafts fixed to bony vault, and a "step off" fixation between spreaders and septal strut.
7) Columellar strut insertion and suture fixation. Tip grafts: shield and cap.
8) DC-F graft (0.6) to the dorsum.
9) Major alar batten grafts to alar rim.
10) DC (4.0 cc) grafts to peripyriform and L maxilla.

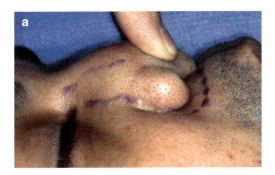
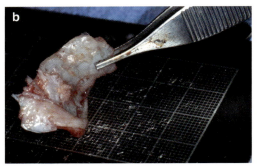
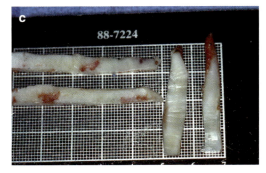
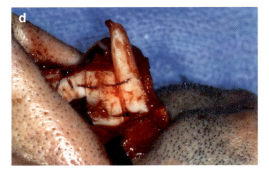

Fig. 9.4 (a–m)

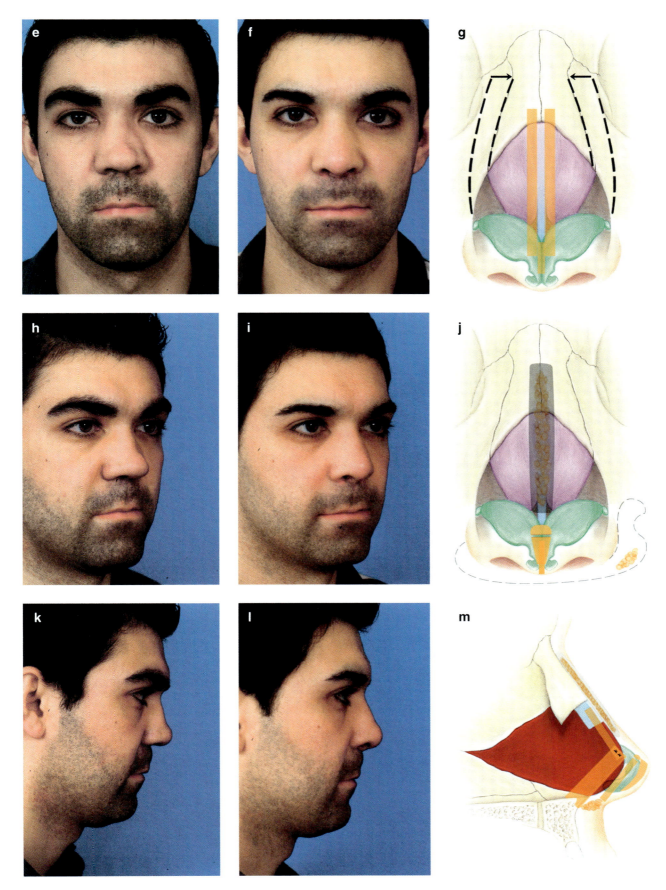

Fig. 9.4 (continued)

Dorsal/Base Disproportion

In analyzing cases with disproportions, it is important to realize that either component can be in excess while the other is either normal or deficient (Fig. 9.5). The fundamental treatment principle is Sheen's adage of "reduce where the structure is excessive, and augment where it is deficient." Although used within the context of secondary supratip deformities, this *balanced approach* is ideal for primary cases where the base is large and the dorsum is normal or hypoplastic. Although relatively rare in Caucasian primaries, it is the fundamental deformity in many ethnic rhinoplasties. Sequentially, one reduces the base as much as possible and then augments the dorsum until the ideal profile is achieved. One does not hide behind the concept of an "irreducible skin sleeve," but rather maximizes lobular reduction and tip definition with structure followed by aggressive alar base reduction. Once the base has been maximally reduced then dorsal augmentation is done to achieve the final result.

Thinning the Skin Envelope. The lobule is ballooned with local anesthesia and undermined via infracartilaginous incisions. Then the open approach is completed and the excess soft tissue excised off the alar cartilages. The undersurface of the skin is never directly defatted as it risks skin loss or scarring.

Structured Columellar and Tip Graft. Using the harvested septal cartilage, large columellar strut, tip, and alar rim structure grafts (ARS) are carved. In these cases, the columellar labial angle is often acute with a retracted columellar. Therefore, the columellar strut is shaped to have a 6–8 mm width which will push down the columellar angle. The alars are advanced high onto the strut and sutured at two points. A full-length structured tip graft is sutured to the alars, often in a projected position with a supporting cap graft.

Alar Base Reduction and ARS. One of the major components of a large base is excess interalar width and flare. If one fails to reduce the base, the nose will always look large. The best method of reduction is a combined nostril sill/alar wedge resection often with the nostril sill component being 2–3 mm, but the alar wedge component being 3–5 mm. In severe cases, the nostril sill component will be deepithelialized and used to cinch the alar base to the ANS. Since many of these cases have "occult alar malposition," ARS grafts are essential and often planned for from the beginning by using a true rim incision rather than the more common infracartilaginous incision. The location of this "rim incision" is where the ARS will be sutured at the time of closure. Nostril splints, followed by taping, are done every night for several weeks.

Dorsal Reduction and Augmentation. Frequently, one has to reduce the convexity of the cartilaginous vault while augmenting the bony dorsum. One often has to excise 1–2.5 mm of the cartilaginous vault in order to achieve a straight dorsum. Subsequently, a straight dorsal profile line becomes the goal and a wide range of dorsal grafts are considered – radix, radix/half-dorsum, or full-length dorsum. These "construct" grafts are fabricated to fill the specific deficit. They are made from fascia and diced cartilage (DC-F). Isolated radix grafts are usually DC+F, whereas longer grafts are DC-F.

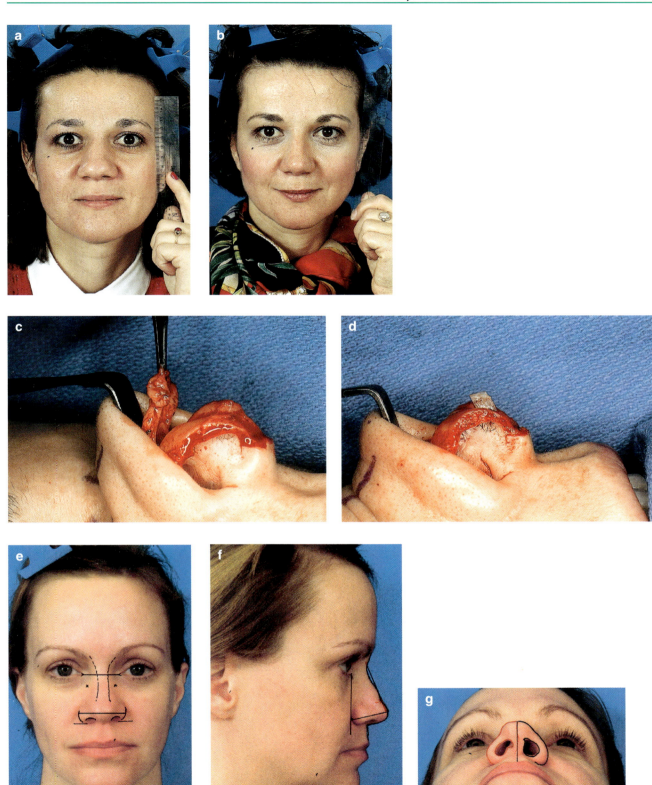

Fig. 9.5 Dorsal/base disproportion, (**a–d**) surgical techniques, (**e–g**) analysis for following case study (Fig 9.6)

Case Study: Dorsal/Base Disproportion

Analysis

This was a very complex nose in which the tip was quite broad and the alar bases even more disproportionate (Fig. 9.6). Her surface measurements were as follows: EN 32, AC 27, AL 38, and AL smiling 43. There was an astounding +11 between AC and AL. The basilar view was even more discouraging and emphasized the severe asymmetry that was present. This case is a classic example of shrinking the base as much as possible and then building up the dorsum. The first step was to narrow the tip significantly and fortunately the alar cartilages responded to suturing. Next, the radix and dorsum were built up using a DC-F graft. The tapered dorsal graft was *cephalically* oriented. Aggressive base excisions were done which further compelled placement of ARS grafts. Unfortunately, I was correct when I told the patient preoperatively that the nostril asymmetry could be made better but not eliminated.

Operative Technique

1) Fascial harvest. Exposure of the septum through a transfixion incision
2) Open approach and creation of 6 mm rim strips
3) Dorsal exposure with rhinion found to be concave. Reduction: bone: 0 mm, cartilage: <1 mm
4) Harvest of septal cartilage. Relocation of caudal septum R to L
5) No osteotomies nor spreader grafts
6) Insertion of columellar strut. Tip sutures: CS, DC, ID, DE
7) Insertion of a radix fascia graft, then a *cephalically* tapered dorsal graft (DC-F: 0.3)
8) Harvest of a retroauricular dermis graft inserted transversely below "allergic line"
9) Closure followed by bilateral combined sill/base resections (R: 3/3, L: 3/3)
10) Insertion of alar rim support grafts

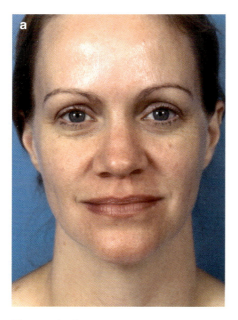
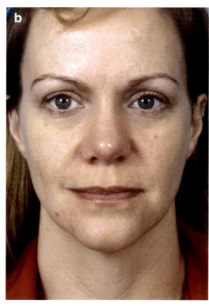
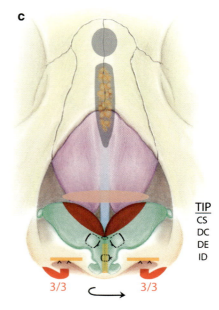

Fig. 9.6 (a–j)

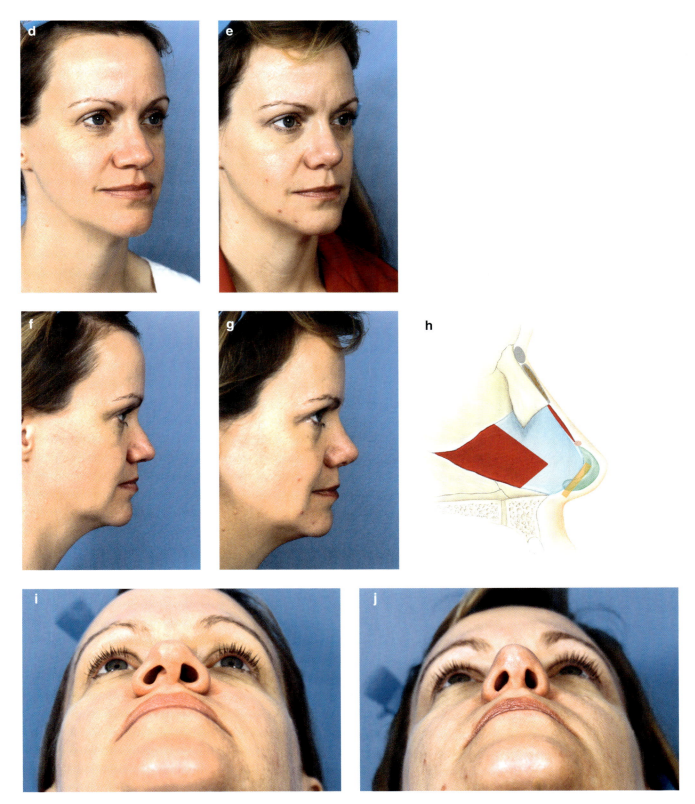

Fig. 9.6 (continuned)

Hispanic Rhinoplasty

The author has extensive experience with Hispanic rhinoplasty and summarized his approach in prior publications (Daniel 2003). Due to the diversity of both their presenting problems and requisite surgical techniques, this group is a microcosm of the Level 1–3 concept. Rather than classify by country of origin, Hispanic noses are best divided into four types based on the presenting deformity which somewhat follows the level of technical difficulty (Fig. 9.7).

Type I: Castilian. These patients are quite similar to the average adolescent nose and require the "Big 3" – reduce the profile, narrow the bony width, and refine the tip. A *functional reduction rhinoplasty* is done. The radix is not grafted. The dorsum is incrementally reduced 1–3 mm. Lateral osteotomies are done. A tip suture will provide the requisite refinement and definition.

Type II: Mexican-American. These cases are challenging as regards analysis and operative planning. They appear to have a convex dorsum whose reduction would solve the problem. Alas, it is a "pseudohump" which is accentuated by a hypoplastic radix and an under-projecting tip. A *finesse rhinoplasty* is required in which the radix area is grafted with DC+F while the tip is projected with tip sutures over a columellar strut. If additional volume is required, add-on grafts of excised alar are inserted. The intervening dorsum may or may not be reduced depending upon its intrinsic excesses. All three types of base reductions may be required.

Type III: Mestizo. The fundamental problem is thick skin with poor tip definition and an extremely wide base. Often this lobular problem is complicated by a dorsal/base disproportion. The solution is an *open structure* strut and tip graft. The critical first step is thinning the skin of the nasal lobule. After judicious injection of local anesthesia in the lobule, bilateral infracartilaginous incisions are made and the skin elevated in the subdermal plane. Then the transcolumellar incision is made and the nose opened. The fibrofatty SMAS tissue is excised off the underlying cartilages. The dorsum is smoothed. The alar cartilages are reduced to 6 mm rim strips. The septal cartilage is harvested through a top-down exposure. A major structural columellar strut and tip graft are carved from the septal cartilage. The excised alar is diced for a probable DC+F graft for the radix. The strut is inserted and the alars advanced onto the strut, often requiring two strut sutures. The shield-shape tip graft is sutured to the tip at the domal notches and a cap graft may be required depending upon the degree of projection. Appropriate osteotomies are done. Frequently, large 3/3 combined nostril sill/alar wedge excisions are necessary which in turn obligate insertion of alar rim support grafts (ARS).

Type IV: Creole. These cases are similar to the African-American or Black nose with tremendous interalar width (>45 mm) mandating aggressive narrowing, an exceedingly flat dorsum which requires augmentation, and an under-projecting tip demanding an open structure tip graft. The necessity for a full-length dorsal augmentation differentiates these cases from the Type III Mestizo. These cases are treated similar to the Black rhinoplasty patient discussed later in this chapter.

Type I: Castilian

Key step: functional reduction
1. Dorsal reduction
    (bone: 2 mm, cartilage: 4 mm)
2. Tip suture
3. Relocation caudal septum

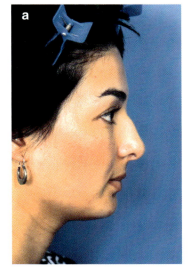 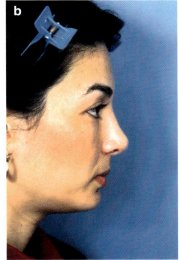

Type II: Mexican-American

Key step: finesse
1. Limited dorsal reduction
    (bone: 0 mm, cartilage: 0.5 mm)
2. Increase tip projection
3. DC-F graft (0.2 cc) to radix/upper dorsum

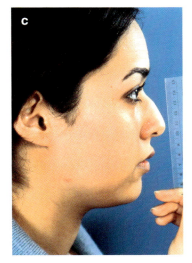 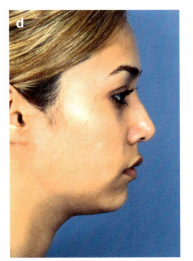

Type III: Mestizo

Key step: balanced approach
1. Soft tissue defatting
2. Open structure tip graft
3. Dorsal reduction (1 mm)
4. Radix graft
5. Combined nostril sill/alar wedge resection

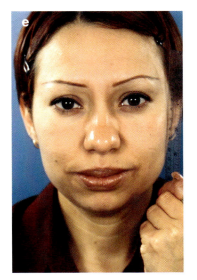 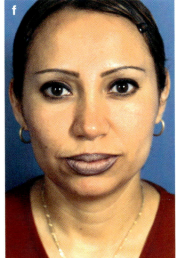

Fig. 9.7 (**a–f**) Hispanic rhinoplasty

Case Study: Hispanic Rhinoplasty

Analysis

A 26-year old of Mexican descent complained of a wide heavy tip with downward drooping on anterior view (Fig. 9.8). Technically, I considered the preexisting inverted-V deformity and hypoplastic upper dorsum a more serious issue. Nostril-tip disproportion can be corrected largely through lengthening the infralobule on the columellar strut. The bony width would be narrowed with osteotomies. The dorsum would be integrated by augmenting the bony area. A DC+F graft consisting of 0.2 cc of diced cartilage was placed beneath the dorsal component of the fascial graft and then molded to fill the defect. The risk of a solid half-length dorsal graft showing at the rhinion is notorious. The harmonious integration of the dorsum as seen on the postop photo confirms the operative plan.

Operative Techniques

1. Harvest of fascia and septal exposure
2. Minimum soft tissue defatting and 6 mm rim strip creation
3. Incremental dorsal reduction: bone: <0.5 mm, cartilage: 2 mm
4. Low-to-high osteotomies
5. Crural strut insertion and tip sutures: CS, DC, ID, DE
6. Ball and apron fascia graft with DC 0.2 below in upper dorsum

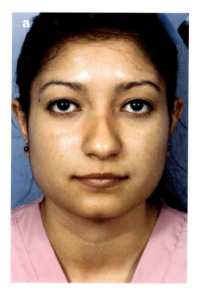
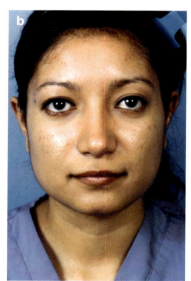
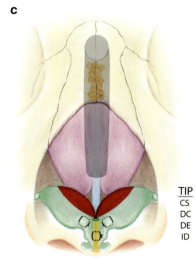

TIP
CS
DC
DE
ID

Fig. 9.8 (a–j)

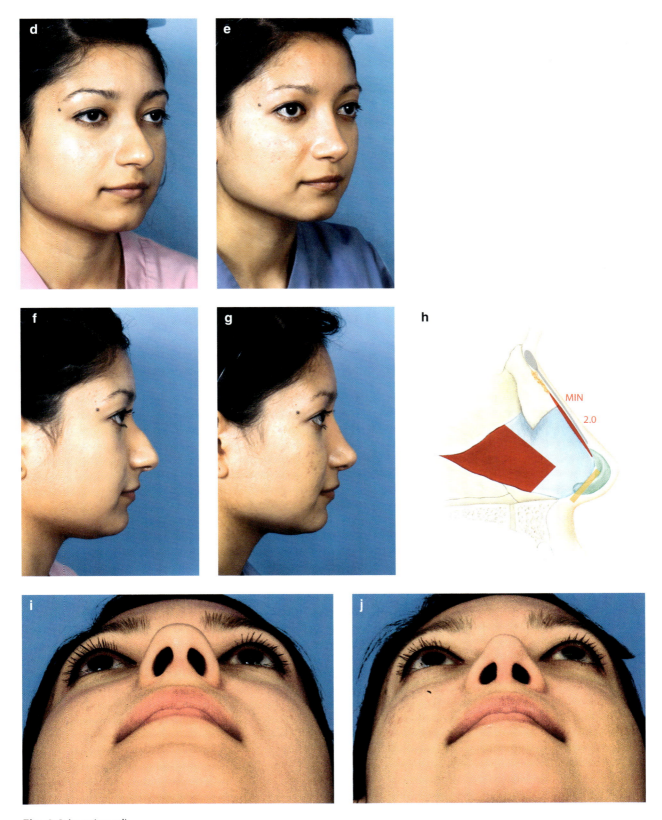

Fig. 9.8 (continued)

Middle Eastern Rhinoplasty

Approximately 20% of the author's practice is of Middle Eastern descent, especially Persian patients. These patients provide an interesting challenge of reconciling operative goals with anatomical reality. In the United States, their goal has gone from a "surgically cute" to "natural" to now "naturally cute" noses. Whenever possible, these patients want their nose to look unoperated (natural), but they expect the dorsum to be slightly curved, the tip rotated and well defined (cute). Obviously, the challenge increases in direct proportion to skin thickness and weakness of the alar cartilages. The author has seen a wide diversity in all the anatomical components including the alar cartilages (Daniel 2009).

Level 1. Approximately one third of the patients have thin skin with a downwardly rotated tip and a beaky aquiline profile (Fig. 9.9a, b). An open approach is highly effective in shifting the tip defining point from the level of the columellar breakpoint to a true 105°The dorsum is lowered incrementally, usually with emphasis on the cartilaginous component, and the upper caudal septum resected for rotation. Tip suturing is done with domal creation sutures at the domal notch and then narrowing of the tip with the interdomal suture. A tip position suture rotates and projects the tip for the desired super tip break.

Level 2. The majority of these patients have a wide nose with a bony hump and a broad dependent tip with no definition (Fig. 9.9c, d). The dorsum is lowered incrementally which requires extensive rasping. A comparable amount of cartilaginous dorsum may be resected. Caudal septum and ANS are often removed to shorten the nose. The osteotomies are often medial oblique and low-to-low. Tip suture is done with significant amount of add-on grafts in both the infralobule and across the domes to create tip definition through the moderately thick skin. Alar base modification most often consists of extended nostril sill excision with alar rim grafts (ARC) for shaping the nostrils.

Level 3. These cases are highlighted by an exceptionally thick skin sleeve, wide nasal bones, and a broad tip with no definition (Fig. 9.9e, f). The skin sleeve is often thinned and is done by raising the entire skin envelop in the subdermal plane followed by resection of the intervening SMAS tissue, from tip to radix, and from one lateral wall to the other. Two 7 FR drains are inserted to drain the nose at the end of the case and to promote "shrink wrapping" of the skin around the underlying framework. Any and all combinations of osteotomies are considered, but maximum narrowing is often necessary. The tip is almost always reconstructed with open structure columellar strut and tip grafts. Aggressive combined nostril sills/alar wedges obligate alar rim support grafts (ARS). Even with this approach, the noses will merely look "better," not great. The patient must be prepared for this outcome.

Level 1

Key steps
1. Dorsal reduction
   (bone: 1.5 mm, cartilage: 4 mm)
2. Caudal septum: 4 mm
3. Tip sutures: CS, DC, ID, TP
4. Asymmetric osteotomies

Level 2

Key steps
1. Defatting lobule
2. Dorsal reduction
   (bone: 2.5 mm, cartilage: 6 mm)
3. Low-to-low osteotomies
4. Tip suture and add-on grafts
5. Alar wedge excision and ARG

Level 3

Key steps
1. Defatting skin envelope
2. Dorsal reduction
   (bone: 2 mm, cartilage: 4 mm)
3. Six osteotomies
4. Open structure tip graft
5. Alar wedge excision and ARG

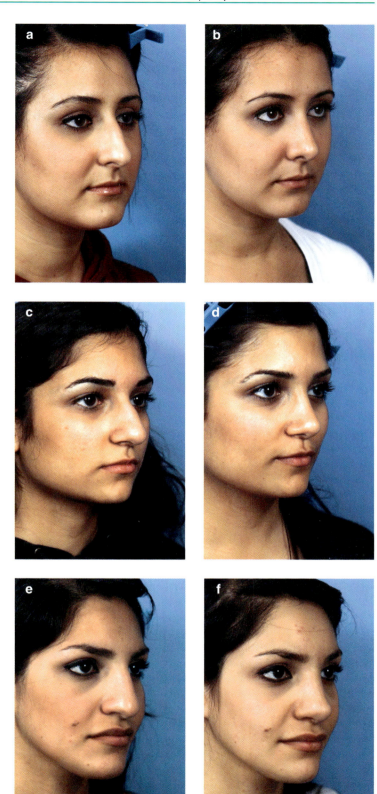

Fig. 9.9 (**a–f**) Middle Eastern rhinoplasty

Case Study: Middle Eastern

Analysis and Commentary

An 18-year-old girl of Persian descent requested a rhinoplasty which would produce a major change in her nose (Fig. 9.10). She wanted a more feminine nose that would be as *cute* as possible. Obviously, I stressed that her skin envelope was thick and its contractility unpredictable. In order to insure clarity of her desire, the patient was given a lateral profile to draw the profiles she wanted. One year after surgery, the patient wanted further narrowing of her bony vault and it was done. The original low-to-low osteotomies narrowed her bony width, but did not change the intrinsic convexity of the bones themselves which was done with double-level osteotomies at the time of revision. The patient is shown at 2.5 years post-op.

Operative Technique

1. Open approach and reduction of alars to 6 mm rim strips
2. Incremental dorsal reduction extending high (bone: 2.5 mm, cartilage 6 mm)
3. Septal harvest and spreader grafts
4. Transverse and low-to-low osteotomies
5. Crural strut and tip sutures: CS, DC, ID, TP, CSp
6. Double-layer domal onlay graft of excised alar to increase definition
7. Alar wedge resection (3.5 mm) and alar rim grafts (ARG)

Note: at 1 year the patient wanted her bones narrowed further and this was done using double-level osteotomies.

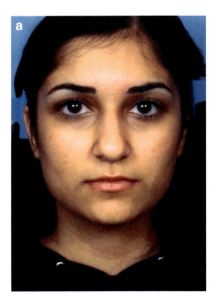
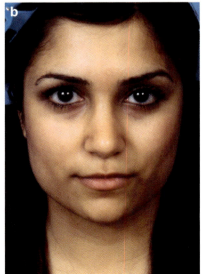
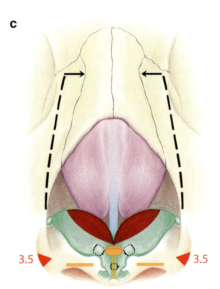

Fig. 9.10 (a–j)

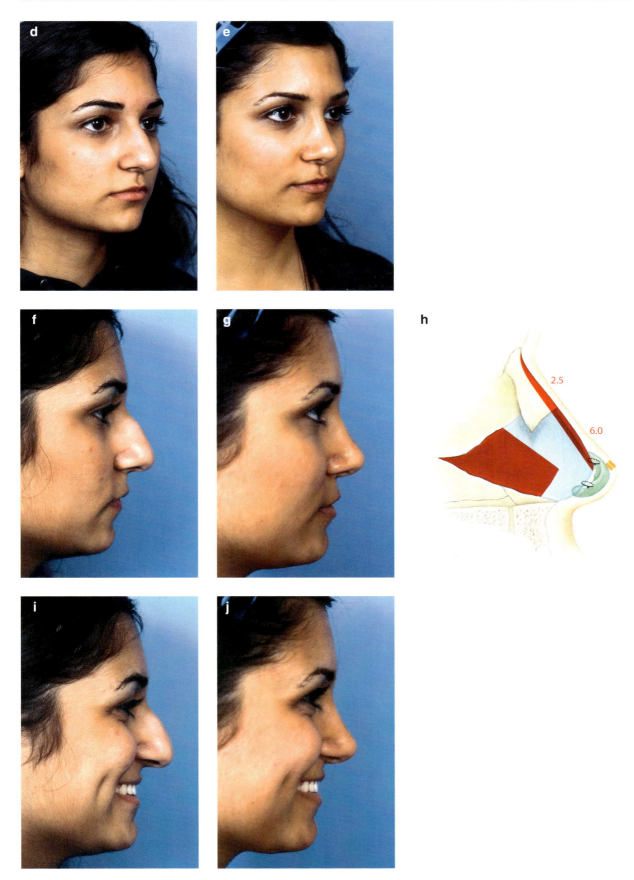

Fig. 9.10 (continued)

Asian Rhinoplasty

As Asian patients become more sophisticated they are faced with a dilemma. They want the nasal refinement provided by a silicone implant, but not the complications. Early in my practice, I did over 75 silicone implants in Asian patients with a very experienced colleague. After seeing the post-op results and dealing with the deviations and dissatisfaction, I swore I would never do another silicone implant. For 15 years, I was faced with a conundrum – the silicone implant provided a much better aesthetic result than autogenous tissue, but the complications were unacceptable. Once I began doing diced cartilage grafts, I was able to obtain excellent aesthetic results which even exceeded those of silicone because of their natural appearance. In contrast to Hispanic and Middle Eastern noses with their wide anatomical variations, Asian rhinoplasty is rather homogeneous Table 9.1 (Fig. 9.11a). One merely adds or deletes certain steps depending upon the patient's anatomy and requests. Despite the broad variation of patients making up the Asian-American community from Cambodia to Korea (think dorsal height), and the Philippines to Vietnam (think skin envelope), the following operation gives excellent results, but does require attention to detail.

Operative Sequence

Graft Harvesting. At the beginning of the operation I harvest a large sheet of deep temporal fascia through a 3 cm incision and conchal cartilage through a retroauricular incision. A tip graft and alar rim support grafts are cut from the conchal bowl. The rest of the conchal cartilage is given to the circulating nurse to dice.

Soft Tissue Defatting. In the majority of cases, the soft tissue envelope of the lobule is defatted beginning with extensive infiltration of local anesthesia (Fig. 9.11b). The skin is elevated in the subdermal plane via the infracartilaginous incisions. Then the transcolumellar incision is made and the entire skin envelope elevated. The SMAS and adipose tissue is carefully excised from the underlying cartilage. Symmetrical 6 mm rim strips are created and the excess flimsy alar cartilage is also diced.

Septal Harvest. Obtaining a large rigid piece of septal cartilage in an Asian patient is both critical and technically demanding. In contrast to the normal septal harvest of cartilage only, a large osseocartilaginous piece of septum is required (Fig. 9.11c). A combined top-down and tip-split approach to the septum is used. A transfixion incision is avoided as the intact membrous septum helps to centralize subsequent insertion of the septocolumellar strut. The entire septum is exposed, especially posteriorly. Since the caudal septum will be reinforced, a 8–10 mm L-shape strut is maintained despite the flimsy septal cartilage which is common in Asian patients. Once the initial cuts are made, a septal scissor is placed parallel to the dorsal strut. The scissors cut across the osseocartilaginous junction. The vertical cut is extended down to the vomer and the cartilage is mobilized. Again the septal scissors are inserted parallel to the vomer and then cut posteriorly across the osseocartilaginous junction. A large piece of osseocartilaginous septum is removed using the septal grasper.

Septocolumellar Graft. The sepal graft is subdivided if possible into a massive 20 × 20 mm piece for the septocolumellar graft, a full-length 15 × 8 mm tip graft, and two alar rim support grafts. Frequently, the septocolumellar graft is composed of cartilage which will be placed

Table 9.1 Asian rhinoplasty – an autogenous tissue operation

Step 1	Fascia and conchal cartilage harvest
Step 2	Soft tissue defatting of lobule
Step 3	Osseocartilaginous septal harvest
Step 4	Septocolumellar graft
Step 5	Open structure tip graft
Step 6	Dorsal graft of DC-F
Step 7	Osteotomies (optional)
Step 8	Alar base modification (optional)

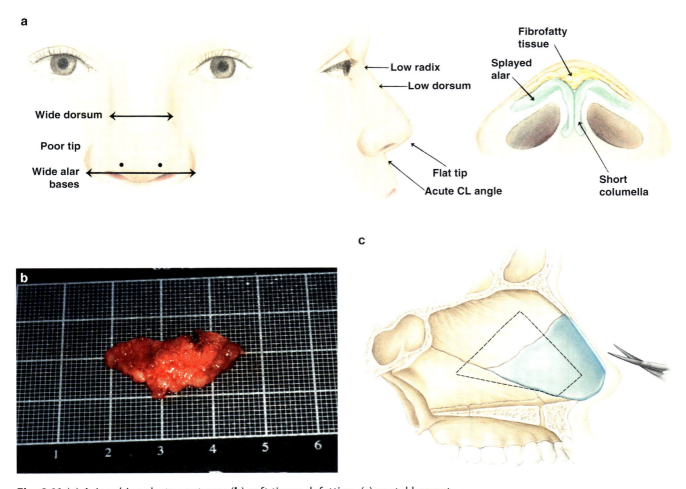

Fig. 9.11 (**a**) Asian rhinoplasty anatomy, (**b**) soft tissue defatting, (**c**) septal harvest

at the top and bone which will rest against the ANS (Fig. 9.11d). Since a "tip split" was done for septal exposure, insertion of the graft is relatively simple and the shaping is done in situ. The graft is placed between the alar cartilages and extends 2–8 mm below the caudal septum depending upon the degree of "columellar show" that one wants to obtain. Once satisfied, #25 needles are placed across the cartilaginous septum and the graft at two points. The caudal border of the graft should rise 6–10 mm above and 6–10 mm caudal to the septal angle. This rigid strut will produce the lengthening and projection that is required in the Asian nose. Three sutures of 4-0 polydioxanone suture (PDS) are inserted at overlapped areas to fix the strut to the caudal septum and dorsal septal cartilage. Final shaping will leave a columellar component that is 5–6 mm in width and the excised cartilage can be used as a rigid tip graft or diced. The final graft looks very much like a "tomahawk."

Tip Graft. Ideally, the tip graft is a long tapered graft of rigid septal cartilage. It is placed in a projecting position above the domes with a cap graft behind it for support (Fig. 9.11e). The reality is that it may be half-length septum or conchal cartilage. The cap graft is essential to maintain tip projection.

Dorsal Grafts. The dorsal graft is a DC-F graft, ranging from 0.7–1.0 cc of a tuberculin syringe (Fig. 9.11g, h). Most Asians will require a dorsal graft of uniform thickness. Currently, I use a separate fascia graft for the radix area and construct the dorsal graft on the back table. These can be either a uniform or tapered construct depending upon the patient's original dorsal deficiency. It is important that the dorsal graft is not done until the maximum tip projection has been obtained. The dorsal graft should not be excessively shortened to create a strong supratip break.

Osteotomies (Optional). I do lateral osteotomies, if the nose is wide. Since the bones are not very high, they are technically low-to-low although I use a curved osteotome. The goal is to narrow the x-width of the bony vault. These are done as indicated despite the fact that the nasal bones are relatively short and there is no open roof.

Alar Base Modifications and ARS/ARG (Usually). Two anatomical realities mandate caution when doing alar wedge resections in Asian patients (Fig. 9.11i, j). First, alar malposition is the "norm" not the exception in Asian patients. Second, the nostril axis ranges dramatically from upward to transverse to even inverted. One of the goals is to change the shape (round to oval) and the axis of the nostrils using alar rim support grafts (ARS). Further complicating the problem is that combined nostril sill excision/alar wedge resections further collapse the alar rim and risk significant scarring. Preoperative discussion must emphasize the limitations of narrowing nostril width, which most patients want, and the risk of scars, which most patients do not expect. Whenever possible, I will do an "extended nostril sill" excision with ARS. Essentially, an angulated nostril sill excision is done which tapers into the true alar crease for 3–4 mm, but is not visible from the profile view.

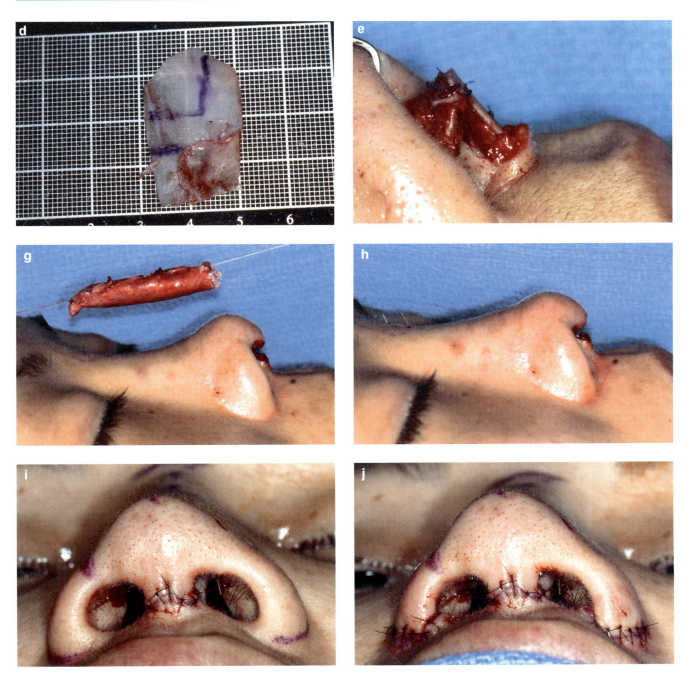

Fig. 9.11 (**d**) Septocolumellar graft, (**e**) tip graft, (**g, h**) dorsal augmentation (DC-F), (**i, j**) alar base excision

Case Study: Asian Rhinoplasty

Analysis

A 32-year-old woman of Chinese descent requested a rhinoplasty (Fig. 9.12). She stated that she did not want an implant as a couple of her friends had problems. The keys to the operation are creation of a more refined projected tip, dorsal augmentation, and narrowing of the alar base. Rigid tip support is critical and thus the "tomahawk septocolumellar strut" was devised. In most Asians, DC-F grafts obviate the need for rib while creating a very natural dorsum – how often do you really need more than 8 mm of augmentation? Since alar malposition is "normal" in the Asian patient, ARS grafts are essential to support the rims and change nostril orientation. At 6 years post-op, the patient has done well and there has been no revisional surgery.

Operative Technique

1) Harvest of fascia and conchal cartilage
2) Open approach with soft tissue defatting of the lobule
3) Tip split with septal harvest of maximum osseocartilaginous tissue
4) Insertion of a columellar pennant graft with bilateral "brace" grafts (short spreaders)
5) Suture of alars over the columellar strut and then addition of a structured tip graft
6) Dorsal augmentation using the entire conchal for a DC-F graft (0.7 cc)
7) Combined nostril sill/alar base excision (2 mm)

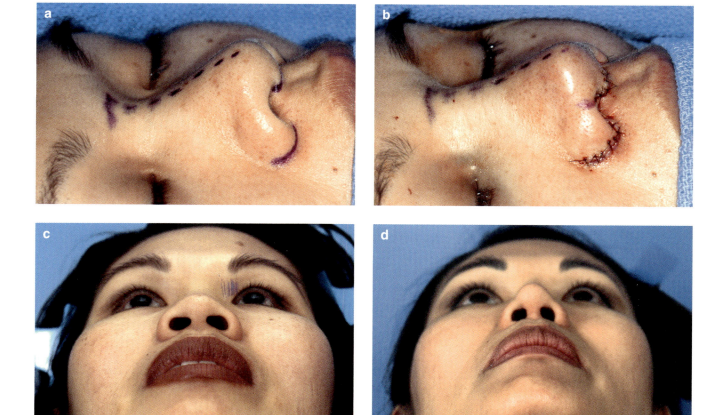

Fig. 9.12 (a–l)

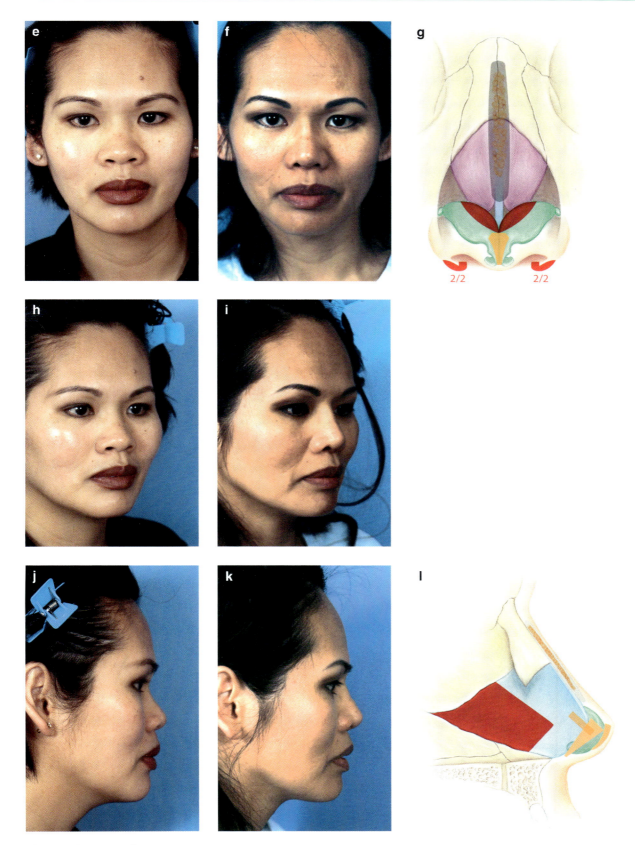

Fig. 9.12 (continued)

Black Rhinoplasty

Despite wide individual variations, the Black nose often comes down to a combination of low dorsum, a bulbous under-projecting tip, and wide alar base plus a retruded columellar labial angle. These cases are technically demanding and one must be willing to make the major commitment required to achieve excellent results. All of the steps used in the Asian nose are required in the Black nose, but to a greater degree (Fig. 9.13). The columellar must be maximally lengthened by advancing the alars on the columellar strut and fixed at two points rather than one. The dorsum may require a true "composite" reconstruction with solid cartilage grafts below and DC-F on top when silicone is not used. The combined alar base/nostril sill excisions may require a *cinch* component.

Note: The surgeon must be sensitive to the patient's desires, their concern for ethnic identity and preservation. Some patients will want minimal refinement, others moderate improvement, and a few maximum change. One should review Matory's (1998) excellant text on Ethnic rhinoplasty.

Surgical Technique

Soft Tissue Defatting. The standard defatting of the lobule is done via the infracartilaginous dissection followed by excision of the soft tissue on the alar surface via the open approach.

Columellar Strut. In most cases, a major columellar strut is inserted first and the medial/middle crura advanced upward to effectively lengthen the columella. Two sutures are used. With the strut in place, the columellar base is advanced upward from the lip and fixed with a #25 needle at the level of the columellar breakpoint. A lower columellar strut suture is inserted. Next, the needle is removed and the alars advanced as high as possible. Then a second CS is placed above the columellar breakpoint.

Tip Graft. A tip graft of solid septal cartilage with sharp edges is placed in a projecting position to achieve tip definition through the thick skin. Often a "backstop" graft of solid cartilage is placed behind it to force the tip graft downward and to provide resistance similar to a cap graft. When the entire infralobule is flat, then I add a shorter tip graft to the infralobule.

Dorsal Graft. Frequently a balanced approach is required with slight excision of the cartilaginous vault (<2 mm) followed by a full-length augmentations using a DC-F graft. In severe cases, a thin (1–2 mm) full-length cartilage graft will be placed first and then a DC-F contour graft on top. The solid graft provides support for the skin envelope and ameliorates the visual separation that one can see between bony and cartilaginous vaults.

Nasal Base. Inevitably, the nasal base is extraordinarily wide in alar flare and nostril sill visibility. If the columellar strut is effective, then the nostrils are often shifted from round to oval and the axis from transverse to 45°. In Black patients, I do not hesitate to do aggressive combined sill/base excisions with 3/6 and 4/8 dimensions being common. One assumes that Keloid scars will remain virtually unreported in the central facial triangle.

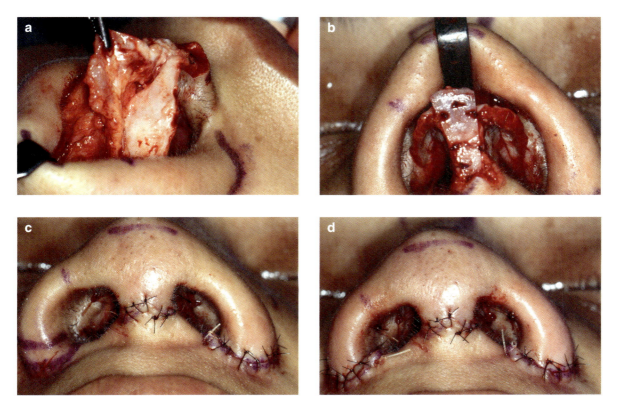

Fig. 9.13 (**a**) Soft tissue defeating, (**b**) tip graft, (**c, d**) combiner nostril sill, alar wedge rectron

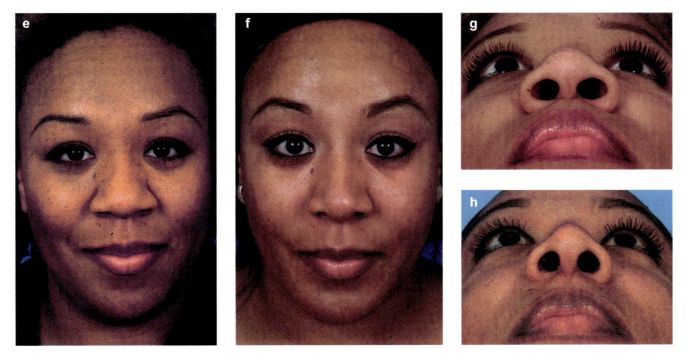

Fig. 9.13 (**e–h**) A 35 year old wanted a major change in her nose

Black Rhinoplasty (Moderate)

Analysis

An 18 year old student felt that her nose was too heavy and too unattractive (Fig. 9.14a-d). She wanted a significant refinement, but within the limits of her ethnicity. The operative highlights were: 1) defatting of the soft tissue envelope, 2) a septocolumellar strut, 3) a structure tip graft, 4) DC-F 0.8cc graft to the dorsum, and 5) a combined sill / wedge resection (3/4). At one year the patient is pleased, but would have accepted even more refinement.

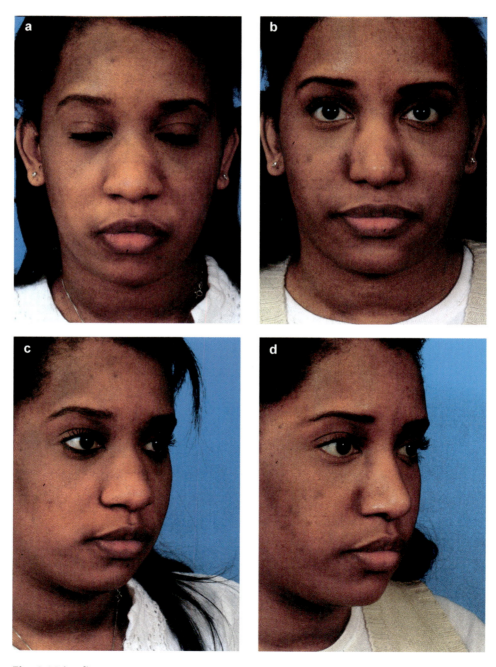

Fig. 9.14 (a–d)

Analysis

A 54 year old wanted to know what could be done to fix her flat, wide nose (Fig.9.14e-h). The interalar width measeured 55mm while her nasal length (N-T) was 28mm. The eventual operative plan included a chin augmentation and submental liposuction plus a central endoscopic forehead lift to move the Nasion higher. The nasal surgery consisted of the following; 1) minimal defatting, 2) rib harvest, 3) columellar strut and structured tip graft, 4) a deep solid dorsal rib graft -6mm thick plus and overlay DC-F graft- 4mm thick, 5) alar cinch excision 4/6, and bilateral composites to alar rims. Postoperatively, the patient stated that she felt pretty for the first time in her life.

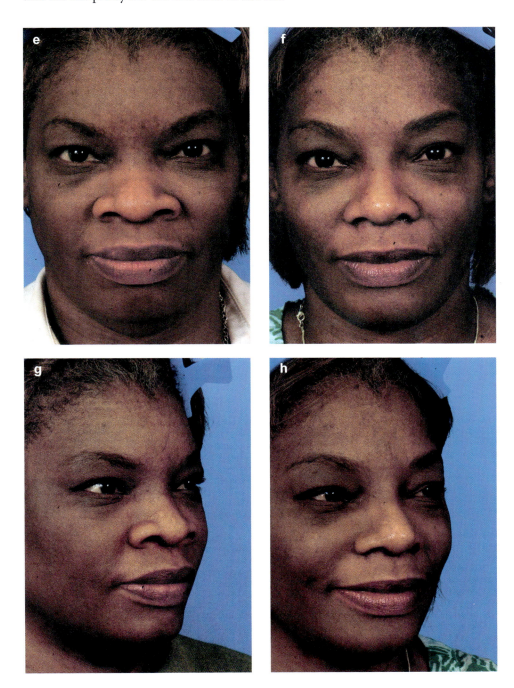

Fig. 9.14 (e–h)

Revision Rhinoplasty

Surgeons do not enjoy revising their own cases as they often feel that it represents a failure to achieve their original goal. I have learned to accept revisions and try to learn from them. At the pre-op visit, I explain to patients that my revision rate is 5–7% by 3 years. I do not charge a surgical fee for most revisions, but ask the patient to pay for OR supplies and/or anesthesia. Why is my revision rate so high? First, I think that I tend to see more difficult primary cases referred by other plastic surgeons and that in most cases I try for maximal aesthetic improvement. Second, I do not try to avoid revisions nor make it difficult for the patient. I would rather have a happy patient recommending me than a disappointed patient disparaging me. Third, I am always curious to know what went wrong since I did my very best at the initial operation. Remember: only you can teach yourself surgical cause and effect and revisions certainly focus your attention. Two examples of what experience has taught me are as follows. With radix grafts, crushed septum was always visible, so I switched to excised alar which had 10% problems and then went to fascia which has a 0% visibility rate. With spreader grafts, the difficulty was an occasional dorsal bump due to the cephalic end of the graft pushing through the open roof. The solution was to suture the graft at two points using an "overlap" suture cephalically.

In preparing this section, I personally reviewed *100 consecutive primary cosmetic* rhinoplasties with a mean follow-up of 18 months. What I found was quite surprising and extremely useful. There were seven revisions which I would classify as follows: (1) one case was supratip fullness following open rhinoplasty, (2) two cases were inadequate tip refinement following closed rhinoplasty, (3) two were dorsal bumps, one from inadequate rasping of the bony vault and the other probably part of a spreader graft, (4) two cases were "laughing struts" (the strut clicked across the ANS only when the patient laughed spontaneously, not when they talked or smiled). All in all, the revision rate was not bad and the degree of difficulty was neither severe nor complicated to fix. The revisions were interesting. The open cases were revised closed while the closed case was revised open. Excision of supratip scar tissue was easily done through intra cartilaginous incisions. The closed tip required a crural strut plus suturing of the previously created symmetrical rim strips (Fig. 9-15). The columellar struts were shortened through the bottom of the transfixion incision. On reflection, I think I could "divide" the bottom of the strut using a #16 needle in the exam room. Dorsal smoothing was done with a rasp via an inter cartilaginous incision. Why go through the trouble of pulling 100 charts and analyzing each one? The reason is that one begins to "see" less than perfect aesthetic results. Specifically, I found that I had not reduced the bony dorsum sufficiently in "high" dorsal humps and probably over resected the caudal septum at its junction with the ANS in long hanging noses. Although painful to see ones deficiencies and revisions, an *annual review* is a crucial learning experience that I highly recommend.

Analysis and Commentary

This patient requested a rhinoplasty, but wanted it to be completely natural. Her primary concern was the profile and not the tip (Fig. 9.15a, d). I did her rhinoplasty closed. After a year, she returned and wanted the tip rotated upward a bit and refined more. An open tip suture technique was done with the following sutures: CS, DC, ID, TP (Fig. 9.15c, f). For me personally, it illustrates all of the advantages of open tip suturing – projection, definition, and tip position.

**Case Study:
Minor Revision**

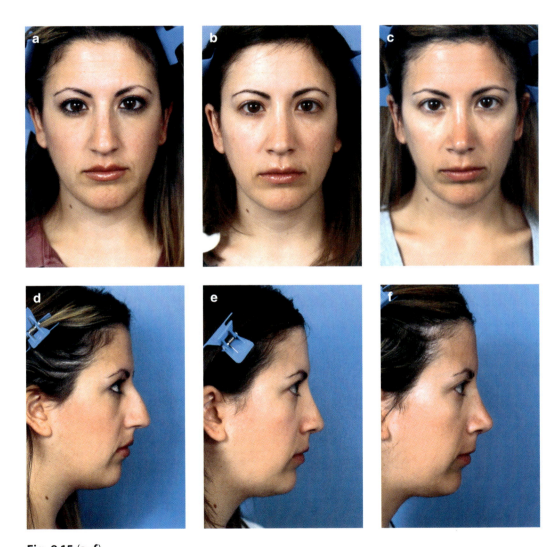

Fig. 9.15 (a–f)

Without question, incorrect patient selection and excessive suturing can produce difficult problems including the "snarl tip" and the upwardly rotated tip. Again, the caveat must be respected – do not tie every suture tight, rather tighten the suture until the desired effect is achieved and then stop. An example is the domal creation suture under thin skin with the resulting sharp point rather than a subtle curve. Yet the most dangerous suture is the tip position suture as it can excessively rotate the tip leading to a very unhappy patient. Although I prefer to wait 1 year, this might be a situation where I would reoperate within a couple of weeks. Excessive infralobular length can be caused by a "lateral steal" technique where the domal creation suture is placed laterally on the crura rather than at the domal notch. One can inadvertently add 4–6 mm to the infralobular length. Errors of omission are often a failure of preoperative analysis and may include not doing osteotomies or nostril sill excisions.

Open tip graft techniques have revolutionized rhinoplasty, but not without a learning curve both for pioneers and followers. One of the first tendencies to avoid is excessive narrowing of the columellar or domes when inserting the crural strut. If the crura are too approximated, then the tip graft will be stuck on the infralobule producing a hanging columella rather than an integrated tip. Also, the projecting tip graft must have a "cap graft" or rigid backstop to resist the folding forces from scar tissue.

When do I do revisions? Usually not before 1 year. The single exception would be obvious displacement of a major dorsal or tip graft. I have reoperated at 10 days for a displaced dorsal graft and was extremely glad that I did. Also, I have done a composite graft to a contracted nostril apex at 6 weeks to appease a very demanding patient. Each revision must be of aesthetic benefit to the patient, and hopefully become a learning experience for the surgeon.

Over the years, one should see a decrease in the complexity of one's revisions and hopefully their frequency. Essentially, the indication should be confined to one area (tip, nostril, etc.) or one major problem (asymmetry) rather than several. Rhinoplasty is not a static operation and with adoption of new techniques there will be a learning curve and new problems to revise. One word of caution – never suggest a revision to a patient, let them ask for it. Revisions only make things "better," never perfect.

Analysis and Commentary

This is the worst result of one of my primary rhinoplasties that I have revised in the last 6 years. At the initial operation, I tried to do this closed, but switched to an open as I could not control the tip cartilages (Fig. 9.16a, d). A columellar strut was inserted and tip sutures done: CS, DC, and DE. At 1 year, the patient was satisfied. However, by 6 years the nasal asymmetry was obvious, especially the tip collapse on right oblique view (Fig. 9.16b, e). A revision was necessary (Fig. 9.16c, f) and consisted of the following:

1) Banked cartilage was removed from the L-temporal area as was temporal fascia.
2) The tip was reopened. The cephalic end of the L-spreader grafts was excised.
3) A "fascial blanket" was inserted under the elevated skin envelope.
4) DC was placed under the fascia in the supratip region.
5) Lateral crural strut grafts were sutured to the lateral crura and along the nostril rim.

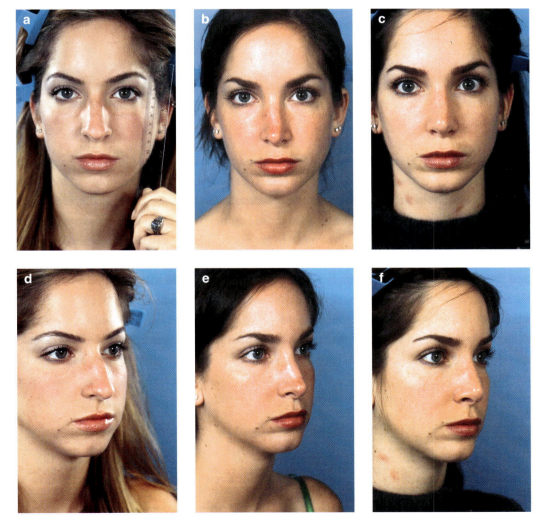

Fig. 9.16 (a–f)

Reading List   Becker H. Nasal augmentation with calcium hydroxyapatite in a carrier-based gel. Plast Reconstr Surg 121: 2142, 2008

Bizrah MB. Rhinoplasty for Middle Eastern patients. Facial Plast Surg Clin N Am 10: 381, 2002

Byrd HS, Salomon J, Flood J. Correction of the crooked nose. Plast Reconstr Surg 102: 2146, 1998

Constantian MB. An alternate strategy for reducing the large nasal base. Plast Reconstr Surg 83: 41, 1989

Daniel RK. Surgical techniques for bulky, boxy, and ball tips. In: Operative Techniques in Plastic and Reconstructive Surgery. Philadelphia: WB Saunders, 2001a

Daniel RK. Rhinoplasty: Large nostril/small tip disproportion. Plast Reconstr Surg 107: 1874, 2001b

Daniel RK. Hispanic rhinoplasty in the United states with emphasis on the Mexican American nose. Plast Reconstr Surg. 112: 224, 2003a

Daniel RK. Asian Rhinoplasty (Video). Alexandria, VA: American Academy of Facial Plastic and Reconstructive Surgery, 2003b

Daniel RK. Middle Eastern update Plast Reconstr Surg 124: 1630, 2009

Dayan SH, Bassichis BA. Facial dermal fillers; selection of appropriate products and techniques. Aesthet Surg J 28: 335, 2008

Jansen DA, Graivier MH. Evaluation of a calcium hydroxyapatite-based implant (Radiesse) for facial soft-tissue augmentation. Plast Reconstr Surg 118: 22, 2006

Flowers RS. Surgical correction of the East Asian nose. In: Daniel RK (ed) Aesthetic Plastic Surgery: Rhinoplasty. Boston: Little, Brown, 1993

Gruber RP, Friedman GD. Suture algorithm for the broad or bulbous nose. Plast Reconstr Surg 110: 1752, 2002

Guyuron B, Ghavami A, Wishnek SM. Components of the short nostril. Plast Reconstr Surg 116: 1517, 2005

Hamra ST. Repositioning the lateral alar crus. Plast Reconstr Surg 92: 1244, 1993

Matory WE Ethnic Considerations in Facial Aesthetic Surgery. Philadelphia: Lippincott-Raven, 1998

McCullough EG, Fedok FC. The lateral crural turnover graft: correction of the concave lateral crus. Laryngoscope 103: 463, 1993

Neu BR. Suture correction of a nasal tip cartilage concavities. Plast Reconstr Surg 98: 971, 1996

Nishimura Y, and Kumoi T. External septorhinoplasty in the cleft lip nose. Ann Plast Surg 26: 526, 1991

Ortiz-Monestaerio F, Olmedo A, Iscoy LO. Rhinoplasty in the Mestizo nose. Clin Plast Surg 4: 89, 1977

Porter JP, Toriumi DM Surgical management of the crooked nose. Aesth Plast Surg 26: 1, 2002

Romo T III, Sclafani AP, Falk AN, et al A graduated approach to the repair of nasal septal perforations. Plast Reconstr Surg. 103: 66, 1999

Roofe SB, Murakami CS. Treatment of the posttraumatic and postrhinoplasty crooked nose. Facial Plast Surg Clin North Am 14: 279, 2006

Rorhrich RJ. External approach to Black rhinoplasty. In: Daniel RK (ed) Aesthetic Plastic Surgery: Rhinoplasty. Boston: Little, Brown, 1993

Rorhrich RJ, Ghavami A. The Middle Eastern nose. In: Gunter JP, Rohrich RJ, Adams WP (eds) Dallas Rhinoplasty: Nasal Surgery by the Masters. QMP, 757–772, 2007

Rorhrich RJ, Gunter JP, Deuber MA, et al The deviated nose: optimizing results using a simplified classification and algorithmic approach. Plast Reconstr Surg 110: 1509, 2002

Sclafani AP, Romo T, Barnett JG, Barnett CR. Adjustment of subtle postoperative nasal defects: Managing the "near-miss" rhinoplasty. Facial Plast Surg. 19: 349, 2003

Toriumi DM. Structural approach in rhinoplasty. Facial Plast Surg Clin North Am 13: 93, 2005

Toriumi DM, and Ries WR. Innovative surgical management of the crooked nose. Facial Plast Clin 1: 63, 1993

Secondary Rhinoplasty: Surgical Techniques

10

Introduction

*C*an secondary rhinoplasty be taught? Three inescapable facts say no: (1) the highly variable normal nasal anatomy is often destroyed by the earlier surgery and distorted by scar contracture, (2) operative plans must be changed radically when intraoperative findings differ markedly from preoperative expectations, and (3) the diversity of cases makes learning surgical cause and effect difficult. Ultimately, secondary rhinoplasty must be based on the fundamental principles of primary rhinoplasty. One simply cannot provide a formula for dealing with the complexities of secondary rhinoplasty. Just as there is a progression from medical school through residency to fellowship, most surgeons should progress from primary rhinoplasty through their own revisions to secondary rhinoplasty over a 3–5-year period. Note: a secondary rhinoplasty is defined as a case where the primary rhinoplasty was performed by another surgeon; a revision is when you reoperate on your own primary case.*

In this chapter, I have emphasized how secondary rhinoplasty differs from primary cases and the advanced surgical techniques that are required. In Chapter 11, I have reviewed the decision-making process and how one selects the appropriate technique. I cannot overemphasize it enough – there are no Level 1 or 2 secondary cases. One must be a competent rhinoplasty surgeon with significant experience in primary cases before taking on secondary cases. The surgeon must be comfortable harvesting and using rib grafts as many patients will not have sufficient septal cartilage available and concha is not structurally adequate. As detailed in Chapter 12, aesthetic reconstructive rhinoplasty has emerged as a separate entity. These latter cases are extraordinarily complex and require even greater surgical skills than secondary rhinoplasty.

Overview   What makes secondary rhinoplasty so hard? While writing this book, I tried to devise a pre-operative "score sheet" for determining the degree of difficulty for secondary cases. Certain factors were obvious – number of prior operations, number of different surgeons, availability of septum, skin thickness, etc. I was becoming convinced that a female patient with an earlier single closed rhinoplasty with a palpable septum would be an easy secondary case. Of course, I then operated on such a patient only to discover that her entire alar cartilages had been excised from the footplates upward thus forcing a total tip reconstruction. The critical issue is that you have no idea of what was done or is available in a secondary case until you open them up. Thus, all secondary rhinoplasties are complex and you must be prepared for any eventuality (Fig. 10.1).

Completing the Primary. From the surgeon's perspective, these are the easiest of secondaries. The patient often complains that the tip does not have enough definition, the bridge looks pinched, the nostrils are too big, and they do not breathe well. If the primary was done closed, then one usually has symmetrical rim strips to work with and a tip suture technique can be done via the open approach. A columellar strut and spreader grafts are often necessary.

Eliminating the Negatives. Many of these patients have a higher degree of nasal complexity and have frequently had a revision by the original surgeon. It is important for the new surgeon to take a "fresh look" while the patient must be able to articulate what they want changed. Most of my patients feel that their nose is still too big and not sufficiently feminine. Often they consider the nose to be a smaller version of the original and not a significant improvement. Technically, one has to be prepared for virtually any problem.

Converting from Operative Look to Natural Nose. Often, these patients feel that their nose looks "done" due to an over-resected bridge, an upwardly rotated tip, retracted nostril, or a tip bossa. The challenge is to create a solid foundation for the nose and improve respiration. Numerous grafts ranging from septal to fascia to concha to composite and even unanticipated rib grafts will be required. Tip surgery can range from tip suture to tip reconstruction, one simply does not know until the nose is opened. All of these cases are done open as one has the option of utilizing the various cartilage remnants and direct observation permits a wide range of techniques. Unfortunately, skin coverage is often a consideration and fascial grafts are used liberally in thin-skin patients. One must be comfortable with dorsal augmentation and the various types of diced cartilage grafts. Nostril retraction or vestibular valve scarring can be so severe that composite conchal grafts have to be utilized. There are no short cuts in managing these cases.

Aesthetic Reconstructive Rhinoplasty. By definition, these are the most difficult of secondaries and require numerous grafts often including rib grafts. The goal is to achieve a natural attractive nose without any indication of prior surgery. One is doing an "aesthetic reconstructive rhinoplasty" to salvage the nose. These cases will be discussed in depth in Chapter 12.

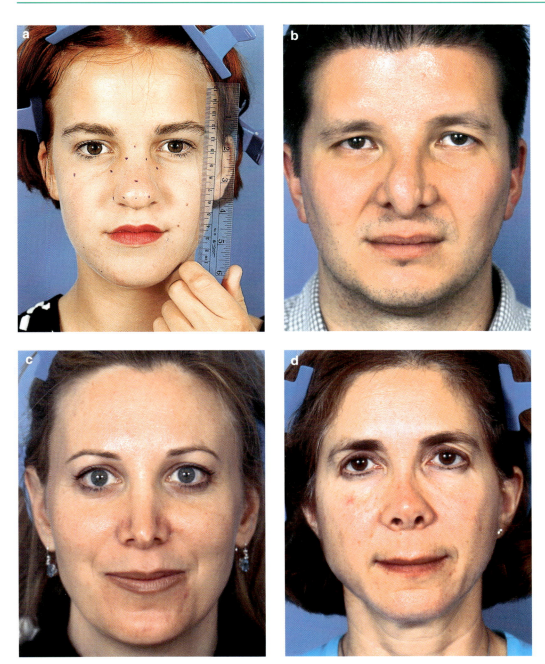

Fig. 10.1 Range of secondary cases, (**a**) completing the primary, (**b**) eliminating the negatives, (**c**) surgical to natural look, (**d**) aesthetic reconstructive rhinoplasty

Case Study: Secondary Rhinoplasty

Analysis

A 22-year-old girl had a rhinoplasty 2 years earlier and hated the result (Fig 10.2). She especially disliked her minimally improved wide bulbous tip and pinched bridge. She had had multiple consultations on the "nose circuit" and been told that she needed a major rib reconstruction. Yet, her goal was still the same small cute nose that had led her to have a rhinoplasty in the first place. I advised her that the donor site progression would be septum to concha to rib. Fortunately, septum proved sufficient and her nose was made more refined and the tip smaller. Her final result is more the "naturally cute nose" that primary patients seek and not a "reconstructed nose" that complex secondary cases often have to accept.

Operative Technique

1) Harvest of temporal fascia. Transfixion incision with confirmation of intact septum.
2) Open exposure revealed alar rim strips following prior transcartilaginous excision.
3) Cartilaginous dorsum lowered 1.5 mm. Bony dorsum smoothed with a rasp.
4) Septoplasty – harvest of the septal body. Caudal septum relocation R to L.
5) Insertion of bilateral spreader grafts.
6) Alar transposition.
7) Insertion of columellar strut plus tip suturing: CS, DC, ID, DE, TP. Add-on graft of excised alar cartilage.
8) Lateral crural strut grafts sutured to lateral crura.
9) Insertion of "fascial blanket" over the dorsum and tip.
10) Lateral crural strut grafts placed into the alar bases (T2), not on nostril margin (T3).

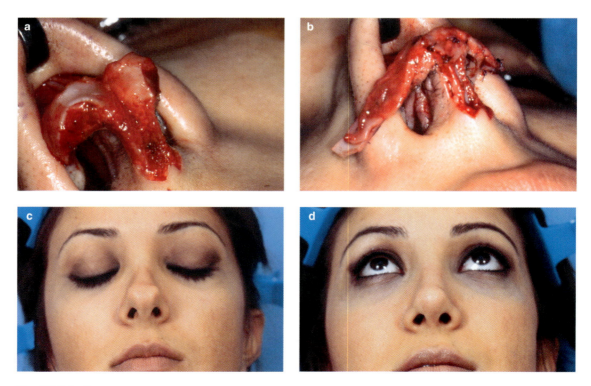

Fig. 10.2 (a–l)

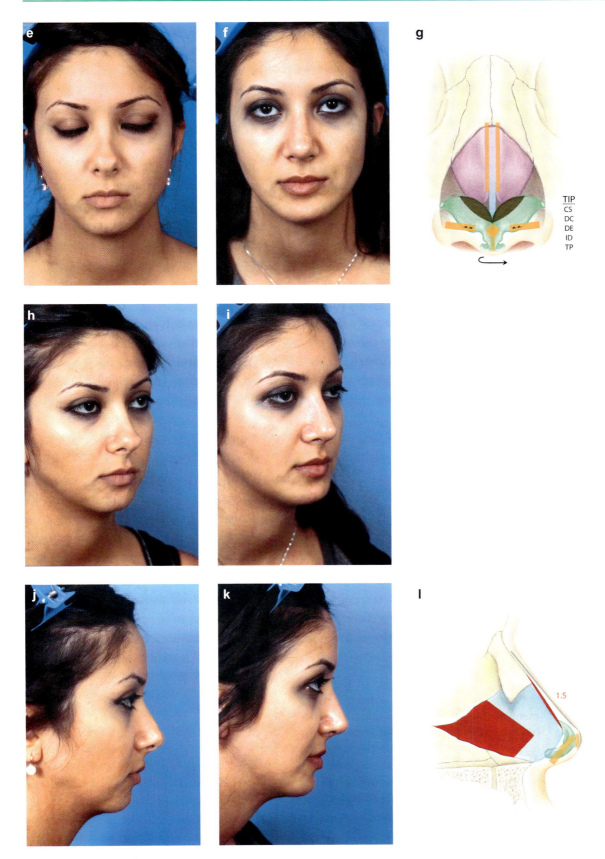

Fig. 10.2 (continued)

Reference Points. The three key components are: three points (nasion, tip, subnasle), three angles (nasofacial, tip, columella inclination), and three lengths (radix height, dorsum, tip projection). Mark the following points: nasion (N), tip (T), subnasale (SN) and alar crease (AC). Draw the following reference lines: (1) Frankfort horizontal, and (2) a vertical line through the alar crease. Draw and measure the following angles: nasofacial, tip, and columella inclination. Measure the following lengths: radix projection (C-N), dorsal length (N-T), and tip projection (AC-T). Once the references are drawn then the ideal is superimposed.

Superimpose the Ideal. Every artist from Leonardo to Wyeth has used grids and canons to define facial relationships. Nasal length is related to midfacial height. A red pencil is used to draw the ideal which in turn defines the patient's deformity. The nasion (N) is the deepest point in the nasofrontal angle. Its level is between eyelashes and alar crease, while its height is $0.28 \times$ midfacial height (MFH). Alternatively, N should be 4–6 mm posterior to the glabellar. The tip (T) is the most projecting point on the lobule as seen on lateral view. The subnasale (SN) is the deepest point in the columella labial angle uniting the columella and the upper lip. The nasofacial angle (NFA) is the intersection between a vertical reference line through the nasion and a straight line drawn from the nasion to the tip (N-T measures dorsal length) with the ideal being 34° for females and 36° for males. The tip angle (TA) is the intersection between a vertical reference line through the alar crease and a straight line from alar crease to tip (AC-T measures tip projection) with the ideal 105° for females and 100° for males. The columella inclination (CIA) is measured between the vertical reference line through the alar crease and a line tangent to the columella with identical ideal values to the tip angle. This inclination has replaced the classic columella labial angle and nasolabial angle in importance. The dorsal length (N-T) is measured from nasion to tip transecting any intervening hump with the ideal being N-Ti = $0.67 \times$ MFH. The tip projection (AC-T) is measured from a vertical reference line through the alar crease to the tip with the ideal being AC-Ti = 0.67 N-Ti. The nasion height (C-N) is measured from a vertical reference line tangent to the cornea out to the ideal being C-Ni = $0.28 \times$ N-Ti, (see Table 2.3, p50).

Operative Alternatives. In most cases, the discrepancy between actual and ideal is quite obvious. However, surgical reality may require acceptance of more limited changes and that is where alternative surgical solutions are best utilized. For example, a major radix augmentation may not be acceptable to the patient and one must determine the impact it will have on planning both dorsal reduction and tip projection. Equally, an obtuse columella labial angle may be soft tissue in origin precluding caudal septal resection. It is this opportunity to evaluate different operative treatments that is of great value.

Obviously, Operative Plan #1 is made by integrating the patient's desires and the surgeon's opinion (Fig. 10.4). Once the examination is completed, one should have a good idea as to the goals, the requisite approach, the necessary changes to each of the four areas, the available graft material, and the functional factors. Photographs, as well as surface measurements, are taken. Then the in-depth study is done working through the progression of actual to ideal to realistic changes finally reaching Operative Plan #2. At the next office visit, I examine the patient asking myself these questions – what is wrong with the nose, what needs to be corrected, and what is possible? I am essentially setting an overall goal (Operative Plan #3) before going through the final step-by-step planning. I ask the patient for input and review any photographs that the patient may have brought. Then, I do yet another internal exam to confirm the functional requirements and check it against the initial evaluation. Each region of the nose is assessed again and one arrives at Operative Plan #4 which will be taken to the operating room. One must consider this as only a *plan* – one that can change dramatically depending on the actual tissues available. In secondary rhinoplasty, the conversion from "operative plan" to "operation" is often a painful lesson in surgical reality.

Operative Planning

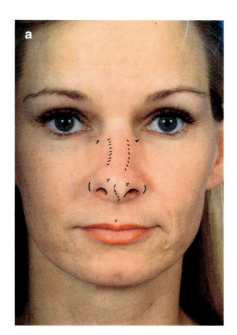
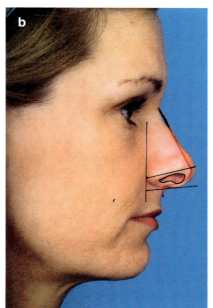
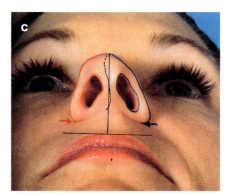

Fig. 10.4 (a–c) Secondary analysis

Skin Envelope

The skin envelope is a major factor in secondary rhinoplasty and determines not only the dissection plane, but often the type of tip surgery.

Thick Skin. The thick-skin envelope has always been considered a major limiting factor for achieving both tip definition and the desired profile line. One must distinguish three characteristics for the skin sleeve: thickness, size, and compliance. The fundamental concept is that, rather than fearing skin contracture, one uses it to reveal the strong structured tip and dorsum which are created during a secondary surgery.

When the supratip area is heavily scarred, I tend to dissect in the subcutaneous subdermal plane rather than in intimate contact with the alar cartilages (Fig. 10.5). The advantage is that it allows me to excise or sculpt the supratip scar while setting the correct thickness of the skin envelope. In most cases, one can resect the soft tissue on top of the alar cartilage without resorting to debulking the undersurface of the skin envelope – a maneuver that risks thinning, distortion, and even slough of the tip skin. In severe cases with minimal alar remnants, the supratip scar is sculpted and a tip graft is sutured directly to the scar tissue. In most cases, the nasal skin is widely undermined over the cartilaginous vault which allows the skin to redrape laterally, avoiding the bunched supratip which occurs with a closed approach. One can even undermine onto the anterior surface of each maxilla for extremely wide undermining. In severe cases, I will insert a 7Fr drain under the skin envelope to evacuate blood and to suction the skin down to the underlying aesthetic structures for 3–5 days.

Thin Skin. Although thick skin receives greater discussion, it is really scarred thin skin that strikes fear in the heart of the secondary rhinoplasty surgeon. The reason is quite simple: every imperfection shows, nothing is hidden. The basic progression is plane of dissection followed by padding. In thin-skin patients, it is critical to dissect in intimate contact with the underlying cartilage (Fig. 10.6). One should see white glistening cartilage if possible. The dissection must be done slowly and meticulously to avoid any skin perforation. I do not hesitate to inject repeatedly with local anesthesia to foster hydrodissection. If a significant skin perforation occurs, close it carefully with skin sutures to get the best possible repair. Do not pretend that it did not happen and allow it to heal secondarily with a terrible scar.

Frequently, one will want additional soft tissue padding and deep temporal fascia is the material of choice, in either single or double layer. For the dorsum, the fascia is folded, sutured along its free edge, and placed underneath the dorsal skin using percutaneous sutures in the radix and direct suturing caudally. When the tip is extremely thin, then a "fascial blanket" is placed beneath the dorsum and over the entire tip lobule. In certain very scarred tips, a dermis graft is sutured over the tip or in areas where a previous skin slough has occurred.

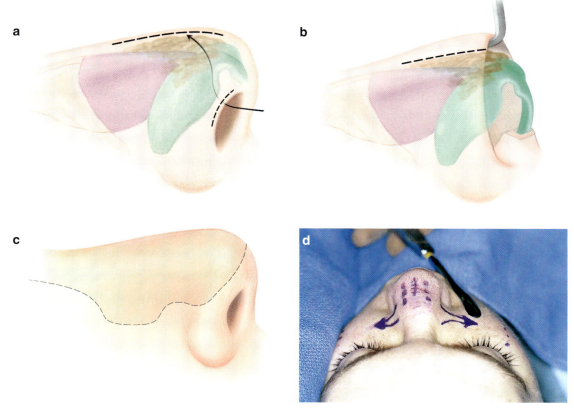

Fig. 10.5 (a–d) Thick skin: (a, b) defatting and (c, d) redraping **DVD**

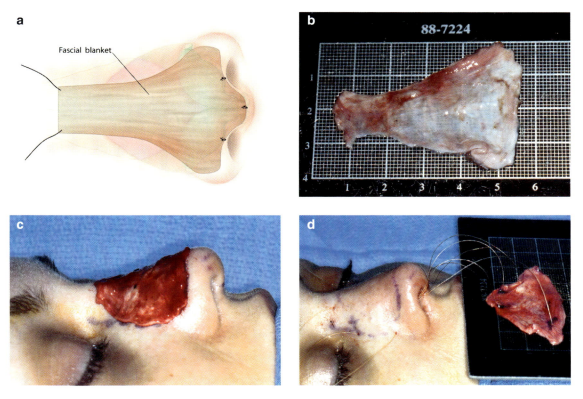

Fig. 10.6 (a–d) Thin skin: Fascial graft coverage **DVD**

Open Approach and Septal Exposure

For the vast majority of complex secondaries, an open approach is the only reasonable method. (Table 10.1). If a prior open approach was done, then the preexisting transcolumellar incision is used, otherwise the inverted-V at the midcolumellar point is preferred. Reopening a prior open rhinoplasty is not a major concern (Daniel, 1995). A bigger problem is skin damage from either steroid injections or too superficial a dissection. The standard infracartilaginous incision is used irrespective of prior incisions. The nasal lobule is injected heavily with local anesthesia to facilitate dissection. The skin is elevated from the incision upward using three point traction with extreme care over the domal points. Careful dissection in intimate contact over the lateral crura is done except in thick-skin patients. The dissection continues up over the dorsum with liberal addition of local anesthesia as necessary.

The septum is exposed through a complete unilateral transfixion incision, with addition of the opposite transfixion as necessary. In most cases, the caudal septum can be exposed "cleanly" and then continue into the dorsum under direct vision. The classic "top down" dissection from the dorsum can be extremely difficult in secondary cases due to scarring from the prior dorsal resection. Using the available "bidirectional approach," the entire septum is exposed. One then determines where and how severely deviated is the septum, how much septum remains for graft material, and how much can the dorsum be safely reduced.

Septal Considerations

1) During injection of local anesthesia, one can assess the resistance and probe for prior septal resections. An endoscope can be of value to document prior septal perforations.

2) It is important to assess the status of the septum prior to dorsal reduction. If the previous surgeon left a 7–8 mm L-shape strut and one is planning to reduce the cartilaginous vault by 3–4 mm, then the risk of septal collapse is very real.

3) The dissection plane may change dramatically as one goes from easy elevation caudally into scarred areas, especially if prior morselization was done. Equally, one can encounter areas of septal overlap with fused layers of perichondrium.

4) In areas of prior resection, one must separate the two mucosal leaflets without tearing them apart. On occasion, there will be a scar layer or even a pseudocartilaginous regrowth of the septum.

5) Harvesting cartilage after prior resections is most often successful in the lower vomerine area as well as superiorly under the dorsal strut near the perpendicular plate (Fig. 10.7).

6) Obviously, one must be able to correct every primary septal deformity which was not treated previously. Also, one may encounter complete disruptions in both the caudal and dorsal portions of the L-shape strut, but often without the advantage of usable septal grafts. Ultimately, the surgeon must be able to fashion both a columella strut and a dorsal graft from either conchal or rib cartilage!

Table 10.1 Open approach to secondary rhinoplasty in 100 consecutive cases

Incisions	Prior open	Old transcolumellar
		New infracartilaginous
Skin	Thin	Hydrodissection
		Dissect on cartilages
	Thick	Subdermal dissection via infracartilaginous
		Transcolumellar dissection upward
		Resect scar tissue on top of alars
Tip analysis	What is the status of each alar cartilage?	
	How much cartilage is resected, incised, or damaged?	
	What was the original tip operation?	
	Will my operative plan work?	

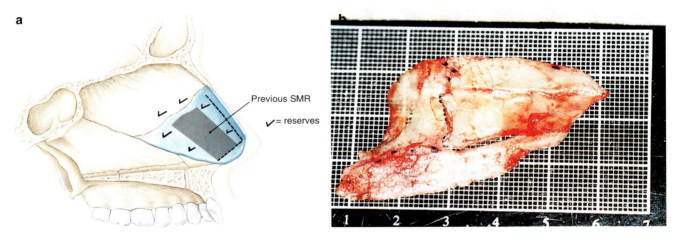

Previous SMR

✓= reserves

Fig. 10.7 (a, b) Secondary septal harvest when prior SMR was done

Dorsal Modification

When planning secondary surgery of the dorsum, one must add straightening, smoothing, and camouflage of the dorsum, to the primary choices of reduction, augmentation, or balance. Frequently, analysis is more complex in secondary cases as none of the cardinal landmarks is ideal and setting each one creates interrelated challenges. Equally, the skin envelope over the dorsum becomes a critical issue, usually revealing thinness over the rhinion or a non-compliant thickness in the supratip area. Further complicating the issue is the number of previous osteotomies with their variable locations and effectiveness. In addition, the prior use of both autogenous grafts and allografts can produce some very difficult intraoperative surprises. The lack of adequate septal material can cause a major problem in dorsal grafting. Fortunately, most cases require dorsal refinement and appropriate osteotomies with dorsal grafting an infrequent necessity.

Secondary Osseocartilaginous Vault Surgery. Based on a review of 100 secondary rhinoplasties, there have been significant changes in the last 8 years (Table 10.2). Excluded from this group are the aesthetic reconstructive rhinoplasties which require rib grafts as well as ethnic noses. The radix area was grafted in 6% of the cases, either as a pure fascia graft or a ball-and-apron fascial graft. The overall approach to the dorsum was reduction (75%), augmentation (21%), and minimal changes (4%). Reduction was divided equally between cartilage-only and combined bone and cartilage. Osteotomies consisted of low-to-high (42%), low-to-low (21%), asymmetric (12%), microoseotomies (6%), double level (3%), and none (16%). Spreader grafts were used quite frequently with bilateral (45%), unilateral (39%), and none (16%). Augmentation was either DC−F or DC+F. Importantly, the choice of augmentation indicated that neither lateral osteotomies nor spreader grafts would be required. Perhaps the most startling change has been the use of fascia. Fascia was used in 81% of the cases in the following ways: dorsal fascia dorsal graft (36%), DC+F (15%), DC−F (6%), and a fascial blanket (24%) interposed between nasal structure and overying skin.

Dorsal Refinement. Many secondary dorsums are a triad of reduction, correction of asymmetries, and spreader grafts (Fig. 10.9). Generalized reduction was done with a rasp for the bony vault and a #11 blade for cartilage vault. The majority of these reductions were in the 1–3 mm range with emphasis on smoothing irregularities. An interesting observation is that a "cartilaginous dorsum only" reduction was done in 42% of the reduction cases. This finding indicates that the bony reduction was done correctly at the initial operation. The critical finding was the use of fascia to pad a thin-skin envelope in 65% of cases. Dorsal fascial grafts could be a isolated dorsal graft or extended over the tip as a "fascial blanket" or combined with a radix graft as a "ball-and-apron graft." When the dorsum was not touched, it obviously indicated that the original surgeon had achieved the ideal dorsal line and the goal was to modify the tip and correct nostril deformities.

Table 10.2 Secondary osseocartilaginous vault surgery in 100 consecutive cases

Radix	Nothing	93%
	Augmentation	6%
	Reduction	1%
Dorsum	Nothing	4%
	Augmentation	21%
	Reduction	75%
Reduction	Bone and cartilage	58%
	Cartilage only	42%
Dorsal grafts	Fascial blanket	24%
	Fascia dorsal	36%
	DC−F	6%
	DC+F	15%
Osteotomies	Low-to-high	42%
	Low-to-low	21%
	Asymmetric	12%
	Microosteotomies	6%
	Double level	3%
	None	16%
Spreader grafts	Bilateral	45%
	Unilateral	39%
	None	16%

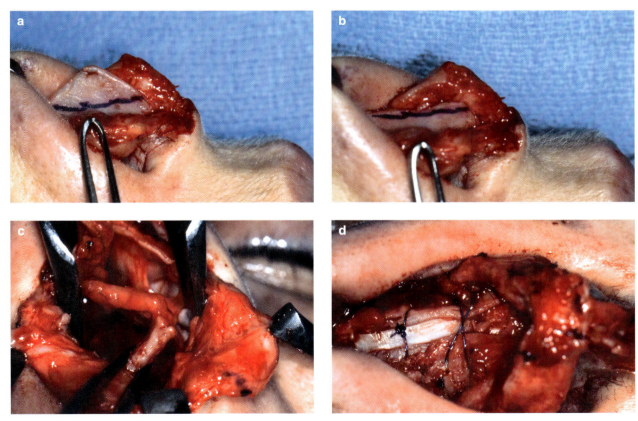

Fig. 10.9 (a–d) Dorsal modification

Secondary Septoplasty and Vestibular Valve

Secondary septal surgery is more difficult than primary surgery for three reasons: (1) the structures are often distorted and scarred from previous manipulation, (2) prior resections may have weakened the critical L-shape strut, and (3) the maximum amount of graft material is needed. The actual indications for septal surgery are somewhat constant: correction of anatomical obstruction and/or harvest of graft material, but with the additional possibility of prior surgical failure and distortion. I did septal surgery in 85% of the secondary cases with 33% of these done solely for harvesting graft material and 67% for the functional reasons with concomitant harvest of graft material. Of tremendous importance, 75% of these secondary cases had a *prior septoplasty* including some resection! Elevation of the mucosal flaps ranged from simple to nightmarish. In addition, 18% or almost one out of five required a total septoplasty to correct the septal deformity. Any thought that one can do secondary rhinoplasty without managing difficult septums is completely naive. As always, one must be prepared to deal with all types of septal deformities including the caudal septum, dorsal deviations, and total septoplasty. Obviously, the prior errors of commission (excessive excision, destabilizing incisions, weakening morselizations) cannot be overestimated. Long-term structural support must be restored.

Caudal Septum. Frequently, the caudal septum will have to be replaced or reinforced due to prior incisions or excisions (Fig. 10.10a). Whenever possible, the replacement graft is sutured into position prior to excising the deformed caudal septum. This allows an accurate replacement without loss of support.

Dorsal Septal Deviation. As always, one straightens the septum first and then uses asymmetric spreader grafts as required (Fig. 10.10b). Rarely, one will need to support the dorsum with a unilateral spreader graft, then divide the dorsal portion of the L-shape strut, and splint it again with a spreader graft on the other side.

Vestibular Valve. These problems are often subdivided into attic and lateral vestibular collapse with careful assessment of mucosal and structural loss (Fig. 10.10c). Vestibular attic webs are classified as thin, which can be treated with Z-plasties or thick, which require composite grafts. In the lateral vestibule, one must answer three questions: (1) Is the lining deficient thereby requiring a composite graft? (2) Does the lateral crura accessory cartilage junction protrude into the airway, thereby necessitating resection?, and (3) How thin and structurally weak is the lateral vestibule? Most often, it comes down to a simple question: Do I have to replace lining with a composite graft or is a conchal cartilage graft sufficient for support?

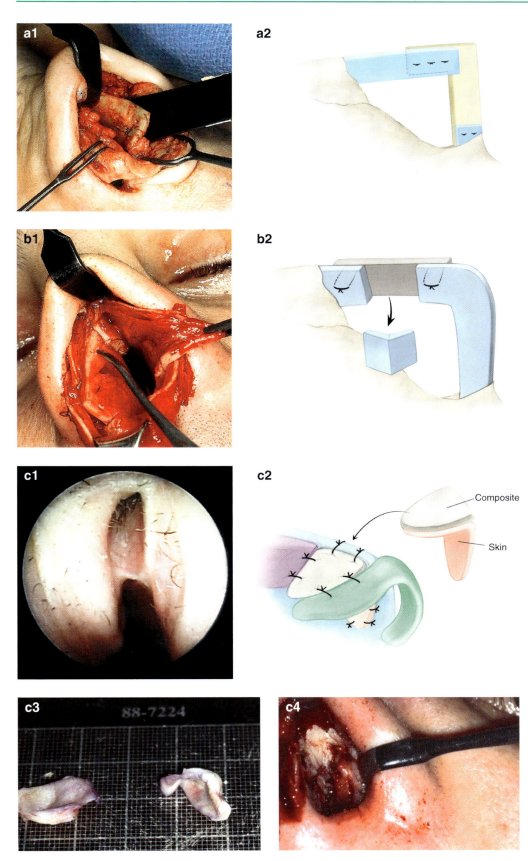

a1

a2

b1

b2

c1

c2

Composite

Skin

c3

88-7224

c4

Fig. 10.10 (**a**) Caudal septal replacement 🅓🅥🅟 (**b**) dorsal septal deviation (**c**) vestibular valve scarring and collapses

Osteotomies and Spreader Grafts

Osteotomies. I find that the majority of secondary cases require osteotomies despite the fact that they were done during the primary rhinoplasty. The need for osteotomies is due to the following: (1) excessive bony width, (2) asymmetries, and (3) bony deformities. Although the usual problem is a wide asymmetric bony vault, standard paired low-to-high or low-to-low osteotomies will usually solve most problems. It is tempting to speculate that the primary osteotomies failed due to a lack of adequate mobilization. When an exceptionally wide dorsum is encountered, then medial oblique, transverse, and low-to-low osteotomies are used (Fig. 10.11a). Small bony asymmetries localized to the keystone area are treated with microosteotomies (Fig. 10.11b). Convex lateral walls can be converted to straight by using double-level osteotomies.

One of the major challenges in secondary cases is the nose with a pinched bony vault. To solve this problem, I have devised a new operation in which the nasal bone is totally mobilized and then stabilized in its normal location (Fig. 10.11c, d). Usually, a combination of medial oblique and low-to-low osteotomies is done. Then using a Boyes elevator the lateral wall is mobilized outward which both moves the wall laterally and converts a vertical wall to an angled wall. Then extra-long spreader grafts are placed as high as possible to stabilize the bone in an outward position. Doyle splints, with the flat superior portion cut off, are sutured high in the airway. The splints force the lateral wall out and are removed at 2 weeks.

Spreader Grafts. I find that less than 5% of secondaries had prior spreader grafts (Fig. 10.11e–h). This omission results in an internal valve that is collapsed and a midvault which is either pinched or asymmetric. In secondary cases, it is essential first to complete the dorsal modification followed by a septoplasty and septal harvest whenever the latter is possible. Also, all osteotomies and mobilization of the lateral walls must be completed prior to graft insertion. Asymmetric spreader grafts are used in almost all secondaries. Rigid septal grafts are only essential when dorsal deviations must be excised and repaired. If graft material is scarce, concha material makes excellent spreader grafts. In primary cases, spreader grafts are directed at opening the internal valve and avoiding a pinched midvault. In secondary cases, spreaders tend to be longer, wider, and inserted higher within the bony vault. These grafts must overcome the deformity and contracture which has occurred following the primary rhinoplasty. In a high percentage of cases, one is actually supporting and aligning the lateral bony wall with these grafts. If the failure to use spreader grafts results in such an obvious form and function liability why do surgeons continue not to use them in primary cases? My conclusion is that most surgeons want to avoid any additional step they can and rationalize that spreader grafts are really not necessary – what a false assumption.

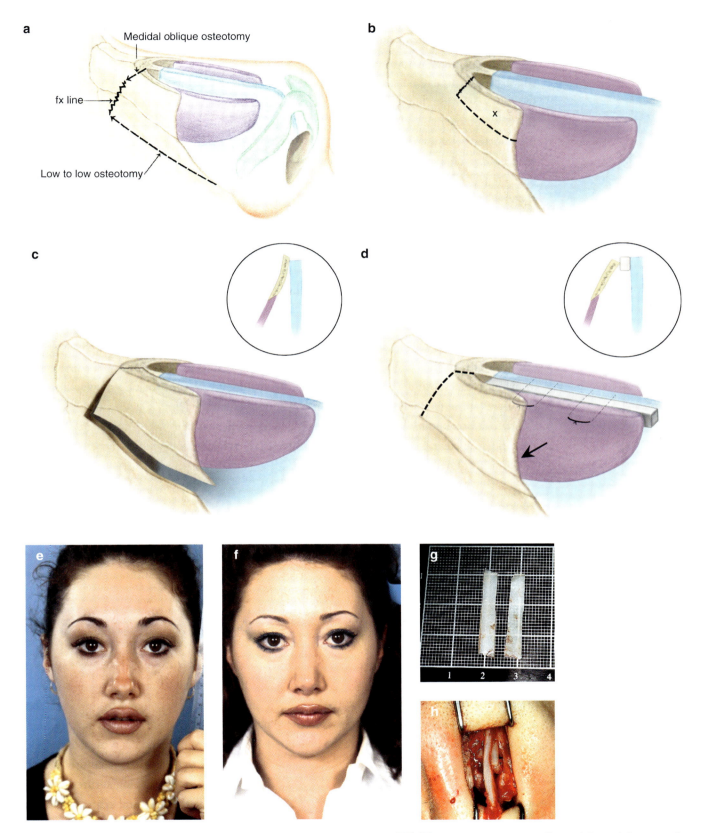

Fig. 10.11 (**a**) Medial oblique osteotomies, (**b**) microosteotomies **DVD** (**c, d**) correcting collapsed lateral bony wall, (**e–h**) spreader grafts in secondary cases **DVD**

Incisions, Divisions, and Bossa

Incisions of lateral crura and domes to weaken their convexity remain an integral part of closed rhinoplasty despite their inevitable tendency to form bossa and distortions. The weaken lateral crura will often require an underlying lateral crural strut to stabilize and reshape them. For some reason, domal division remains popular for narrowing the wide tip among endonasal surgeons despite its ineffectiveness, especially under thick or thin skin. Fortunately, these divisions can be repaired after insertion of a columellar strut and the domal segments sutured. Sharp pointed bossa or prominences are usually excised and the edges sutured with 5–0 PDS. Coverage with a concealer grafts is frequently necessary to insure a smooth tip.

Tip Sutures

Suturing a secondary tip is somewhat similar to the techniques used in primary tips (Fig. 10.13a–c). The first step is to release the scar contracture and then analyze the remaining alar remnants. Symmetrical rim strips are created by appropriate excision of any excesses or asymmetries. I delay any repair of previous transections or excision of deformed segments until the columellar strut is in place. After columellar strut insertion, the domal creation sutures are done. Usually, the cartilages remain sufficiently malleable, and one can create a tight domal convexity with adjacent lateral crura concavity. An interdomal suture is inserted to narrow tip width and to equilibrate domal height. The skin is redraped and the tip evaluated. Frequently in secondary cases, it will be necessary to add a tip position suture to achieve the desired supratip break. The addition of lateral crural convexity sutures is essential for minimizing lateral convexities or excessive tip width.

Tip Sutures Plus Add-On TRG Grafts

Once tip suturing is completed, add-on TRG grafts are used liberally to increase definition and projection (Fig. 10.13d–f). Excised lateral crura are the material of choice. Skin thickness will dictate the number of layers while aesthetic goals will dictate graft placement. Single infralobular concealer grafts are necessary under thin skin, whereas double-layer onlay domal grafts are common under thicker skin.

Lateral Crural Deformities

Deformities of the lateral crura are very real in secondary cases. They may require either excision, sutures, or grafts with transpositions an occasional necessity. Surprisingly, decisions regarding the lateral crura are just as complex as the domes and the role of lateral crural strut grafts cannot be over emphasized.

Structured Tip Grafts

In most secondary cases, a structured tip graft is not done for subtle changes of definition or projection (Fig. 10.13g–i). Rather, the grafts are designed to show a distinct change in the tip and to overcome a scarred or thick-skin envelope. A strong solid shield-shape tip graft is the graft of choice. The tip graft is fixed in a higher position of projection with a cap graft behind it. The first step is to prepare the alar cartilages for the structured tip graft. A combination of

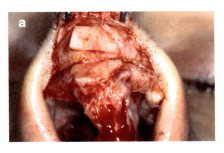
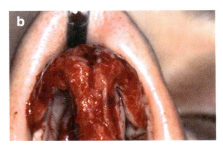
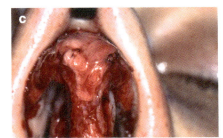

Fig. 10.13 (**a**) Prior tip graft with thin skin, (**b**) alars sutured, (**c**) fascia coverage

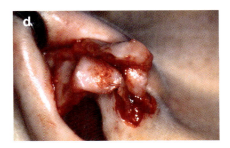
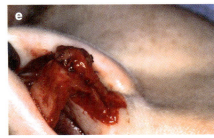
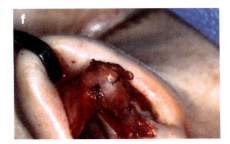

Fig. 10.13 (**d**) Prior delivery procedure, (**e**) alars sutured, (**f**) diamond shaped add-on TRG graft

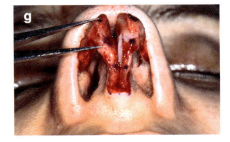
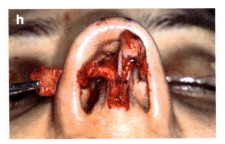
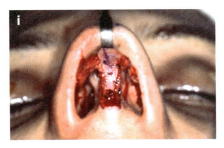

Fig. 10.13 (**g**) Persistant over projection of tip, (**h**) 6 mm domal segmant excision, (**i**) rigid structure tip graft

Reading List   Constantian M. Four common anatomic variants that predispose to unfavorable rhinoplasty results. Plast Reconstr Surg 105: 316, 2000

Constantian MB, Clardy RB. The relative importance of septal and nasal valvular surgery in correcting airway obstruction in primary and secondary rhinoplasty. Plast Reconstr Surg 98: 38, 1996

Daniel RK. Rhinoplasty: Creating an aesthetic tip. Plast Reconstr Surg 80: 775, 1987. Follow-up: Daniel RK. Rhinoplasty: A simplified, three-stitch, open tip suture technique. Part I: Primary rhinoplasty, Part II: Secondary rhinoplasty. Plast Reconstr Surg 103: 1491, 1999

Daniel RK (ed). Aesthetic Plastic Surgery: Rhinoplasty. Boston: Little, Brown, 1993

Daniel RK. Rhinoplasty and rib grafts: Evolving a flexible operative technique. Plast Reconstr Surg 94: 597, 1994

Daniel RK. Secondary rhinoplasty following open rhinoplasty. Plast Reconstr Surg 96: 1539, 1995

Daniel RK. Rhinoplasty: Septal saddle nose deformity and composite reconstruction. Plast Reconstr Surg 119: 1029, 2007

Daniel RK. Diced cartilage grafts in rhinoplasty surgery: current techniques and applications. Plast Reconstr Surg 122: 1883, 2008

DeRosa J, Watson D, Toriumi D. Structural grafting in secondary rhinoplasty. In Gunter JP, Rohrich RJ, Adams WP (eds) Dallas Rhinoplasty: Nasal Surgery by the Masters. QMP, 719–740

Gunter JP. Secondary rhinoplasty: The open approach. In: Daniel RK (ed) Aesthetics Plastic Surgery: Rhinoplasty. Boston: Little, Brown, 1993

Gunter, JP, Rohrich, RJ. The external approach for secondary rhinoplasty. Plast Reconstr Surg 80: 161, 1987

Gunter JP, Rohrich RJ, Friedman RM. Classification and correction of alar-columellar discrepancies in rhinoplasty. Plast Reconstr Surg 97: 643, 1996

Juri J. Salvage techniques for secondary rhinoplasty. In: Daniel RK (ed) Aesthetic Plastic Surgery: Rhinoplasty, Boston: Little, Brown, 1993

Kim DW, Toriumi DM. Nasal analysis for secondary rhinoplasty. Facial Plast Surg Clin North Amer 11: 399, 2003

Kridel RW, Konior RJ. Controlled nasal tip rotation via the lateral crural overlay technique. Arch Otolaryngol 117: 441, 1991

Meyer R. Secondary and Functional Rhinoplasty – The Difficult Nose. Orlando: Grune and Stratton, 1988

Peck GC. Techniques in Aesthetic Rhinoplasty. (2nd ed.) Philadelphia: JB Lippincott, 1990

Rohrich RJ, Sheen JH. Secondary rhinoplasty. In: Grotting J (ed) Reoperative Plastic Surgery. St. Louis: Quality Medical Publishing, 1994

Rohrich RJ, Sheen JH, Burget O. Secondary Rhinoplasty. St. Louis: Quality Medical Publishing, 1995

Sheen JH. Achieving more nasal tip projection by the use of a small autogenous vomer or septal cartilage graft. A preliminary report. Plast Reconstr Surg 56: 35, 1975

Sheen JH. A new look at supratip deformity. Ann Plast Surg 3: 498, 1979

Sheen JH, Sheen AP. Aesthetic Rhinoplasty (2nd ed.) St. Louis: Mosby, 1987

Sheen JH. Tip graft: A 20-year retrospective. Plast Reconstr Surg 91: 48, 1993a

Sheen JH. Balanced rhinoplasty. In: Daniel RK (ed) Aesthetic Plastic Surgery: Rhinoplasty. Boston: Little, Brown, 1993b

Tabbal N. The alar sliding graft for correcting alar collapse and expanding the nasal tip. Aesth Surg J 20: 244, 2000

Toriumi DM. New concepts in nasal tip contouring. Arch Facial Plast Surg 8: 156, 2006

Toriumi DM. Augmentation rhinoplasty with autologous cartilage grafting. In Park JL, ed. Asian Facial Cosmetic Surgery, Philadelphia: Elsevier, 2007, pp. 229–252

Toriumi DM, Johnson CM. Open structure rhinoplasty: featured technical points and long-term follow-up. Facial Plast Clin North Am 1: 1, 1993

Toriumi DM, Hecht D. Skeletal modification in rhinoplasty. Facial Plast Surg Clin North Am 4: 413, 2000

Secondary Rhinoplasty: Decision Making

11

In a primary rhinoplasty, a great deal of decision making goes into the operative plan, which is then executed with minimal changes in 90% of cases. When modifications are required, it is usually a single step moved up or down the scale; i.e., a combined sill base excision rather than a pure nostril sill excision. In contrast, the operative plan for a secondary case is complex and a challenge to figure out. Intraoperatively, the best conceived plan serves merely as a guide, the execution of which requires constant decision making and often radical changes to its fundamental components. An example of constant decision making is elevating the skin envelope – a relatively straightforward step in a primary case, but stressful in a scarred thin secondary case. A radical change in the operative plan can be the creation of symmetrical rim strips. In a primary case, the surgeon knows that a 6 mm alar rim strip is possible, only in rare cases will the lateral crura need to be relocated (alar malposition) or flipped (severe concavity). No matter how much experience the surgeon has, no one knows for sure what the alar cartilages will be like in a secondary case and the same goes for the septum. Thus, every secondary rhinoplasty is a surprise, often bad, and one must be prepared for significant intraoperative stress. The three requirements most essential for doing secondary rhinoplasty are the following: (1) know exactly what the patient dislikes about their nose and what they want, (2) do photographic analysis and write out an operative plan, but stay flexible as major changes will be required, and (3) the more surgical techniques you have experience with the better. This chapter is an attempt to guide you through the decision-making process of secondary rhinoplasty, which will hopefully teach the reader to recognize the challenges ahead of time and deal with them intraoperatively.

Decision Making: Skin Envelope

In the majority of secondary cases, the skin envelope can be dealt with employing the techniques learned in Level 3 primary cases – controlled defatting for thick skin and fascial coverage for thin skin. The critical difference is that in primary cases failure to correct the skin challenges merely downgrades the final result. In difficult secondary cases, the skin envelope can lead to failure often with the final result looking like a smaller, more distorted version of the pre-op nose, but on a very unhappy patient.

Thick Skin: Secondary

The two critical components are defatting of the skin envelope and providing strong structural support to the lobule. In these cases, maximal defatting of the lobular skin is done and occasionally the entire skin envelope (Fig. 11.1). The lobule is injected with sufficient local anesthesia to facilitate the dissection. The skin is elevated first in the subcutaneous plane via the infracartilaginous incisions. Then, the transcolumellar incision is made and the skin elevated toward the domes. Elevation is completed in the superficial plane, which leaves the subcutaneous tissue on the underlying alar cartilages. One is not elevating the skin at the cartilage level as done in primary cases. Next, subcutaneous and scar tissues are excised by dissecting in contact with the cartilage. Intraoperative drains (#7 Fr) are used when extensive resection is done, especially when muscle is resected in the radix area. Serial casting is done for 2–3 weeks. It consists of replacing the acrylic cast at 1 week with a soft foam-lined cast, which remains on for another week. Although skin envelope defatting is important, structural support is essential. The columellar struts are long (25–35 mm) and rigid (septum or rib, not concha). Solid structural tip grafts rather than add-on grafts are employed and placed in the projected position. Frequently, isolated tip grafts are obligate necessities due to prior weakening or resection of the lateral crura.

Thin Skin: Secondary

As previously shown, fascia is used in 60% of secondary cases either as an isolated dorsal graft or as a fascial blanket to reline the entire nasal skin envelope (Fig. 11.2). Fascial grafts to the dorsum can be either single or double layers. A double layer of fascia is used underneath the thin dorsum to pad the skin and to prevent a "shrink rap" effect. If the skin on the tip is also thin, then a continuous sheet of fascia for dorsal and tip coverage becomes a "fascial blanket" for the entire undermined area. If a bossa has dangerously damaged the dermis, then a specific ball of fascia is sewn directly over the domes. An "interpositional fascial graft" is used in cases with severe steroidal damage or early reoperation to release skin folds created by metallic splints. The skin is released and raised followed by insertion of the fascial graft using numerous percutaneous guide sutures. In severe cases, one has to decide whether to use dermis or fascia grafts. The answer seems to be dictated by loss of dermis. Small dermis grafts are placed beneath depressed areas or sites of prior skin loss. Furrows are treated by wide undermining and tailored dermis grafts fixed percutaneously beneath the furrow. Certain cases will have such severely damaged or destroyed skin that an open approach is precluded and a staged approach is favored. The first stage is to raise the skin and place a dermis graft widely beneath the damaged area. One then waits 6–9 months before raising the skin or resecting the small scarred area.

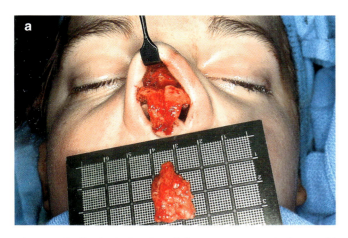
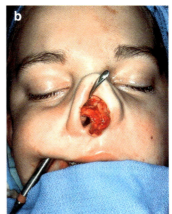

Fig. 11.1 (a, b) Thick skin (see following case study for result)

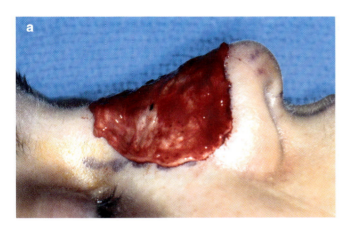
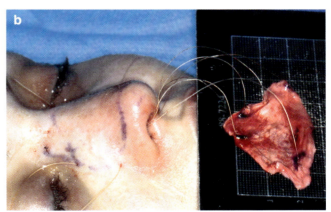
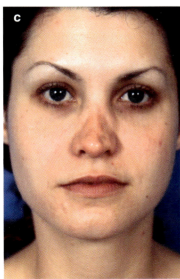
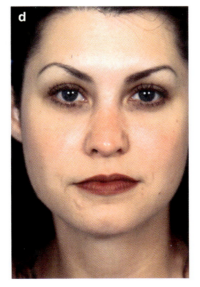

Fig. 11.2 (a–d) Thin skin. Result at one year following only insertion of a fascia graft

Case Study: Thick Skin Sleeve

Analysis

A 15-year-old presented for a secondary rhinoplasty 1 year after her primary. She felt that her nose was still too wide and the tip too bulbous (Fig. 11.3). The skin envelope was extremely thick and the tip indeed quite wide. Since her profile was acceptable, the osseocartilaginous vault would be narrowed *dorsally* and at the *base bony width* without changing the profile. At 1 year post-op, the patient was pleased with the result. The tip changes were achieved by aggressive deffating of the skin envelope via a subcutaneous dissection followed by direct excision against the alar cartilages not by direct thinning of the skin (intraops see Fig. 11.1). At *15 years post-op*, (Fig 11.3 right) the skin envelope shows relatively little change from 1 year post-op, thereby confirming that no dermal damage had occurred.

Operative Technique

1) Infracartilaginous incisions with subcutaneous dissection. Extensive defatting and excision of supratip scar tissue.
2) Septal harvest.
3) Dorsal width narrowing using 6-mm wide paramedian osteotomies.
4) Base bony width narrowing with transverse and low-to-low osteotomies.
5) Excision of redundant upper lateral cartilage and suture repair of dorsum.
6) Insertion of columellar strut with 7 mm width at SN point.
7) Crural strut suture followed by 4 mm domal segment excision.
8) Insertion of a rigid curved structure tip graft.
9) Wide skin undermining over nose and maxilla from nasal and intraoral incisions.

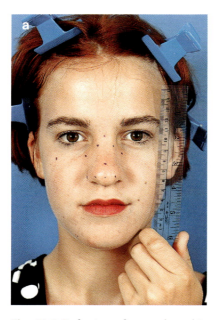 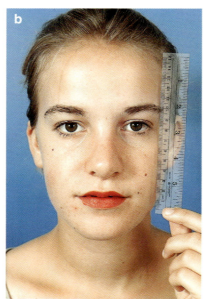 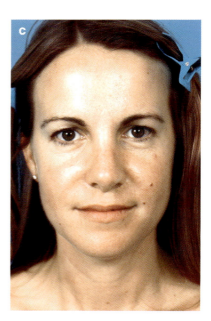

Fig. 11.3 Defatting of secondary skin envelope: (**a**) preop (**b**) 1 year postop (**c**) 15 years postop

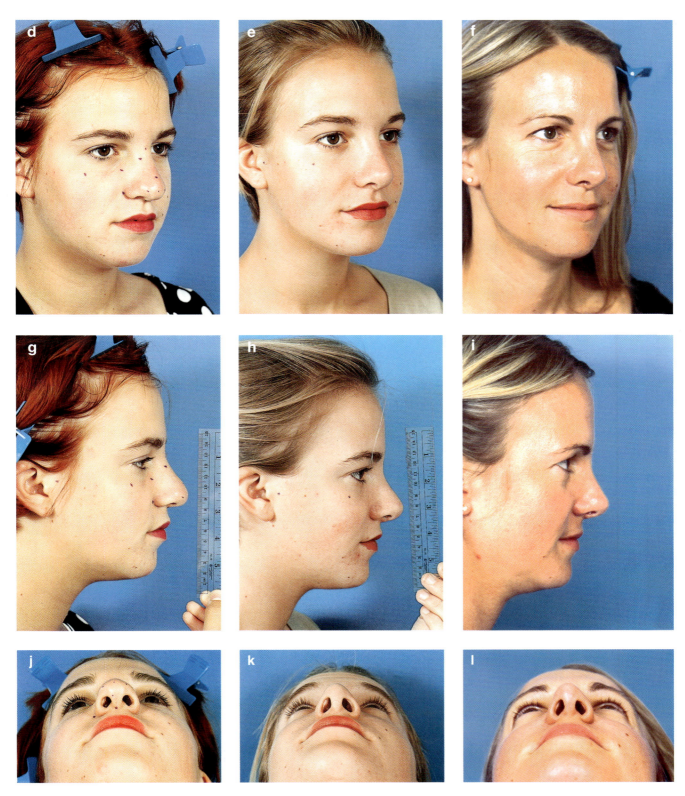

Fig. 11.4 (d–l)

Case Study:
Thin Skin

Analysis

A 39-year-old woman had had a rhinoplasty at age 15. Eventually, she got tired of not being able to breath and having a "nose job" look (Fig. 11.4). Her nostrils collapsed completely on deep inspiration. The septum was deviated into the left airway. Aesthetically, she felt that her nose was too pointy, too long, too done. Technically, the skin was paper thin with the cartilages showing through. Bilateral asymmetric spreaders opened the internal valves while the lateral crural strut graft supported the external valves. Resection of a 5 mm junctional segment of lateral crura and A1 accessory cartilage was necessary to eliminate the deep lateral depressions. The lateral crural strut graft provided support. A "fascial blanket" was placed between the elevated skin and incorporated into the suture closure all the way down to the transcolumellar incision.

Operative Techniques

1) Septal exposure and confirmation of severe deviation into L airway.
2) Open approach with visualization of previous bilateral domal division.
3) Dorsal exposure. Bidirectional approach to septum. Cartilaginous dorsum smoothed.
4) Septal body resection correcting deviation and providing graft material.
5) Insertion of spreader grafts: R: 2 mm, L: 2.5 mm.
6) Undermining of lateral crura with segmental excision of lateral crura – A1 junction.
7) Suture of lateral crural strut graft toward the pyriform aperture (Type I).
8) Insertion of a crural strut plus tip sutures (CS, plus domal division repair).
9) Application of a "concealer graft" of excised alar cartilage to hide suture repair.
10) Insertion of a "fascial blanket" to cover all undermined areas, especially the lobule.
11) Note: no bony vault surgery or osteotomies.

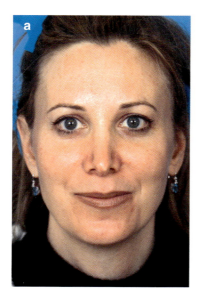 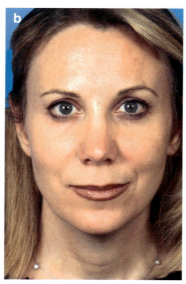 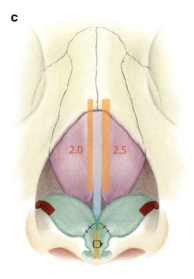

Fig. 11.4 (a–j)

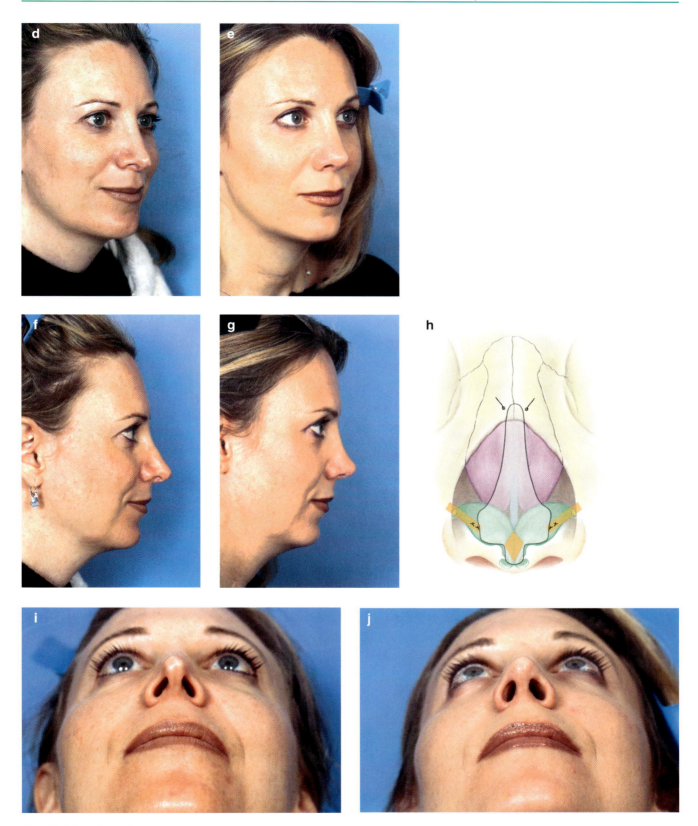

Fig. 11.4 (continued)

Decision Making: Dorsal Modification and Osteotomies

As previously noted, the secondary dorsum can be improved in many cases with the triad of smoothing the bony dorsum using a rasp, reducing the cartilaginous dorsum, and correcting the inverted V with spreader grafts. Many secondary noses remain wide and a high percentage of low-to-low osteotomies are required. All of these steps are a part of routine primary rhinoplasties and do not represent a greater degree of complexity. The most challenging issues are straightening the deviated asymmetric dorsum, augmenting the bridge, and realigning the bony base.

The Deviated Nose. Correcting the deviated asymmetric nose begins with the septum – check for deviations caudally and dorsally. Caudal deviations are obvious, but whether the dorsum is intrinsically straight will only be revealed once the upper laterals are detached from the dorsal septum. Asymmetric osteotomies are often done with all combinations possible. The encountered problems can be due to errors of omission or commission, as well as intrinsic bony asymmetries. Microosteotmies of the nasal bones just beneath the keystone area are often necessary. Once the osteotomies are completed, then dorsal deviations of the septal strut are addressed by splinting the nondeviated side first, resecting the deviation, and placement of a second spreader graft. Asymmetric spreader grafts are often essential (Fig. 11.5a–d).

Camouflaging and Augmenting the Bridge. Despite our best attempt at straightening the bridge, the dorsum can remain asymmetric and camouflage is one solution. Obviously, every effort is made to achieve true structural straightness before resorting to concealment. The DC−F graft is the easiest way to restore a natural dorsal contour and to *camouflage* any persistent deformity. One inserts a double-layer dorsal fascial graft and then places small amounts of finely dice cartilage in the areas of deficiency. Another entity is the over-resected bridge, which requires *augmentation*, either partial or full length. In these cases, one has to choose between a DC−F or a DC+F graft. I prefer the DC+F graft for localized or highly tapered augmentations. As the dorsal augmentation exceeds 2 mm and becomes less tapered, then the DC−F graft becomes the choice. Essentially, the fascial container is the same as a double level fascial graft, but now the diced cartilage is placed inside the sleeve rather than beneath it.

Realigning the Bony Base. A significant number of secondary cases have markedly different bony bases on the two sides caused by prior osteotomies (Fig. 11.5e–h). Most frequently, one lateral wall is outwardly displaced and the other is inwardly displaced. Low-to-low and transverse ostetotomies are used on both sides. The outwardly displaced wall is mobilized toward the midline often using the leverage of the osteotome against the maxilla to force the wall inward. The inwardly displaced wall is mobilized outward often by placing a Bois elevator in the nose and carrying the wall outward beyond the bony base. Careful palpation will confirm a successful mobilization. It is then important to inset a full-length spreader graft up into the open bony vault on the previously concave side to stabilize the bony wall (see Fig. 10.11d, p. 369).

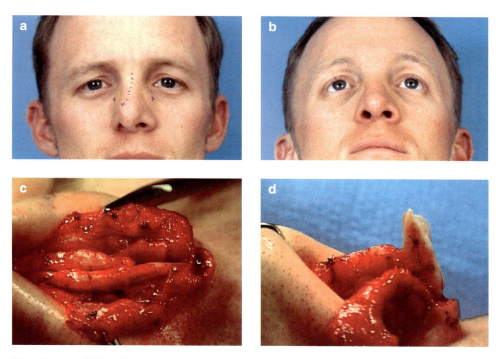

Fig. 11.5 (a–d) The deviated secondary nose

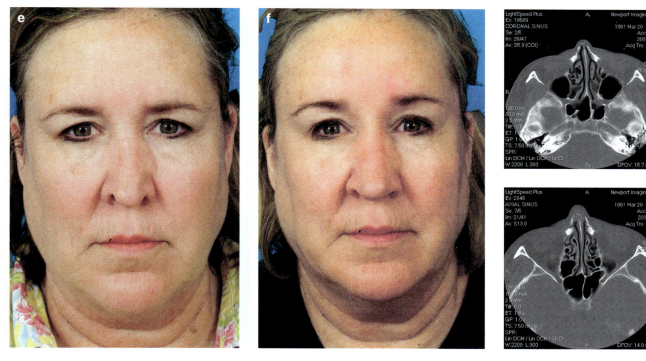

Fig. 11.5 (e–h) The deviated secondary nose, realigning the bony base and opening the bony vault

Case Study: Secondary Dorsal Deviation

Analysis

A 27-year-old male presented with a history of nasal trauma plus a prior attempt to straighten the nose including a septoplasty (Fig. 11.6). The internal exam indicated that the septum was severely deviated to the left caudally, but to the right cephalically. There were numerous synechiae plus enlarged inferior turbinates. The dorsal deviation was most apparent in the "head down" position. The combination of prior trauma and nasal surgery is a recipe for unpredictable difficulties. Once the septum was exposed, it became obvious that there had been a partial resection and a totally displaced swinging door septoplasty. The options were either to fabricate an L-shaped replacement graft or obtain a rib graft. Fortunately, it was possible to achieve rigid support for the nose using a total septoplasty.

Operative Techniques

1) Division of synechiae using a cautery.
2) The septal mucosa was elevated, but extensive morselization made it challenging.
3) Open approach with bidirectional septal exposure. Partial prior resection.
4) Prior "swinging door" septoplasty created a "crossover" blockage of both airways.
5) Asymmetric osteotomies. R: transverse and low to low. L: low to low.
6) Lowering of cartilaginous dorsum 3 mm.
7) Total septoplasty. Reinsertion of a two piece L-shaped strut.
8) Columellar strut followed by advancement of alar cartilages over strut.
9) Add-on grafts: transdomal insufficient then shield shape. ARG on R.
10) Bilateral partial inferior turbinectomy.

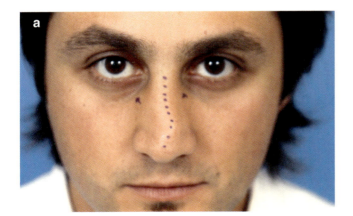 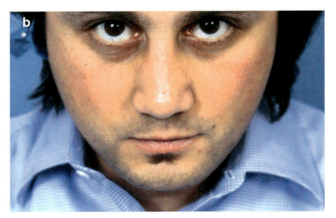

Fig. 11.6 (a–j)

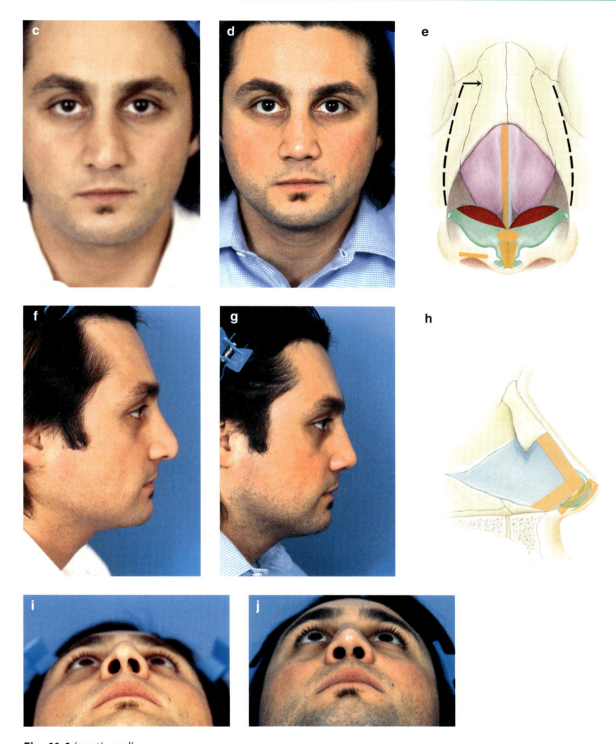

Fig. 11.6 (continued)

Case Study: Dorsal Augmentation

Analysis

A 52-year-old woman had been unhappy with the result of her primary rhinoplasty for 30 years (Fig. 11.7). The intranasal exam revealed severe vestibular scarring (>66%) that would require bilateral composite grafts. The septum was deviated into the left airway. Externally, the nose was a classic bony saddle deformity due to over resection of the dorsum, probably from using an osteotome for the hump reduction. The open approach revealed that there were *no alar cartilage remnants* – nothing to work with and thus total tip reconstruction became a priority. The tip graft was made from a "shave" of outer rib cartilage. Vestibular stenosis was reduced by using bilateral composite grafts. At 4 years post-op, the patient has done very well and the 6 mm dorsal augmentation has been maintained. The criticism that DC–F grafts do not produce "dorsal lines" is visually invalid.

Operative Techniques

1) Harvest of cartilaginous portions of the 9th and 8th ribs. Fascial harvest.
2) Open approach revealed total resection of the alar cartilages, nothing was left.
3) Bidirectional exposure of septum due to heavy scarring. Septal harvest.
4) Splitting of the vestibules with recreation of massive vestibular mucosal defects.
5) Insertion of a "septal brace" to support the caudal septum.
6) Unilateral low-to-low osteotomy on the L.
7) Columelar strut insertion and then a shield tip graft of rib.
8) Composite graft harvest. Suturing of composite grafts into vestibular defects.
9) A DC–F graft (0.8 cc) placed in the dorsum to help spread the internal valves.

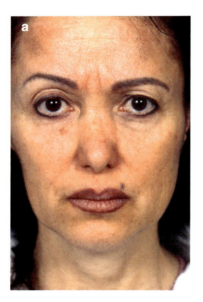 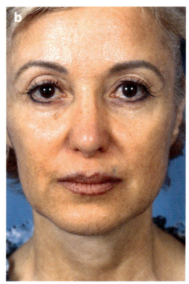 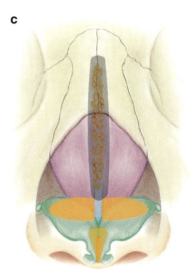

Fig. 11.7 (a–j)

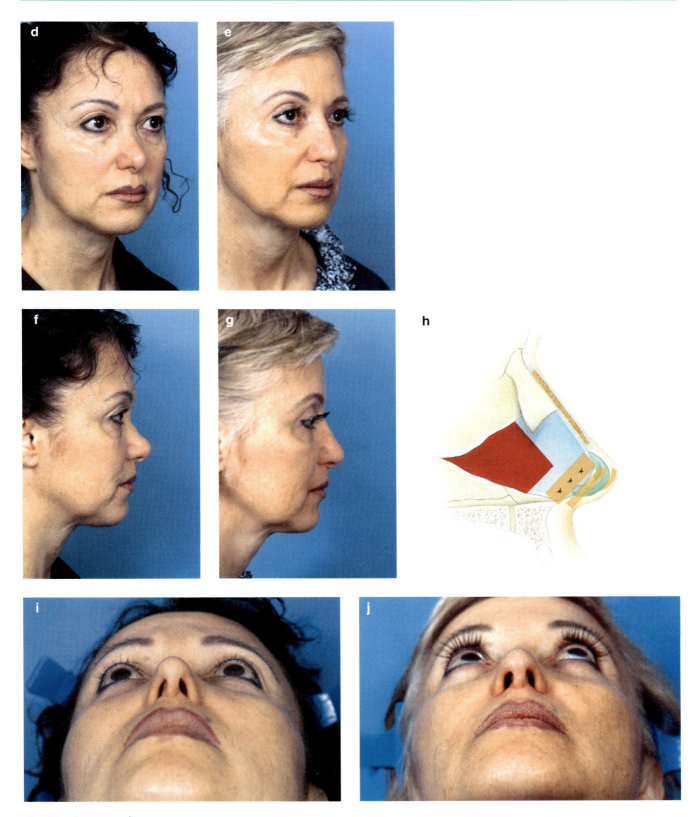

Fig. 11.7 (continued)

Decision Making: Secondary Septum and Valves

Secondary septal surgery requires greater skill as to exposure and management of persistent deviations and surgical sequelae. Elevation of the mucosal leaflets can be difficult as 75% of my secondary cases have had prior septal surgery. Despite the original surgeon's attempt at fixing deviations, one often finds persistent caudal deviations and bony deflections. The greatest challenges are prior incisions that have destabilized the L-shaped strut. From a frequency perspective, it is the internal valve that predominates in primary cases, whereas it is the nostril and vestibular valves that pose the greatest technical challenge in secondary cases.

Secondary Septal Surgery. What makes the secondary septum difficult is destabilization with loss of structure, and inadequate septal tissue for reconstruction thereby mandating a rib graft (Fig. 11.8a–d). External and internal exams reveal persistent deviations plus a void over the septal body and, most alarming, a lack of septal support for the tip. When one confirms a lack of septal support and a probable prior septal resection, then permission for a rib graft is essential. The operation begins with an open approach plus a transfixion incision, which allows *bidirectional septal exposure*. The degree of septal compromise and available graft material are readily obvious. If a rib graft is necessary, then it is harvested at this time and the appropriate spreader grafts and struts are carved. The grafts are placed in saline to allow any warping to occur. The nasal surgery is continued and the osteotomies are completed. Whatever portion of the septum remains deviated or structurally weakened is definitively corrected. Then the spreader grafts and a *septal strut* are inserted to rebuild the essential L-shaped strut.

Septal Perforations. The open approach allows easy mobilization of the mucosal lining and direct suture of perforation edges together. Then a large disk of fascia is placed in-between the mucosa and actually sutured at four corners to serve as a scaffold if the mucosa does not heal properly. In general, I only close perforations of 2 cm or smaller.

Valvular Surgery in Secondary Rhinoplasty. Valvular problems are usually a result of surgical commission (vestibular webs), or surgical omission (external valve) or both (internal valves) (Fig. 11.8e–g). Whenever possible the solution is to provide structural support with restoration of mucosal lining an occasional necessity. Spreader grafts are used 85% of the time with the majority being asymmetric. The external valve is supported with the spectrum of ARG, ARS, and lateral crural strut grafts. When in doubt, the scarred heavy tissues of secondary cases make ARS grafts preferable to ARG. Due to its technical complexity, most surgeons want to avoid treating vestibular stenosis if possible. The first step is to recreate the defect, but with dissection of the lining from lateral to medial. This step allows the thicker composite portion of the graft to be put laterally. Then the thinner skin portion is sutured to the septal defect thereby avoiding any bulk in the narrow valve angle.

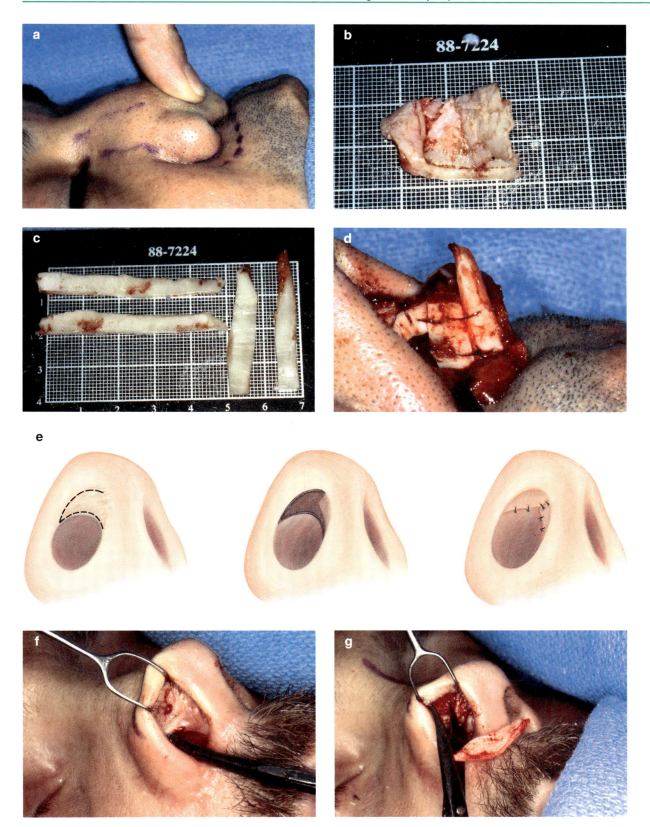

Fig. 11.8 (**a–d**) Secondary septal surgery, (**e–g**) secondary valvular surgery

Case Study: Secondary Septal Surgery

Analysis

A 33-year-old patient had a functional septoplasty after which she noted a dip on her profile and that her tip was drooping (Fig. 11.9). Her original surgeon told her that she had a 2 cm septal perforation. As with most saddle nose patients, the acute deterioration of their appearance, literally in front of their eyes, drive their desire to accept a rib reconstruction. No attempt would be made to close the septal perforation. Since the cartilage vault was intact, it could be elevated onto a rigid columellar strut. The spreader grafts were fixed cephalically to the cartilaginous vault and then "walked-up" the columellar strut until the desired profile line was achieved. The columellar strut with its fixation to the ANS supported both the tip and the cartilage vault.

Operative Techniques

1) Harvest or cartilaginous portions of the 9th and 8th rib.
2) Open approach and exposure of normal alar cartilages.
3) Septal exposure revealed *a vertical division in the dorsal portion of the L-shaped strut.*
4) Gingival incision, exposure of ANS, then a drill hole through ANS.
5) Insertion of a columellar strut, split vertically to fit over ANS, and sutured to ANS.
6) Insertion of spreader grafts with a "step off" fixation to columellar strut.
7) Advancement of alars onto and over strut with tip suturing: CS, DC.
8) Ball and apron fascia graft with placement of DC (0.1 cc) in the radix area (DC+F graft).

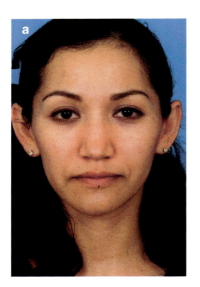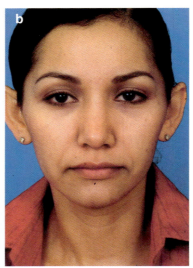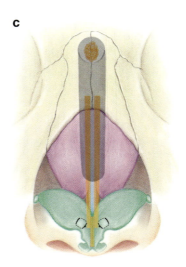

Fig. 11.9 (a–j)

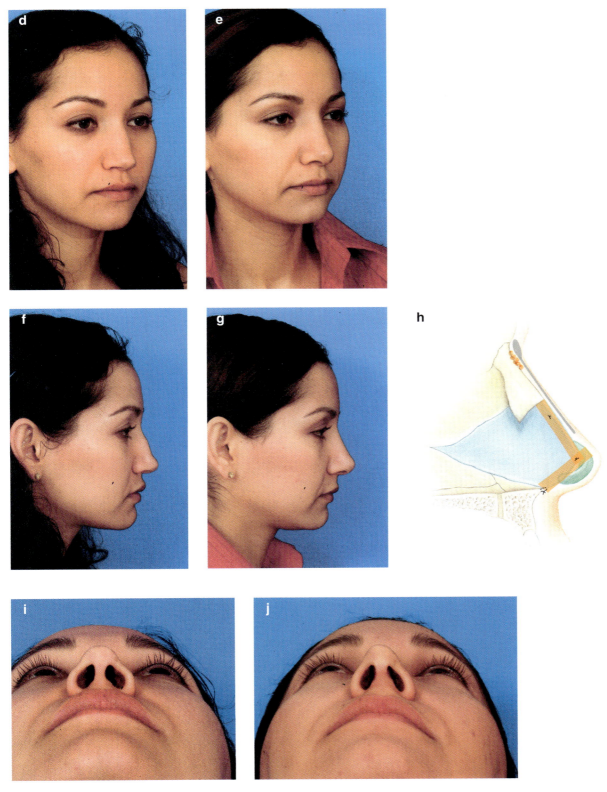

Fig. 11.9 (continued)

Decision Making: Secondary Tip Surgery

In secondary surgery, selection of the appropriate tip operation is guided by what is left of the alar cartilages to work with, the degree of columellar support, and the thickness of the skin envelope. Preoperatively, the surgeon and patient must answer two questions. (1) What do we not like about the tip? (2) What type of tip do we want to achieve? If there is one guiding principle, it is the need to provide *structure* to the tip and the entire nose. This section will be discussed as a series of sequential intraoperative questions.

1) *What will be the plane of dissection?* In thin skin patients, I dissect in direct contact with the cartilages and inject copious amounts of local anesthesia to facilitate the dissection. In thick skin patients, I will dissect in the subdermal plane leaving as much subcutaneous tissue and scar tissue on top of the alar cartilages as possible.

2) *What is the status of the septum?* The septum provides support to the nasal lobule and influences the columellar. By exposing the septum, I will know four things: (1) What is the degree of septal obstruction? (2) Can I safely reduce the cartilaginous dorsum? (3) How much graft material can be harvested? (4) What needs to be done to the caudal septum?

3) *What is the status of the alar cartilages?* Once exposure is completed, one should take a "time out" to analyze the alar cartilages remnants. Obviously, the range is from minimal to total resection. Yet, the reality is that 75% of secondary tips can be sutured if one includes the use of add-on grafts. The problem is at either extreme – a deficient 5% where there is virtually no middle or lateral crura left and the excessive overprojected tip that the original surgeon was too afraid to reduce. In between, an array of difficult tips exists where the lateral crura are divided at the domes or mangled by excessive suturing. It is helpful to answer the question – what was the original tip operation and what can I do to either complete the primary operation or undo its consequences?

4) *Will my original operative plan work?* This is a critical question and one that must be answered honestly and realistically. One must remain flexible and ready to switch to an alternative procedure. It is also time to consider prepping other donor sites for eventual graft harvest. The most important question is – can I suture these alars or do I have to excise a portion of them and insert a tip graft? Surprisingly, the lateral crura are often problematic and one has to decide whether to reinforce, transpose, or recreate. In many cases, the alars must be mobilized, which is achieved by *release of scar tissue* in-between the crura in the columellar, between the domes and the septal angle, and then between the lateral crura and the upper lateral cartilages. One must make a decision and decide on a specific tip operation. At this point, the rest of the secondary septorhinoplasty is done ranging from dorsal profile to septoplasty to osteotomies, to spreader grafts. One then returns to the tip.

5) *What type of columellar strut?* The columellar strut is the foundation for the tip and is used in all cases. These struts tend to be slightly larger and stronger than those used in primaries as they need to resist contracture forces. It is not uncommon to use two strut sutures, one above and one below the columellar breakpoint, to fix the alar remnants to the strut. Frequently, an acute columellar labial angle is present and it can be corrected with a wider strut or a plumping graft or both.

6) *Tip suturing in Secondaries versus Primaries?* In 50% of cases, the original surgeon created symmetrical rim strips and one just begins at this point and sutures the tip. Once the scar tissue is released, the only variation is that the alars may be more rigid and the sutures might need to be tied a bit tighter. Essentially, creation of the tip diamond is quite comparable to a primary case. Once the ideal tip configuration is achieved, one needs to redrape the skin and assess tip shape. Insertion of a single suture in the transcolumellar incision may be required. Under thicker contracted skin, there will be greater need for tip position sutures to achieve ideal projection as well as add-on grafts for definition. Thin skin often dictates increased smoothing and perhaps a fascial graft.

7) *What can be done to the Domal Segment?* The alternatives with the domal segment is whether it can be shaped with sutures, repaired with sutures, or excised. If the original surgery was done closed, then shaping the domal segment with sutures is the first choice. Occasionally, a prior domal division would have been done, which can be repaired and then covered with a concealer graft. If the tip is overprojected then direct excision of the domes is done, the divided edges repaired, and an open structure tip graft inserted.

8) *What must be done to the Lateral Crura?* An easy exam question is – what portion of the tip is the most operated upon? The lateral crura is the obvious correct answer. Ideally, the lateral crura would either be the correct width or underresected. Overresection or transection is a common finding. Both deformities require support using lateral crura strut grafts. Alar rim structure grafts (ARS) are often sutured into the closure to strengthen the rims with composite grafts used to lower the retracted rims. Lateral crura transposition is reserved for correcting a persistent alar malposition.

9) *What is the role of add-on TRG grafts?* Excised alar cartilage obtained from reducing the lateral crura can be used as a concealer graft to cover infralobular bifidity or to add volume to the infralobule. Transverse grafts can cover suture repairs of the domal segments. These grafts are often essential under thin skin. However, they are often ineffective in secondary cases under thick skin in achieving definition or projection.

10) *When do you go to a structure tip graft?* A structure tip graft is done to create a new tip following excision of deformed or overprojecting domes or even with when no domes remain. They are also used to achieve projection under thick noncompliant skin envelopes.

11) *What are the implications of an isolated tip graft?* When the lateral crura have been excised completely, then an isolated tip graft, preferably of septal cartilage is sutured to a major columellar strut inserted between the crural remnants. In these rare cases, major ARS grafts or alar battens of concha can be sutured along the nostril rims and create an attractive tip. In thin skin patients, true alar replacement grafts of conchal cartilage may be necessary to avoid shrink wrapping of the skin envelope around the tip graft.

Case Study: Secondary Tip

Analysis

This 39-year-old patient had had two prior rhinoplasties (Fig. 11.10). The number of problems with this nose was overwhelming, but it essentially came down to creation of a normal tip. The skin was thick with a scar from a previous surgical tear. At 3 years post-op, the result far exceeds both mine and the patient's original expectations. The reason for this success was the creation of a defined tip point (T). On the pre-op oblique photo, the distance from the columellar breakpoint (C') to tip (T) approaches 15 mm with the tip being poorly defined. In the post-op oblique, we see T as a distinct entity crowning the nose. On anterior view, the three leaf clover deformity is gone and the more balanced nose even reduces the visibility of the patient's facial asymmetry.

Operative Technique

1) Open approach. Alar analysis indicated prior domal division and "verticalization."
2) Septal exposure. Prior SMR done with no cartilage available.
3) Prior dorsal graft exposed and removed. Dorsal reduction (bone: 1, cartilage: 3)
4) A 3.5 mm caudal septum excision.
5) Harvest of conchal cartilage. Insertion of conchal spreader grafts.
6) Columellar strut made from excised dorsal graft. Suture fixation to alar remnants.
7) Repair of prior domal division. Tips sutures: CS, DC, TP.
8) Conchal tip grafts: infralobular over laid by full-length graft.
9) Bilateral composite grafts to support nostril rims.

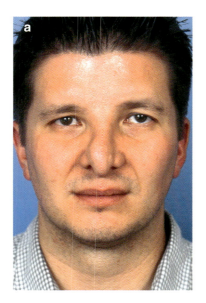 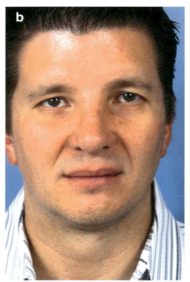 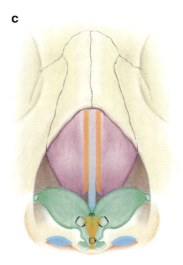

Fig. 11.10 (a–j)

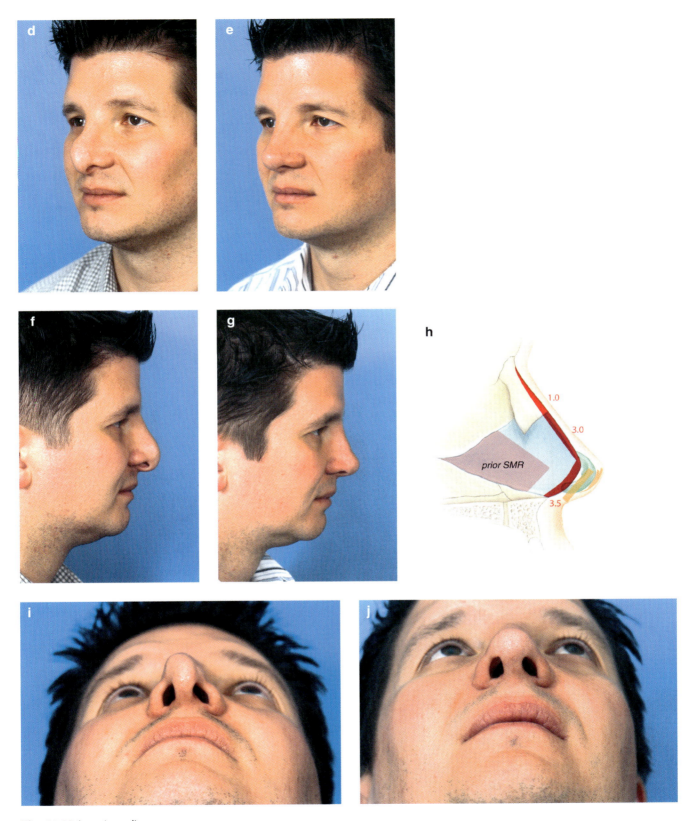

Fig. 11.10 (continued)

**Case Study:
Secondary
Rhinoplasty**

Analysis

A 52-year-old woman had had a rhinoplasty at age 17 and hated the result right away. A revision 1 year later did not improve it (Fig. 11.11). Her respiration was significantly impaired. The vestibular and internal valves were collapsed. The nasal tip was extremely pointy with a sharp bossa and the dorsum had a ski slope curvature. Intraoperatively, every secondary rhinoplasty is a surprise, which requires flexibility. Reversing the Goldman tip and covering the suture repair with a concealer graft were devised out of necessity. The lateral crural strut grafts provided vestibular support. The paucity of donor graft material led to a rib harvest. As seen at 4 years post-op and without any revisions, the dorsum looks natural with its "dorsal lines" and has maintained its 4–5 mm of augmentation from day 1 without any absorption of her DC-F graft (see DVD).

Operative Technique

1) Septal assessment and prior partial SMR found.
2) Open approach. Tip injected repeatedly to allow safe skin elevation.
3) Tip "time out." Analysis revealed a prior Goldman tip.
4) Cartilaginous dorsal reduction (3 mm). Septal harvest.
5) Columellar strut insertion. Repair of divided alars at the dome.
6) Lateral crural strut grafts with T2 location into alar bases. ARG on L.
7) Concealer graft to tip in the infralobular position.
8) Harvest of cartilaginous portion of 5th rib. DC–F graft (1.0 cc) fabricated.
9) Insertion of dorsal grafts (DC–F).
10) A 2 mm nostril sill excisions. Footplate grafts to columellar base.

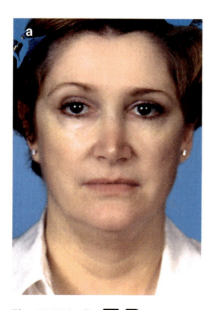 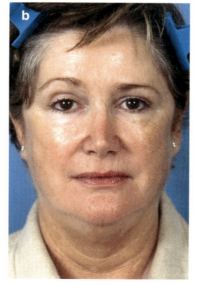 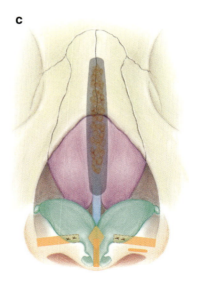

Fig. 11.11 (a–j) **DVD**

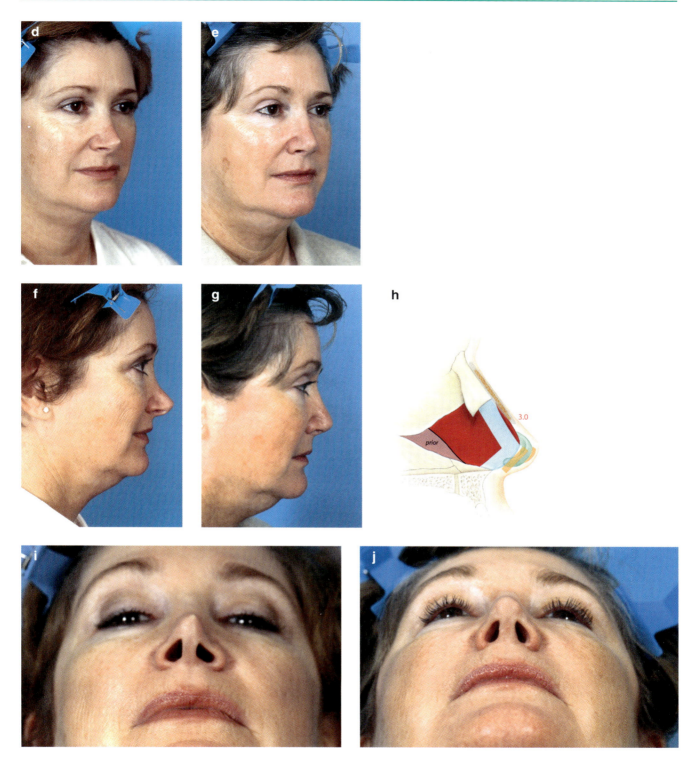

Fig. 11.11 (continued)

Decision Making: Base and Nostrils

In secondary cases, nostril distortions can be a visible stigmata of a prior rhinoplasty and their correction is obligatory, not optional. Equally, the types of procedures required are technically demanding and often require excision and replacement of scarred tissues. Analysis of secondary base deformities can be very complicated (Fig. 11.12a). The following questions must be answered.

Will the usual techniques work? Nostril base surgery is surprisingly common in secondary surgery because the vast majority of surgeons are not comfortable with nostril excisions and are not as compulsive in their execution as they should be. They tend to find a reason not to do the excision rather than maximizing the result at the primary surgery. Essentially, nostril sill, alar wedge, and combined excisions are utilized whenever there was an error of omission at the time of the original surgery. Obviously, nasal base changes secondary to a rhinoplasty can also occur creating the need for excisions. Also, one must carefully inspect the nose for prior excisions and take them into account when designing future excisions. A frequent occurrence is to design a combined excision following a prior nostril sill excision. The sill scar is opened, but continued into a new alar wedge excision. The closure will correct the retracted scar in the nostril sill from the prior surgery as well as reduce alar flare.

What about the nostril rims? The most common sequela is a "visual break" or notch in the nostril rim, which can give a "three leaf clover" appearance to the tip. Suturing ARS grafts along the nostril rims is highly effective at restoring support to the rims. In secondary cases, an ARS is superior to an ARG. It is important to realize that septum is two to four times as thick as alar cartilages. Thus, the ARS grafts must be shaped and thinned before being sutured into the rim incision. ARG grafts placed in pockets are used for intraoperative weakness rather than correcting contracted secondary problems.

What to do about the retracted nostril rim? When the nostril rim deformity extends beyond weakness or notches to a truly retracted nostril rim with significant visibility into the nose, then the solution is a composite graft from the concha. One needs to differentiate between the "retracted nostril" and the "retracted nose/retracted nostril." The distinction is very important.

Retracted Nostril Rim. Composite conchal grafts are effective for lowering isolated nostril retraction (Fig. 11.12b). Infraoperatively, the surgeon will reinforce or transpose the alar cartilages which stabilizes and correctly localizes the alar cartilages. It is at this point that the true deficiency of the nostril defect becomes apparent and the composite graft must be used to fill the defect.

Retracted Nose. When the entire nose is involved, then lengthening of the nose and pulling down the nostril rims is indicated (Fig. 11.12c). If there is heavy scarring between the lateral crura and upper lateral cartilages, it may be necessary to incise the area and insert a composite graft to force the alars downward. Once the alars are lowered maximally, then the persistent nostril retraction is treated with either ARS or composite grafts.

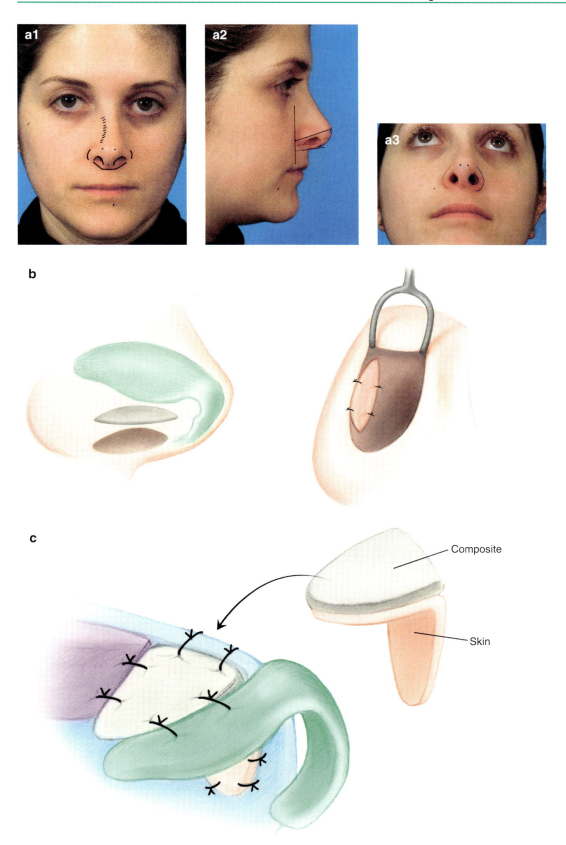

Fig. 11.12 Secondary nasal base surgery, (**a**) analysis and planning for the case study that follows, (**b**) composite strip graft, (**c**) internal valve area composite graft

Case Study: Secondary Base and Nostril

Analysis

A 26-year-old sought improvement in the nasal appearance following two prior open rhinoplasties (Fig. 11.13). She did not like her droopy columellar or the crookedness on anterior view. The nostril rim retraction and long infralobule on oblique view made me suspicious that she had had extensive "midline" sutures, which had pulled the alar rims upward. This case illustrates why I consider multiple midline sutures between the alar cartilages to be a terrible technique for most surgeons. Secondary correction required transection of the sutures and the restrictive scar tissue. Composite grafts are often necessary to lower the nostril rims. These are "sliver" grafts that are sutured first to the caudal rim, then contoured in place, and sutured cephalically. Nostril splints are worn at night for at least 2 weeks.

Operative Technique

1) Fascial harvest followed by septal exposure, no prior septal surgery.
2) Open approach with exposure of extensively sutured tip and prior domal division.
3) Dorsal smoothing, then 3 mm excision of caudal septum and ANS contouring.
4) Septal harvest. Insertion of asymmetric spreader grafts (R: 2.5 mm, L: 1 mm).
5) Removal of all prior tip sutures and mobilization of alar cartilages.
6) Insertion of columellar strut and repair of domal divisions. Isolated tip graft.
7) Insertion of a laterally draping dorsal graft of fascia plus a fascial ball at the tip.
8) Closure of all incisions. Nostril sill excisions (R: 2 mm, L: 2.5 mm).
9) Sliver composite grafts sutured into nostril rims.

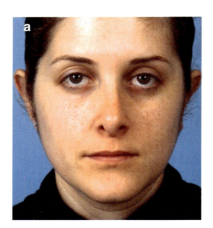 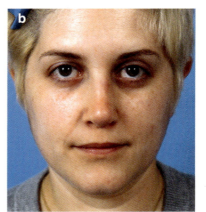 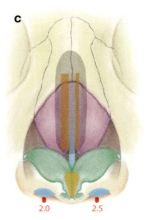

Fig. 11.13 (a–j)

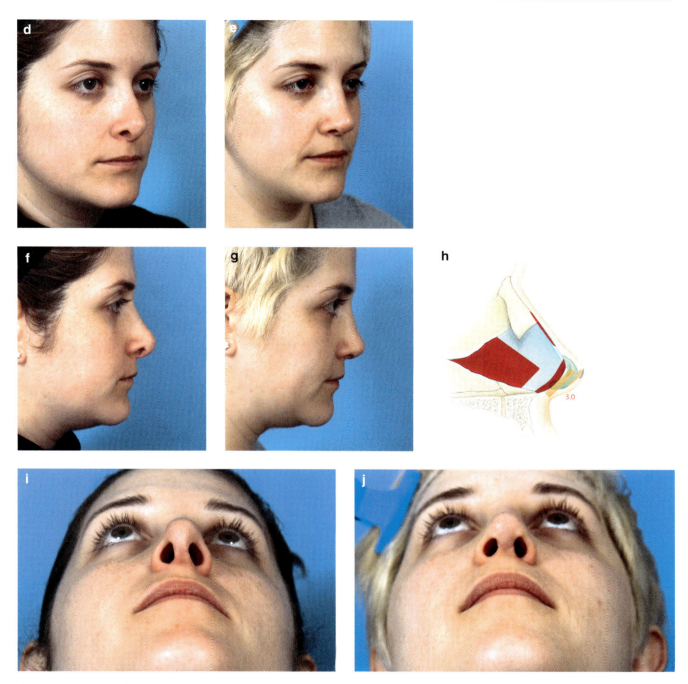

Fig. 11.13 (continued)

Reading List   Aiach O. Atlas of Rhinoplasty. St. Louis, MO: Quality Medical Publishing, 1996 (2nd ed. in press)

Boccieri A, Marco C. Septal considerations in revision rhinoplasty. Facial Plast Surg Clin 14: 357, 2006

Constantian MB. Distant effect of dorsal and tip grafting in rhinoplasty. Plast Reconstr Surg 90(3): 405, 1992

Daniel RK. (ed) Aesthetic Plastic Surgery: Rhinoplasty. Boston, MA: Little, Brown, 1993

Daniel RK. Rhinoplasty: An Atlas of Surgical Techniques. Berlin: Springer-Verlag, 2002

Daniel RK. Tip refinement grafts: the designer dorsum. Aesth Surg J 29: 528, 2009

DeRosa J, Toriumi DM. Role of septal extension grafts in tip contouring. In: Gunter JP, Rohrich RJ, Adams WP (eds) Dallas Rhinoplasty, 2nd ed. St. Louis, MO: Quality Medical Publishing, 2007

Fry HJH, Interlocked stresses in human septal cartilage. Br J Plast Surg 19: 276, 1966

Gibson T, Davis WB. The distortion of autogenous cartilage grafts; its cause and prevention. Br J Plast Surg 10: 257, 1958

Gruber RP. Lengthening the short nose. Plast Reconstr Surg 91: 1252, 1993

Gunter JP, Clark CP, Friedman RM. Internal stabilization of autogenous rib cartilage grafts in rhinoplasty: A barrier to cartilage warping. Plast Reconstr Surg 100: 161, 1997

Gunter JP, Rohrich RJ, Adams WP (eds). Dallas Rhinoplasty: Nasal Surgery by the Masters, 2nd ed. St. Louis, MO: Quality Medical Publishing, 2007

Johnson CM Jr., Toriumi DM. Open Structure Rhinoplasty. Philadelphia, PA: W.B. Saunders, 1990. Additional information in Johnson CM, Wyatt CT. A Case Approach to Open Structure Rhinoplasty, 2nd ed. New York: Elsevier, 2006

Juri J, Juri C, Grilli DA, et al Correction of the secondary nasal tip and of alar and /or columellar collapse. Plast Reconstr Surg 82: 160, 1988

Kridel RWH, Soliermanzadeh P. Tip grafts in revision rhinoplasty. Facial Plast Surg 14: 331, 2006

Maring VP, Landecker A, Gunter JP. Harvesting rib cartilage grafts for secondary rhinoplasty. In: Gunter JP, Rohrich RJ, Adams WP (eds) Dallas Rhinoplasty, 2nd ed. St. Louis, MO: Quality Medical Publishing, 2007, 705

Menick FJ. Anatomic reconstruction of the nasal tip cartilages in secondary and reconstructive rhinoplasty. Plast Reconstr Surg 104: 2187, 1999

Meyer R. Secondary Rhinoplasty. Berlin: Springer, 2002

Millard DR. The alar cinch in the flat, flaring nose. Plast Reconstr Surg 40: 669, 1980

Sheen JH. Secondary rhinoplasty. Plast Reconstr Surg 56: 137, 1975

Sheen, JH. Secondary rhinoplasty surgery. In: Millard DR Jr (ed) Symposium on Corrective Rhinoplasty. St. Louis, MO: Mosby, 1976

Sheen JH, Sheen AP. Aesthetic Rhinoplasty, 2nd ed. St. Louis, MO: Mosby, 1987

Suzuki S, Muneuchi G, Kawai K, et al Correction of atrophic nasal ala by sandwiching an auricular cartilage graft between para-alar and nasal floor retrogressive flaps. Ann Plast Surg 51; 513, 2003

Tardy ME. Rhinoplasty: The Art and the Science. Philadelphia, PA: W.B. Saunders, 1997

Toriumi DM. Structural approach to rhinoplasty. Facial Plast Surg Clin North Am 13: 93, 2005

Aesthetic Reconstructive Rhinoplasty

12

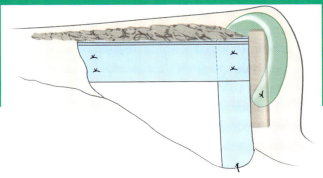

During the past decade, a new sophisticated level of nasal surgery has emerged – aesthetic reconstructive rhinoplasty. It has its origins from two sources. The first is the incredible aesthetic results achieved in nasal reconstruction by Burget (1994) and Menick (1999). These advances are to nasal reconstruction what Tessier's contribution was to facial reconstruction. The second is the dramatic improvement in the results of secondary rhinoplasty beginning with the balanced approach of Sheen and then followed by the correction of the nasal foundation using the open approach. The critical factors are the insertion of structure and the goal of achieving true aesthetic natural results rather than mere "improvement." However, these advances have not come without an equally dramatic increase in requisite surgical skills including the use of rib grafts. One only has to think of the three Cs – clefts, cocaine, and catastrophes to realize the difficulty of both the problems and the corrections. In many cases, the solution will be the new concept of "composite reconstruction" in which a deep structural foundation layer is inserted first and then overlaid with an aesthetic contour layer (Daniel 2007). The advantage of this technique is that one can maximize the reward while minimizing the risk. For the experienced surgeon seeking the greatest challenges in rhinoplasty surgery, these cases represent an extension of techniques perfected in secondary rhinoplasty rather than a completely new operation with a prolonged learning curve. Yet a word of caution is necessary. These are neither hopeless cases nor can a beginning surgeon justify doing them because the expected improvement is minimal. These patients have suffered a great deal in their lives and deserve the best possible result.

Introduction

Step #6. The next step is the *deep foundation layer* which *is a replication of the L-shape septal strut*. The spreader grafts replace the dorsal component and a true *septal strut* replaces the vertical component. I expose the ANS through a gingival incision and drill a hole through the ANS. If the ANS has been resected, then I use a burr to make a central groove in the midline and then drill holes through the pyriform lip on either side. I pass a 4–0 polydioxanone suture (PDS) suture through the drill hole and leave it.

Step #7. I insert the spreader grafts high underneath the bony vault. It is important to assess the width and avoid making the nose too wide. Once satisfied, the grafts are held in place with #25 needles and then multiple five-layer sutures of 4–0 PDS are inserted. On occasion, it may be necessary to place drill holes through the bony vault to fix the spreader grafts. Next, the alar cartilages are separated from top down and the precut *septal strut* is passed from the dorsum down to the ANS. The septal strut is either split vertically in its lower 10 mm to straddle the ANS or placed in a groove. Once the septal strut is seated, then the preplaced 4–0 PDS is used to fix the strut rigidly to the ANS. It is important to realize that this is a *septal strut* and not a sepal extension graft designed to influence the columellar – they are not the same!

Step #8. The classic tongue-in-groove overlap of spreader grafts on either side of a strut is not used because it is too bulky and can block the internal valve angle. Rather, a "*step-off*" configurations is used. One spreader graft is kept long as an overlap brace and the other is cut shorter to act as a midline abutment against the strut. They are sutured together with 4–0 PDS. At this point, one has a rigid L-shaped septal replacement which becomes the foundation for the nose.

Step #9. The *aesthetic layer* is comprised of the tip support and the dorsal contour. A standard columellar strut (25 × 3) is inserted between the alar cartilages. As usual, the alars are advanced upward, fixed with a #25 needle, and sutured with 5–0 PDS. Frequently, the alars might have been damaged and there will be a need for either add-on or structure tip grafts. Essentially, these maneuvers are the ones done in secondary cases.

Step #10. Once the tip is finalized then a custom "made to measure" DC-F dorsal graft is constructed on the back table. Variations in length, width, and thickness can be controlled. The graft is guided into place with cephalic percutaneous sutures and then sutured at the septal angle.

Step #11. Frequently, the peripyriform area is contracted and will require support using diced cartilage. Pockets are made beneath each alar base and onto the maxilla via the gingival incision. The DC is packed into the pockets and the incision closed with 4–0 chromic.

Step #12. Fascial grafts and rib perichondrium are often used in thin-skin patients. Perichondrium should not be used indiscriminately throughout the nose as it diminishes definition. It is useful for padding, whereas fascia is preferred for filling.

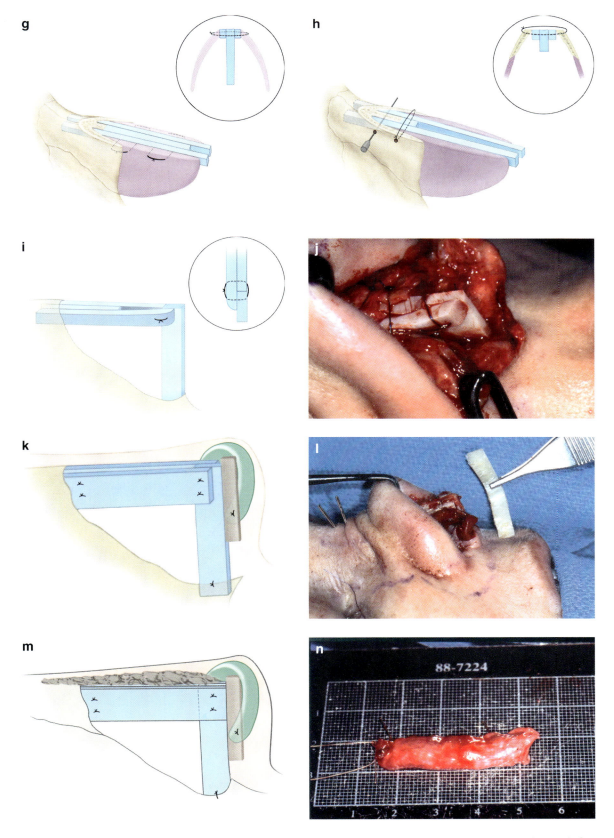

Fig. 12.1 Spreader graft fixation to (**g**) cartilage vault or (**h**) bony vault, (**i, j**) septal strut to spreader graft fixation using a step-off (**k, l**) Insertion of a columellar strut to support the tip **DVD** (**m, n**) dorsal augmentation with a DC-F graft **DVD**

Case Study: Composite Reconstruction

Analysis

A 32-year-old woman was totally obstructed despite two prior septorhinoplasties including an open procedure (Fig 12.2). The CT-scan showed severe septal deviation plus severe bony vault deformity/angulation. She also had a septal perforation and no structural support. Rib graft reconstruction was the only option.

Operative Technique: Step By Step

1) CT-scan revealed severe bony and septal deviation.
2) Harvest of the Ninth and Eighth Ribs.
3) Exposure at subdermal level. Alar cartilages intact.
4) Spreader, septal, and columellar grafts cut. Rest of cartilage diced.
5) Deformed septal remnants removed, leaving no septal support. Medial oblique and transverse osteotomies done.
6) Spreaders fixed to *bony vault* with sutures thru drilled holes.
7) Septal strut fixed to ANS with split straddle and suture.
8) Step-off fixation of septal strut to spreader grafts.
9) Columellar strut and tip sutures: CS, DC, ID.
10) Uniform 3 mm thick DC-F graft (0.5 cc) inserted to dorsum.
11) Nostril sill excision (R 2.5, L 3.0)

Note: There is a critical difference between a septal strut to restore stability and a columellar strut that projects the tip above the dorsal line (Fig. 12.2b).

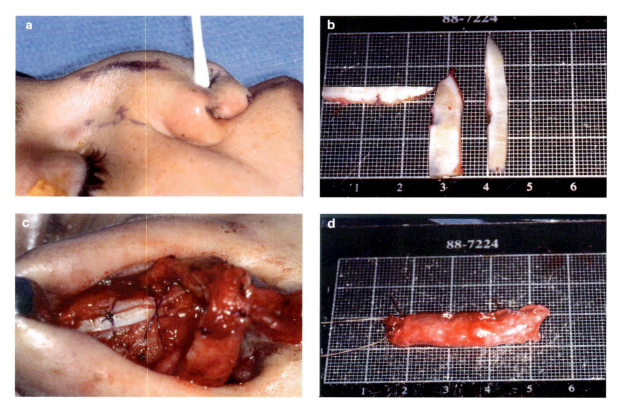

Fig. 12.2 (a–l)

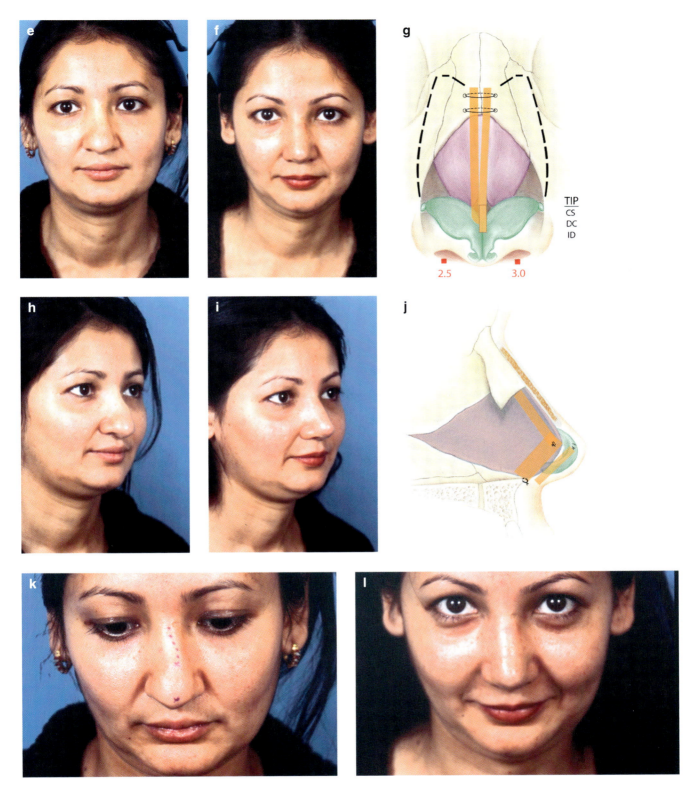

Fig. 12.2 (continued)

Case Study: Over-Resected Nose

Analysis

This 50-year-old patient had undergone a single rhinoplasty as a teenager. She finally decided that it was time to get rid of her "Miss Piggy nose job look" (Fig. 12.3). Due to the prior excessive excision and need for structure, rib cartilage was essential. The tip would need to be forced downward and the dorsum augmented. Fortunately, the nasal lining was not constricted thus allowing mobilization, downward rotation, and fixation on a septocolumellar strut. Dorsal augmentation using a DC-F graft provided a capstone to the midvault which had been widened by the spreader grafts. Despite the very thin skin, the DC-F graft has not shown in the patient at 5 years post-op.

Operative Technique

1) Harvest of the ninth rib cartilage. Fascia harvest.
2) Open approach with exposure of a prior "universal" tip.
3) Exposure and excision of septal body.
4) Insertion of 3 mm wide extended spreader grafts.
5) Insertion of a "tomahawk" septocolumellar graft pushing the tip downward 8 mm.
6) Repair of the alar domal divisions then covered by a concealer tip graft.
7) Dorsal augmentation with a DC-F graft (1.0 cc).
8) Nostril sill excisions followed by insertion of alar rim structure graft (ARS) grafts.

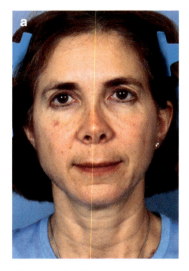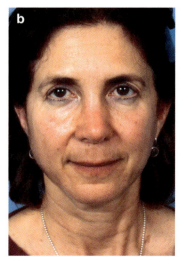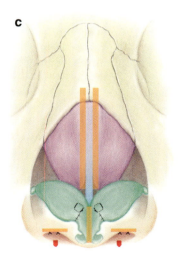

Fig. 12.3 (a–j)

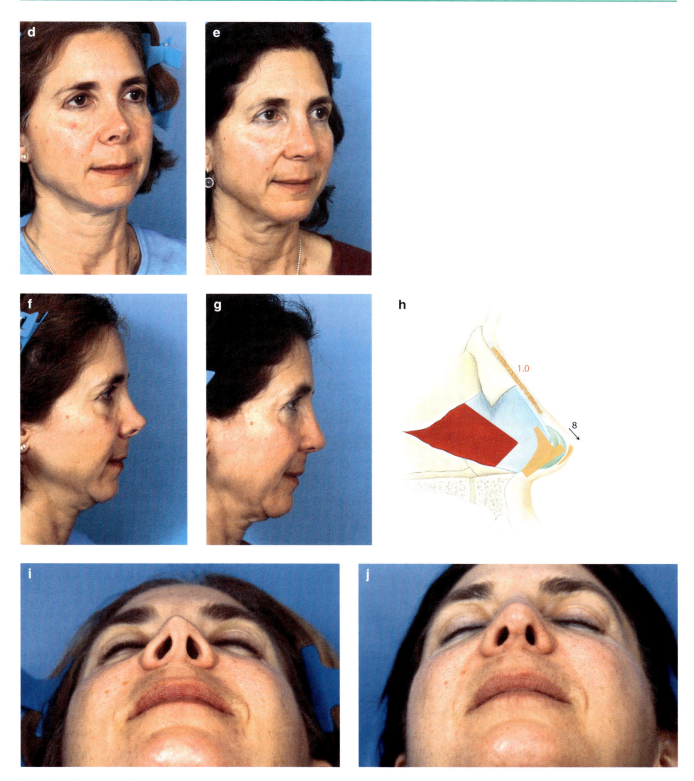

Fig. 12.3 (continued)

Case Study: Septal Saddle Nose

Analysis

I did a primary rhinoplasty on this patient at age 22. It was done closed and there was no septal surgery. She returned 4 years later with an obvious septal saddle collapse (Fig. 12.6). I was devastated that this could have happened. However, intranasal exam revealed a 4 cm septal perforation and the patient admitted to substance abuse. I used a "two strut" approach to the problem – a septal strut to restore the L-shaped septal support and a columellar strut to project the tip above the dorsal line. DC is often placed in the peripyriform area to overcome contracture, see lateral views (Fig 12.6f, g).

Operative Technique

1) Harvest of the cartilaginous portions of the ninth and eighth ribs.
2) Open approach with tip split to expose a weakened collapsed septum.
3) Low-to-high osteotomy on R side.
4) A 20 × 10 mm septal strut was fixed in a groove to the ANS.
5) Extended spreader grafts fixed to cartilage vault and then to the septal strut using a "step-off" configuration.
6) Columellar strut inserted with alar advancement onto strut.
7) Domal onlay tip graft from rib cartilage with perichondrial cover.
8) Fascial graft to dorsum for smoothing.
9) Insertion of 4.0 cc of DC to peripyriform area.
10) Nostril sill excisions. Alar battens of split rib to alar rims.

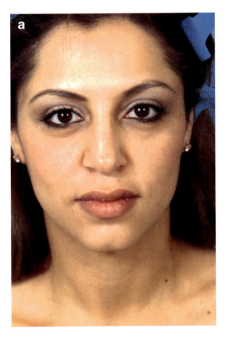
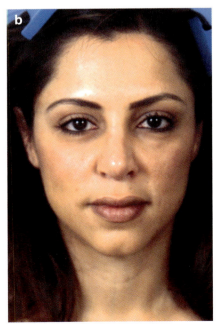
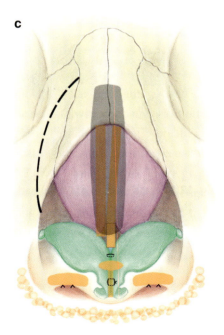

Fig. 12.6 (a–j)

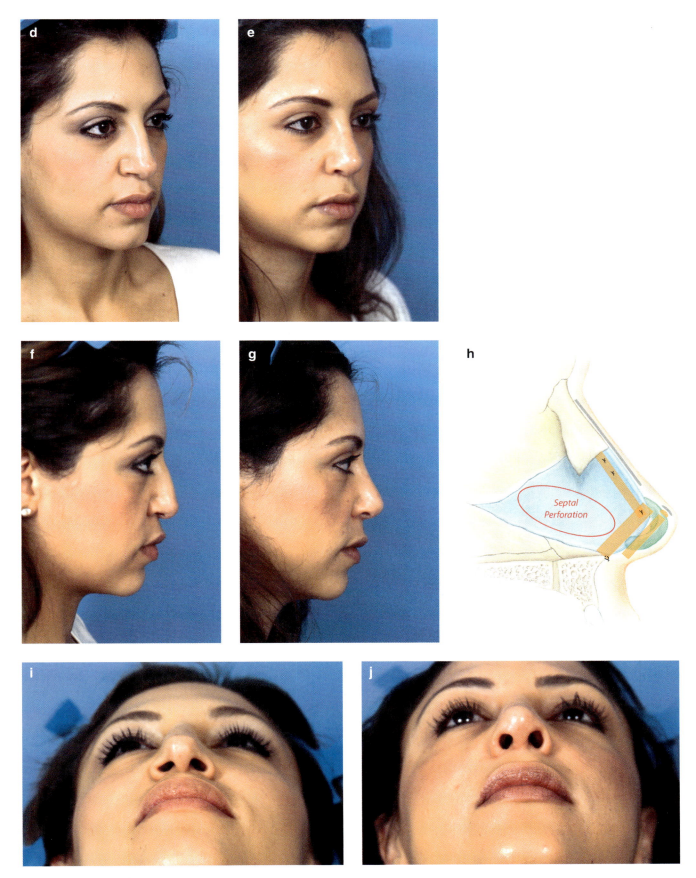

Fig. 12.6 (continued)

Cocaine Nose   Cocaine eats through the septum, erodes the nasal lining, penetrates the maxillary sinuses and can even vaporize the upper lateral cartilages. The progression is from septal perforation to loss of septal support to contracture of the mucosal lining and ultimately to compromise of the skin envelope itself. Put simply, all cocaine noses are difficult. The range is from dorsal collapse correctable with composite reconstruction to severe midvault collapse necessitating an osseocartilaginous dorsal graft, and eventually severe intranasal lining contracture requiring intraoral mucosal flaps.

Surgical Correction. The timing of surgical correction requires that the patient be "clean" of cocaine for at least a year. Structural support is critical when the lining is contracted. No attempt is made to close the septal perforation.

1) *Nasal Lining Release.* The nasal lining can be released using the Meyer (2002) "sleeve" technique where the lining is released high up under the bony vault and then dragged downward leaving the donor area to heal by secondary intention. In severe cases, it may be necessary to excise the heavily scarred mucosa in the upper lateral area to allow derotation of the tip. All mucosal tears must be repaired until it is water tight to minimize infection.

2) *Dorsal Support.* I prefer an osseocartilaginous rib graft for the dorsum and a cartilage graft for the columella strut (Fig. 12.7). The two are joined in a tongue-in-groove fashion to force the tip downward. Since most cocaine patients have not had a prior rhinoplasty, the alar cartilages can be advanced over the strut. Due to the contracted skin sleeve, one should plan on a single strut and advance the tip above the dorsal line. Very thin tip grafts made from rib are frequently utilized. Closure of the columellar incision can be difficult. It may require V-Y techniques and even skin grafts on the internal incisions.

3) *Nostril Support.* Vestibular contracture and nostril collapse are two problems requiring extensive grafting. Alar batten grafts extend into the alar base to provide support to the contracted mucosa (Fig. 12.8). One combination used in a severe contracture (see Fig 12.9) was the following: (1) a true lateral wall graft (20 mm high × 15 mm wide) along the caudal border of the bony vault, (2) a composite graft (15 mm high × 8 mm wide) to release the contracted vestibule, and (3) an alar batten graft (15 mm high × 10 mm wide) of thin rib cartilage to support the nostril rim. Nostril splints are inserted deep into the nose, sutured, and left for 3–4 weeks if possible.

4) *Peripyriform Grafting.* As the nasal lining contracts in the cocaine nose, the nasal base sinks inward towards the pyriform aperture. Surgeons have recommended relining the nose with nasolabial flaps. This procedure is unnecessary and creates irreparable facial scarring – do not do it. One can easily move the nasal base forward by widely undermining the peripyriform area and maxilla followed by insertion of diced cartilage grafts (3.0–5.0 cc).

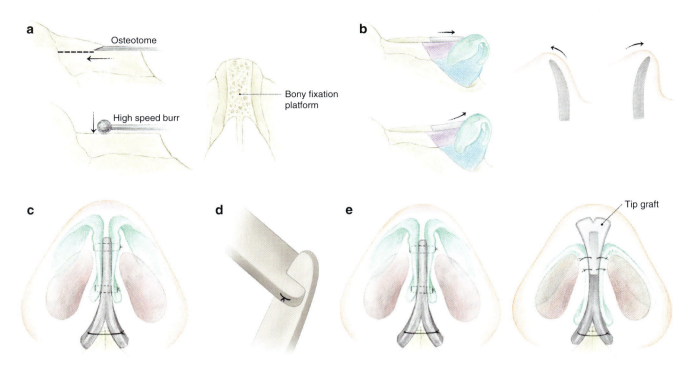

Fig. 12.7 (a–e) osseocartilaginous reconstruction

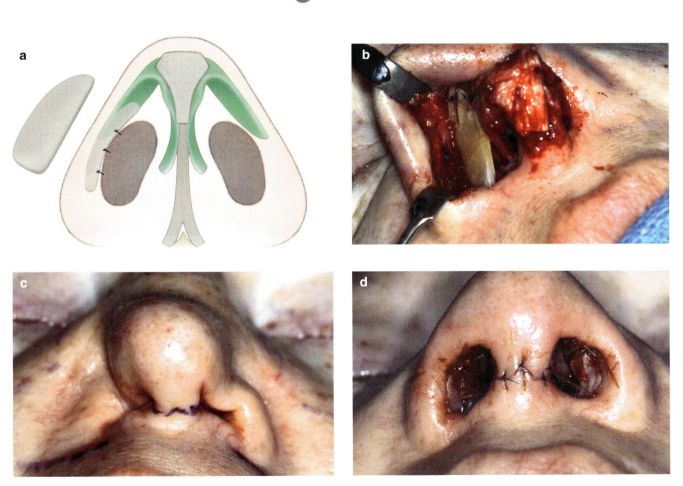

Fig. 12.8 (a–d) Nostril/alar base support

Case Study: Cocaine Nose

Analysis

A 48-year-old woman presented with a history of cocaine abuse and had been "clean" for 5 years (Fig. 12.9). She felt that her nose was continuing to collapse and felt that surgery was necessary because of total nasal airway obstruction. A 4–5 cm septal perforation was present. Traction on the columellar indicated severe restraint. Due to the restricted nasal lining, a total "mucosal sleeve advancement" was done. Once, mobilized, a deep foundation layer of spreader grafts and a true septal strut provided support. The aesthetic contour was created with alar advancement over the columellar strut and then aesthetic dorsal augmentation with a DC-F graft. Support of nasal base was achieved with massive (15 × 9 mm) composite grafts placed in the vestibules.

Operative Technique

1) Harvest of the cartilage portion of the ninth and eighth rib.
2) Open approach with tip split exposing a collapsed caudal septum.
3) Total mobilization of mucosal lining including the upper lateral cartilage (ULC).
4) Spreader grafts fixed in a "step-off" fashion to septal strut.
5) Columellar strut inserted with alars advanced over it. Structured tip graft with perichondrial coverage.
6) Dorsal augmentation using a DC-F graft (0.3 cc).
7) Composite grafts to "vestibular release" defect.
8) Diced cartilage (1.0 cc) to each peripyriform area.

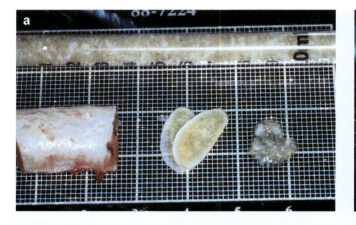
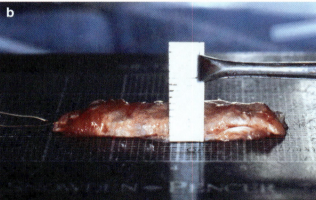
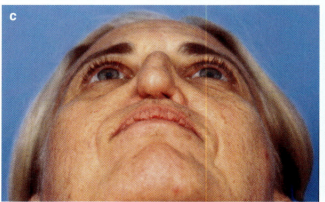
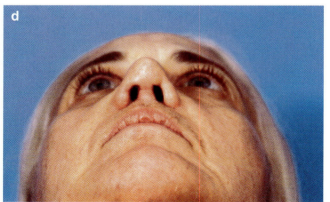

Fig. 12.9 (a–l)

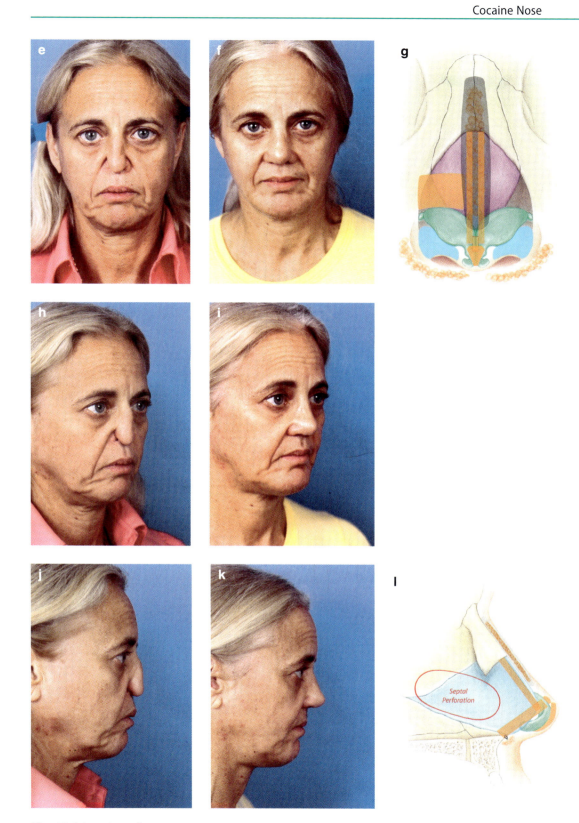

Fig. 12.9 (continued)

Implant Disasters

Nasal implant extrusion is usually heralded by focal redness followed by ulceration and exposure. If the infection decompresses internally, patients will try to ignore the problem. If it erupts externally, surgery is sought immediately.

Staged Reconstruction. In most cases, the implant is removed intranasally and any external skin wound allowed to heal by secondary intention. This approach is strongly recommended for those cases with infected Porex implants due to mark tissue in growth and the difficulty of removing all of the implant. I will insert a dermis graft to maintain some contour and revitalize the damaged skin.

Early Reconstruction. The problem with delayed reconstruction is skin contracture and a severe deformity for the patient (Fig. 12.10). One option is to remove the implant and place the patient on appropriate antibiotics. Early reconstruction at 7–10 days in a clean wound is done with limited risk. At that time, one has the option to proceed or delay depending upon the degree of infection. The benefit to the patient is an early return to near normality.

Immediate Reconstruction. A high-risk option is to remove the implant and do immediate reconstruction. It is considered only for those with silastic implants and willing to gamble on complete loss of the reconstruction due to persistent infection (Fig. 12.11). Do not do this operation in patients with infected Porex implants. Repeated consultations and detailed informed consent are essential.

1) *Open Approach.* An open approach is used irrespective of the skin ulceration site. The implant, including its capsule, is removed and the wound cultured again. The wound is profusely irrigated with antibacterial solution. The feasibility of the operative plan is reassessed.
2) *Graft Harvest.* The usual grafts are rib, fascia, and dermis with the latter necessary under any skin ulceration.
3) *Columellar and Tip.* A major structural columellar strut is inserted and fixed to the ANS. The alar cartilages are then advance upward on the strut and fixed at two points. A full-length tip graft is placed in the projected position and cap grafts added.
4) *Dorsum.* A full-length DC-F graft is inserted with an optional radix graft of fascia to build up the glabellar region. If possible, a new plane of insertion is developed between the nasal SMAS and the dorsum.
5) *Dermis Graft.* If the tip skin is compromised or the grafts exposed, then a dermis graft with minimal fat is inserted with the dermis side up beneath the ulceration. The ulceration is allowed to heal by secondary intention. One can expect a tip defect to heal within 6 weeks. The scar will be 50% smaller than the original defect and probably 75% smaller than an excisional closure. A simple scar revision can be done at 6 months if requested.

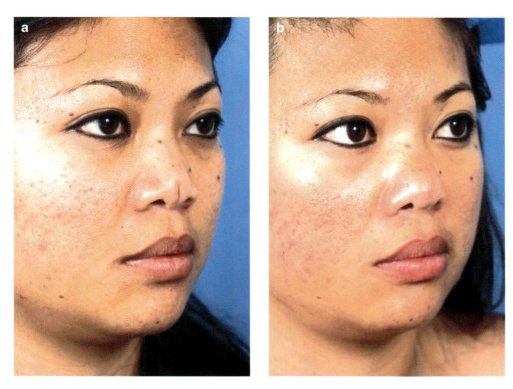

Fig. 12.10 (a, b) Early reconstruction at 8 weeks with composite reconstruction and a dermis graft *DVD*

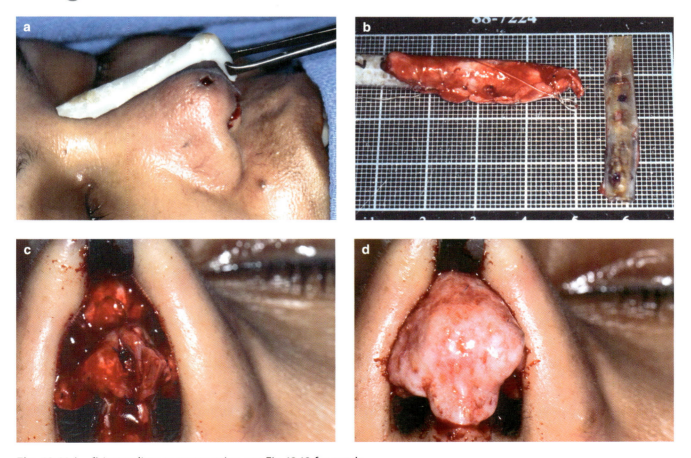

Fig. 12.11 (a–d) Immediate reconstruction see Fig 12.12 for result

Case Study: Infected Implant

Analysis

A 50-year old of Filipino descent presented with an infected nasal implant 23 years after its insertion. The implant had been exposed for 2 months (Fig. 12.12). All cultures were negative. The patient was given a choice of three options for reconstruction – staged, early, or immediate. Given her work schedule, she opted for immediate reconstruction despite the significant risk of infection. Due to the extensive damage to the tip skin, immediate closure was not planned. At 9 months postop, the underlying dermis graft has allowed the skin to contract and avoid a depressed tip scar (intraop photos Fig. 12.11). The patient was able to avoid a 6–12-month period of abnormal appearance and the difficulty of fixing a contracted skin sleeve.

Operative Technique

1) Harvest of cartilaginous portions of the ninth and eighth ribs.
2) Removal of the implant and its capsule thru an open approach.
3) Profuse irrigation of the wound with antibiotic solution.
4) Insertion of a structural columellar strut fixed to ANS.
5) Simple advancement of the alar cartilages over the strut.
6) Dorsal augmentation with a DC-F graft (0.9 cc).
7) Coverage of the lobule with a dermis graft from suprapubic area.
8) No closure of the tip wound.

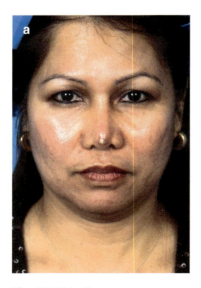 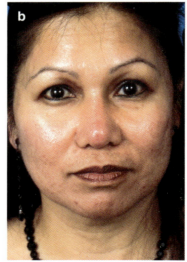 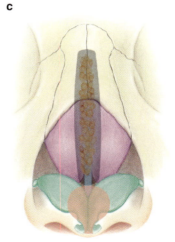

Fig. 12.12 (a–j)

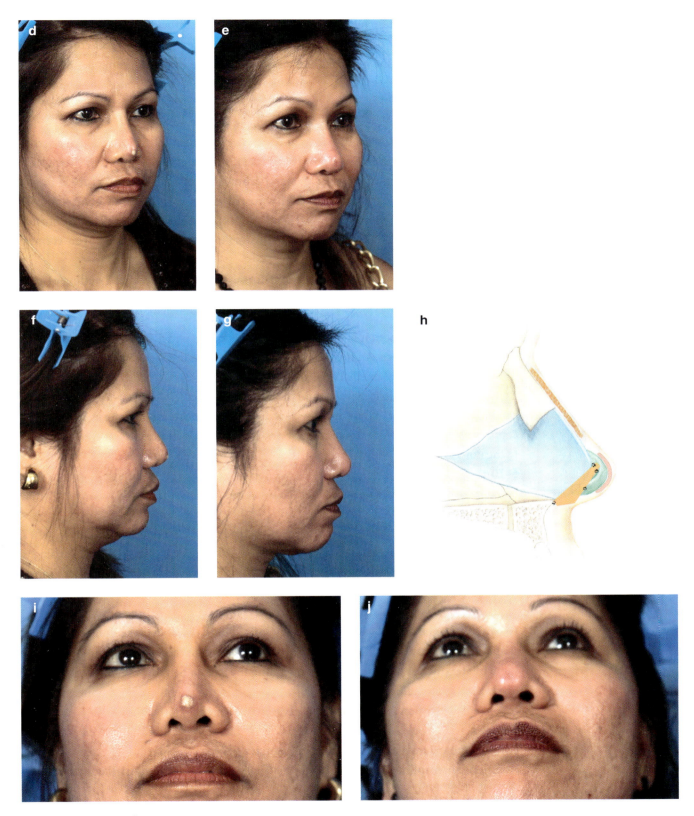

Fig. 12.12 (continued)

Case Study: Unilateral Cleft Nasal Deformity

Analysis

A 14-year old presented for repair of her unilateral left cleft lip nasal deformity (Fig. 12.15). The septal body was severely deviated and totally blocked the left airway while the caudal septum was deviated to the right. Correction required resection of fixed deformities and structural support throughout the L-strut. Subtle maneuvers would not work. Due to her normal skin thickness, add-on grafts were effective. Multiple attempts to adjust nostril size were not effective. Alas, the nostril dilemma was nothing new. I always tell the patient the following: "Our goal is to give you an attractive natural appearing noncleft nose. The contour of the nose is more important than the nostrils."

Operative Technique

1) Open approach via a staggered columellar incision. Alar cartilages normal.
2) Incremental dorsal reduction (bone: 0.5 mm, cartilage: 1.0 mm).
3) Septal exposure revealed severe deviation with need for a "temporary L-strut."
4) Resection of septal body. Creation of a "tomahawk" septocolumellar graft.
5) Insertion of strut with fixation to ANS and dorsal septum. Resection of severely deviated caudal septum. Addition of spreader grafts with five-layer dorsal fixation.
6) Transverse and low-to-low osteotomies.
7) Advancement of the alars onto the strut and then cap and shield add-on tip grafts.
8) Alar rim graft (ARG) on left. Composite graft and multiple cartilage grafts on right.
9) Partial inferior turbinectomy on left.

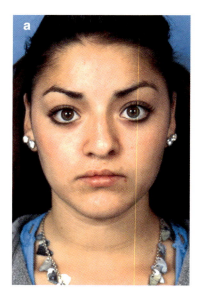 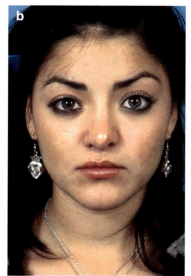 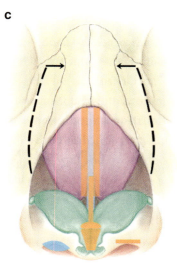

Fig. 12.15 (a–j)

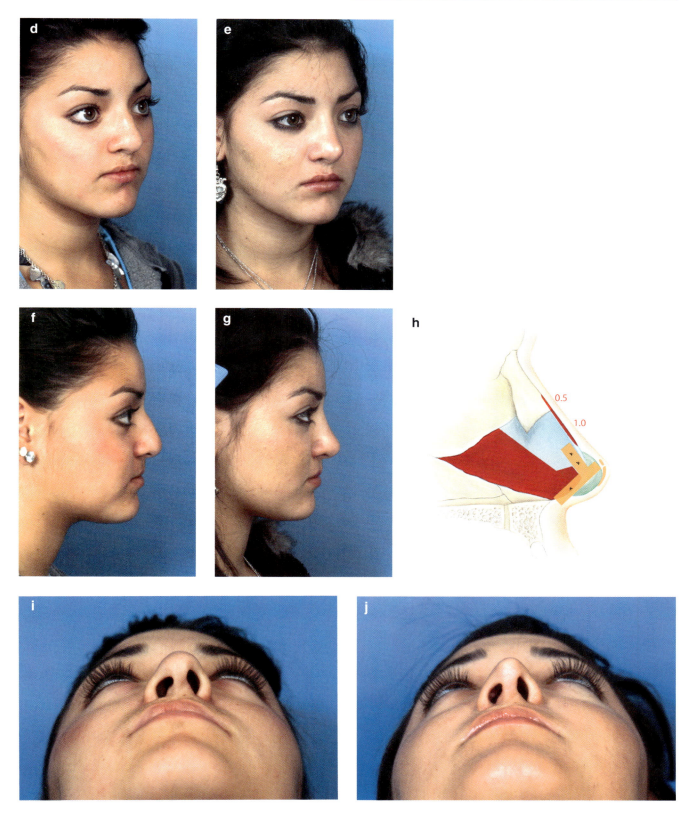

Fig. 12.15 (continued)

Bilateral Cleft Lip Nose

The pathology of bilateral cleft nasal deformity is different than the unilateral deformity (Fig. 12.16). These cases are extremely difficult and require a wide variety of cartilage grafts. Equally, the scarred restricting skin envelope and major functional problems increase the demand for surgical expertise. One major difference from the literature is that I have not found the short columella to be a limitation in the majority of bilateral cleft patient. Composite grafts to the columella and banked forked flaps are not necessary.

Surgical Techniques. As in all cleft nasal deformities, structure is critical in providing support and achieving an aesthetic result (Fig. 12.16). Whenever possible, I use the standard inverted-V and infracartilaginous incisions placed low on the columella, but never in the columella labial angle. However, preexisting scars may force modifications.

Septal Surgery. In the majority of bilateral cases, the septum is deficient in its distal third, but not severely deviated. The septum is approached through a "tip split" thereby preserving the membranous septum integrity. This maneuver allows for more control of the septocolumellar support graft. A major harvesting of the septal body is done. A septocolumellar graft linking caudal septum and columella provides support and prevents secondary distortion. These grafts are often massive (25 × 20 mm) which achieves both lengthening (10–15 mm) and projection (5–8 mm). The graft is placed with percutaneous needles as a unilateral spreader graft juxtaposed to the caudal septum. Suture fixation with 4–0 PDS is done first at the ANS and then to the septum at multiple points. The turbinates may be markedly enlarged as the flat broad tip confers a platyrrhine configuration. Judicious reduction is done as indicated.

Tip Creation. The alar cartilages are advanced upward on the septocolumellar graft using a double-skin hook placed in the nostril apices. Strong traction will determine whether it is necessary to undermine the collumelar base and mobilize additional skin out of the upper lip. The alar cartilages are advanced on the strut beginning with the footplates, then the collumella breakpoint, and ultimately the middle crura. Next, the alar cartilages are refined with domal creation sutures and approximated over the top of the strut. In most cases, the skin is so thick that a rigid tip graft is used to gain the desired tip definition.

Closure/Alar Bases. All of the incisions are closed and tension is rarely a problem due to the prior upward advancement of the columella base. In virtually all bilateral cases, alar base narrowing is a necessity and a combined nostril sill/alar wedge excision is the usual solution. In asymmetric cases, it is important to do the more severe side first and to vary the amount of excision. I reserve the alar cinch maneuver for those rare cases where the nostril size is small or the sill is of limited width.

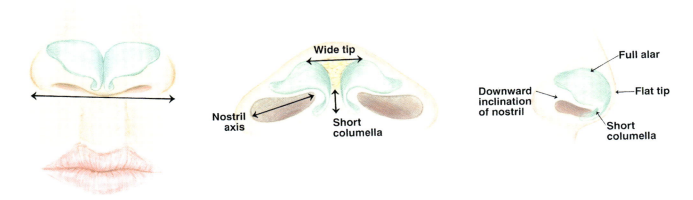

Fig. 12.16 Pathology of the bilateral cleft lip nasal deformity

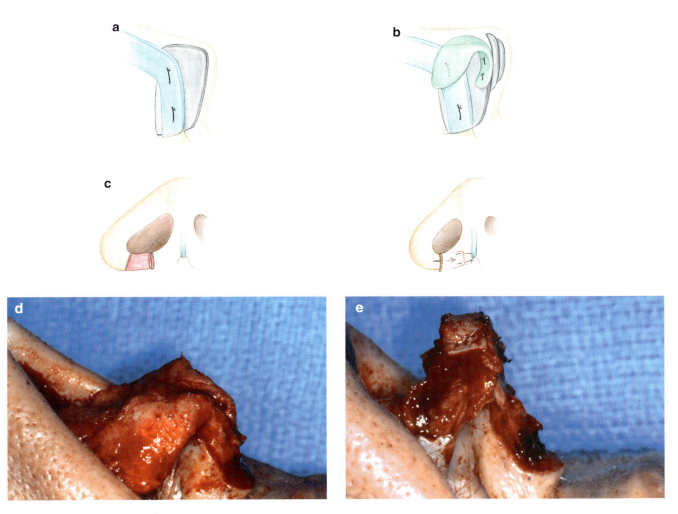

Fig. 12.17 (a–e) Surgical techniques

Case Study: Bilateral Cleft Nasal Deformity

Analysis

A 34-year-old patient had undergone numerous operations (>20) for his bilateral cleft lip deformity including three on his nose (Fig. 12.18). The patient stated that he had "a blob" for a nose and would be grateful for anything that could be done. The skin sleeve was incredibly thick and noncompliant. At 2 years, the result was a significant improvement for a nose that was a true deformity. The columellar strut and onlay tip grafts created a tent pole effect which triangulated and supported the tip (intraop photos Fig. 12.17d, e). Serendipitously, a drain was inserted into the nose to reduce blood accumulation following the radix reduction. As soon as the suction bulb was compressed, the entire nasal skin dramatically "shrink wrapped" around the tip.

Operative Technique

1) Harvest of the cartilaginous portion of the ninth rib.
2) Open approach with skin elevation in a subdermal plane.
3) Excision of a 9 mm thick supratip scar ball.
4) Thick radix reduction (4 mm). Dorsal width measured 17 mm.
5) Dorsum narrowed from 17 to 7 mm using paramedian, transverse, and low-to-low osteotomies.
6) Major columellar strut inserted.
7) Alar rim remnants excised and replacement with alar battens.
8) Double thickness domal onlay grafts from rib cartilage.
9) Nasal drain (7 Fr) inserted with shrink wrapping effect on skin.

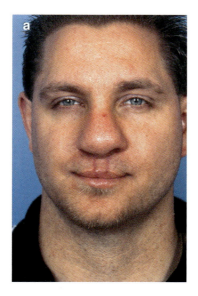
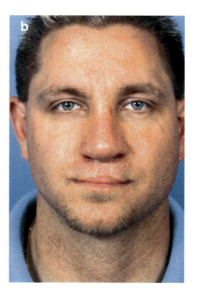
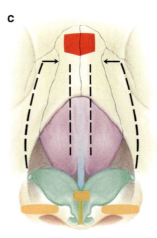

Fig. 12.18 (a–j)

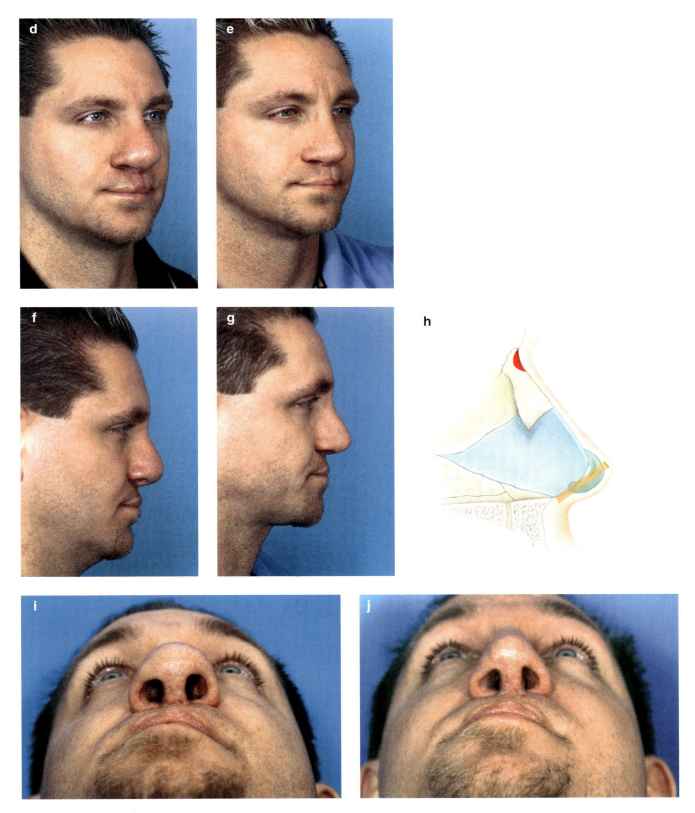

Fig. 12.18 (continued)

The Practice of Rhinoplasty: A Summation

I am frequently asked by visiting surgeons if I have always done just rhinoplasty surgery. I tell them yes with a smile and say that it was my father who was a pioneer in reconstructive microsurgery as well as a researcher into the blood supply of the skin, electrical burns, and hand transplantation. My 30-year progression from reconstructive microsurgeon to rhinoplasty surgeon seems to fade in the intense focus required to do that particular rhinoplasty at that particular moment. After "experiencing" 5,000 rhinoplasties, what advice do I have for the younger surgeons wanting to become a rhinoplasty surgeon?

Step #1. No one emerges from their residency or fellowships being very good at rhinoplasty surgery. The requisite expertise is lacking. One does not have experience with a diverse range of patients nor an understanding of surgical cause and effect. It is what you learn and what your commitment is in your practice that will determine whether you become a good rhinoplasty surgeon. The slate is clean, it is commitment that counts.

Step #2. If learning rhinoplasty surgery is so difficult, why bother? The answer is simple – creativity and challenge for the surgeon, a profound life-changing event for the patient. There is no other surgical procedure that will fascinate and challenge you throughout your entire surgical career.

Step #3. Where to begin? The first step is to assess your core competence and confidence in rhinoplasty. Your residency and fellowship training will have exposed you to certain techniques. Plan to master these techniques first within the outline of the basic rhinoplasty operation (Chapter 2). Defining Level 1 cases and operating within your comfort zone are critical in the first year or two of practice. Your goal is to become comfortable with the entire perioperative course of rhinoplasty surgery, from consultation through long-term follow-up. Also, it establishes your reputation for competency in the community. Despite being cautious, you will misjudged certain cases and end up doing a few Level 2 cases, thus inadvertently expanding your comfort zone.

Step #4. Every rhinoplasty you do is a learning experience – so maximize it! Take photos of every nose consult and do a three-step analysis. Write out an operative plan. If they come back, they will be impressed with your preparation and you can check your initial assessment. Refine your operative plan – record what changes are necessary intraop. Take tip photos before closing. Write out your "three questions." See the patient frequently post-op and always look at your op diagram. Reread the Section of "Teaching Yourself Surgical Cause and Effect" in Chapter 1.

Step #5. Read everything you can on rhinoplasty surgery. Attend as many meetings as possible, both local and international. You learn a lot not only from the lecturers, but also from talking with other attendees. Do not hesitate to go to multispeciality or different specialty meetings. I find DVDs are extraordinarily valuable for understanding the details of specific techniques. If possible, find a course with cadaver dissections.

Step #6. Find a mentor or visit several surgeons who do a lot of rhinoplasties. The older and more established the surgeon, the more likely they are to help you out. For 1 year, I spent every

Thursday morning in the operating room with Dr. Paule Regnault and then every Thursday afternoon doing my own cases. The experience was incredible. Once a year, I go and spend 2–3 days in the OR with a colleague. I always learn an enormous amount.

Step #7. Identify your weaknesses and correct them. Due to my plastic surgery background, I needed to strengthen my knowledge of managing nasal obstruction early in my practice. I did the following: (1) took the 3-day Cottle Rhinology Course, (2) went to the Mayo Clinic Rhinology Course and spent a clinical week with Dr. Eugene Kern, (3) operated with an ENT colleague for 6 months, and (4) had a Resident spend a year developing a "localized rhinomonometry" system.

Step #8. As you develop greater confidence, then expand your comfort zone to Level 2 cases and eventually Level 3 cases. Be forewarned – you will have problems and unhappy patients. What to do? Try and be objective. Will a revision make a difference? Should you arrange a consultation for the patient with a colleague? Learn from your revisions. Early on, I was as excited about one of my revisions as I was about a primary as I got to see what I did wrong. Although I do not enjoy revisions, it is still fascinating to truly understand what went wrong.

Step #9. Decision time. Realize that you will reach a point when you need to reassess your commitment to rhinoplasty surgery and at what Level you wish to remain. If you have a broad interest in your primary surgery specialty, you may wish to remain at Level 1 and enjoy straightening crooked male noses and eliminating the bumps on cute teenage girls. The surgery is fun and the stress limited. Some will want to take on the challenge of Level 2 cases consisting of more difficult primaries and ethnic rhinoplasties which will require competency with a large number of grafts. Realistically, only about 10% of the surgeons will enjoy doing Level 3 cases and infinitely difficult secondary rhinoplasties with their requisite rib grafts. It is important to operate within your comfort zone. There is no need to give up doing rhinoplasty just operate within your comfort zone.

Step #10. A rhinoplasty practice is a career journey, not a destination. I am convinced that few surgeons would want or could deal with an exclusive rhinoplasty practice for more than 10 years. Although the majority of patients are appreciative and delighted with their result, there is a minority whose unhappiness and anguish erodes one's soul. As has been said "be careful of what you wish for, you just might get it." Yet, I still continue to suffer from "nose lust" and the curiosity of how to correct challenging nasal deformities. I am both cursed and blessed to have had this affliction for the last 25 years – it has been delightful.

Reading List   Burget GC, Definitive Rhinoplasty for Adult Cleft lip nasal deformity. In Losee, JE, Kirschner RE Eds Comprehensive Cleft Care, New York: McGraw Hill, 499-523, 2008

Burget GC, and Menick IJ. Aesthetic Reconstruction of the Nose. St. Louis: Mosby, 1994

Byrd HS, Van der Werff JF, Stevens HP, et al Primary correction of the unilateral cleft nasal deformity. Plast Reconstr Surg 106: 1276, 2000

Byrd HS, El-Musa KA, Yazdani A. Rhinoplasty in the cleft lip nasal deformity. In Gunter JP, Rohrich RJ, Adams WP eds Dallas Rhinoplasty. 2nd ed, St. Louis: QMP, 1261, 2007b

Calvert JC, Brenner KB, DaCosta-Iyer M, Evans GRD, and Daniel RK. Histological analysis of human diced cartilage grafts. Plast Reconstr Surg 118: 230, 2006

Daniel RK. Rhinoplasty and rib grafts: Evolving a flexible operative technique. Plast Reconstr Surg. 94: 597, 1994

Daniel RK. Composite Reconstruction (Video). Alexandria, VA: American Academy of Facial Plastic and Reconstructive Surgery, 2003

Daniel RK. Discussion. Velidedeoglu H, Demir Z, Sahin U, et al Block and Surgical-wrapped diced solvent-preserved costal cartilage cartilage homograft application for nasal augmentation. Plast Reconstr Surg 115: 2081, 2005

Daniel RK. Rhinoplasty: Septal saddle nose deformity and composite reconstruction. Plast Reconstr Surg 119: 1029, 2007

Daniel RK. Diced cartilage grafts in rhinoplasty surgery: current techniques and applications. Plast Reconstr Surg 122: 1883, 2008

Daniel RK, Calvert JC. Diced cartilage in rhinoplasty surgery. Plant Reconstr Surg 113: 2156, 2004

Daniel RK, Brenner KA. Saddle nose deformity: a new classification and treatment, Facial Plast Surg Clinics 14: 301, 2006

Daniel RK. Rhinoplasty: dorsal grafts and the designer dorsum. Plast Surg Clin 2010

DeRosa J, Toriumi DM. Role of septal extension grafts in tip contouring. In Gunter JP, Rohrich RJ, Adams WP eds Dallas Rhinoplasty 2nd ed, St. Louis: QMP, 597, 2007

Goodman, WS External approach Rhinoplasty. Can J Otolayrgol. 2: 207, 1993

Guerrerosantos J, Travanino C, Guerrerosantos F. Multifragmented cartilage wrapped with fascia in augmented rhinoplasty.117; 804, 2006

Gunter, JP, Clark, CP, Friedman RM. Internal stabilization of autogenous rib cartilage grafts in rhinoplasty: a barrier to cartilage warping. Plast Reconstr Surg 100: 162, 1997

Gunter JP, Clark CP, Friedman RM, Hackney FL Internal stabilization of large autologous rib cartilage grafts to avoid warping in rhinoplasty. In Gunter JP, Rohrich RJ, Adams WP eds Dallas Rhinoplasty. 2nd ed, St. Louis: QMP, 705, 2007

Guyuron B, Varghai, A. Lengthening the nose with a tongue-and-groove technique. Plast Reconstr Surg 111: 1533, 2003

Guyuron B, Afrooz PN. Correction of cocaine –related nasal defects. Plast Reconstr Surg 121: 1015, 2008

Heller JB, Gabbay JS, Trussler A, et al Repair of large nasal septal perforations using facial artery musculomucosal (FAMM) flap. Ann Plast Surg 55: 456, 2005

Kelly MH, Bulstrode NW, and Waterhouse N. Versatility of diced cartilage-fascia grafts in dorsal augmentation. Plast Reconstr Surg 120: 1654, 2007

Kim DW, Shah AR, Toriumi DM. Concentric and eccentric carved costal cartilage: a comparison of warping. Arch Facial Plast Surg 8: 42, 2006

Menick, FJ. Anatomic reconstruction of the nasal tip cartilages in secondary and reconstructive rhinoplasty. Plast Reconstr Surg 104: 2187, 1999

Meyer R. Secondary Rhinoplasty. Berlin: Springer, 2002

Pribaz JJ, Weiss DD, Mulliken JB, et al Prelaminated free flap reconstruction of complex central facial defects. Plast Reconstr Surg 104: 357, 1999

Raghavan U, Jones NS, Romo R III. Immediate autogenous cartilage graft in rhinoplasty alter alloplastic implant rejection. Arch Facial Plast Surg 16: 192, 2004

Sheen JH. Aesthetic Rhinoplasty. St. Louis: Mosby, 1978

Subject Index

Printing and Binding: Stürtz GmbH, Würzburg

Return or exchange
only possible when packaging unopened